Extrahepatic Manifestations in Liver Diseases

FALK SYMPOSIUM 69

Extrahepatic Manifestations in Liver Diseases

EDITED BY

R. Schmid
Department of Medicine
University of California School of Medicine
San Francisco, CA 94143
USA

W. Gerok
Medizinische Universitätsklinik und Poliklinik
W-7800 Frieburg-im-Breisgau
Germany

L. Bianchi
Institüt für Pathologie der Universität
CH-4003 Basel
Switzerland

K. P. Maier
Medizinische Klinik
Fachbereich Gastroenterologie
Stadtische Krankenanstalten
W-7300 Esslingen
Germany

Proceedings of the 69th Falk Symposium held in Basel, Switzerland, October 15–17, 1992

KLUWER ACADEMIC PUBLISHERS
DORDRECHT / BOSTON / LONDON

Distributors

for the United States and Canada: Kluwer Academic Publishers, PO Box 358, Accord Station, Hingham, MA 02018-0358, USA
for all other countries: Kluwer Academic Publishers Group, Distribution Center, PO Box 322, 3300 AH Dordrecht, The Netherlands

A catalogue record for this book is available from the British Library

ISBN 0-7923-8996-4

Library of Congress Cataloging-in-Publication Data

Falk Symposium (69th: 1992: Basel, Switzerland)
Extrahepatic manifestations in liver diseases: proceedings of the 69th Falk Symposium held in Basel, Switzerland, October 15–17, 1992/edited by R. Schmid ... [et al.].
p. cm.
Includes bibliographical references and index.
ISBN 0-7923-8821-6 (casebound)
1. Liver—Diseases—Complications—Congresses. I. Schmid, Rudi, 1922–
II. Title.
[DNLM: 1. Liver—physiopathology—congresses. 2. Liver Diseases—physiopathology—congresses. WI 700 F191e 1992]
RC846.F35 1992
616.3′6207—dc20
DNLM/DLC
for Library of Congress 93-15126
CIP

Published in the United Kingdom by Kluwer Academic Publishers, PO Box 55, Lancaster, UK.

Kluwer Academic Publishers BV incorporates the publishing programmes of D. Reidel, Martinus Nijhoff, Dr W. Junk and MTP Press.

Typeset in Great Britain by Technical Keying Services, Manchester.
Printed and bound in Great Britain by Hartnolls Ltd., Bodmin, Cornwall.

Contents

List of Principal Contributors

L. BIANCHI
Institüt für Pathologie der Universität
Schönbeinstr. 40
CH-4003 Basel
Switzerland

L. M. BLENDIS
Toronto Hospital, General Division
200 Elizabeth St
Toronto
Ontario M5G 2C4
Canada

J. BOSCH
Unidad de Hepatologia
Hospital Clinico y Provincial
Villarroel, 170
E-08036 Barcelona
Spain

T. D. BOYER
Division of Digestive Diseases
Department of Medicine
Emory University School of Medicine
PO Drawer AL
Atlanta
GA 30322
USA

M. BROTMAN
Department of Medicine
CPMC, California Campus
Ground Floor, 3700 California St
San Francisco
CA 94118
USA

F. CALLEA
Department of Pathology
Giannina Gaslini Institute
Largo G. Gaslini 5
I-16148 Genova
Italy

M. H. DAVIES
Birmingham Liver Unit
Queen Elizabeth Hospital
Edgbaston
Birmingham
B15 2TH
UK

N. FAUSTO
Department of Pathology and Laboratory Medicine
Brown University School of Medicine
Box G
Providence
RI 02912
USA

P. FERENCI
Universitätsklinik für Innere Medizin IV
Gastroenterologie und Hepatologie
Allgemeines Krankenhaus der Stadt Wien
Währinger Gürtel 18–20
A-1090 Wien
Austria

P. GENTILINI
Istituto Clinica Medica Generale e Terapia Medica II
Viale Morgagni, 85
I-50134 Firenze
Italy

W. GEROK
Medizinische Universitätsklinik und Poliklinik
Hugstetter Str. 55
W-7800 Freiburg im Breisgau
Germany

O. HAMBERG
Rigshospitalet A-2152
Division of Hepatology
Blegdamsvej 9
DK-2100 Copenhagen
Denmark

H. HARTMANN
Department of Medicine
Division of Gastroenterology and Endocrinology
University of Göttingen
Robert-Koch-Str. 40
W-3400 Göttingen
Germany

D. HÄUSSINGER
Abteilung Innere Medizin II
Medizinische Universitätsklinik und Poliklinik
Hugstetter Str. 55
W-7800 Freiburg im Breisgau
Germany

B. LAUNOIS
Clinique Chirurgicale
Hopital de Pontchaillou
Rue Henri Le Guilloux
F-35033 Rennes Cedex
France

D. LEBREC
Laboratoire d'Hemodynamique Splanchnique
INSERM U-24 et Service d'Hepatologie
100 Boulevard du General Leclerc
F-92118 Clichy Cedex
France

J. LINDENBAUM
Department of Medicine
Columbia University
630 West 168th Street
New York
NY 10032
USA

K. P. MAIER
Medizinische Klinik
Fachbereich Gastroenterologie
Städtische Krankenanstalten
Hirschlandstr. 97
W-7300 Esslingen
Germany

U. A. MEYER
Department of Pharmacology
Stanford University School of Medicine
Stanford
CA 94305-5332
USA

K. H. MEYER ZUM BÜSCHENFELDE
I. Medizinische Universitätsklinik
Johannes Gutenberg Universität
Langenbeckstr. 1
W-6500 Mainz 1
Germany

M. J. MIHATSCH
Institut für Pathologie der Universität
Schönbeinstr. 40
CH-4003 Basel
Switzerland

R. K. OCKNER
Liver Center
University of California San Francisco
San Francisco
CA 94143-0630
USA

J. REICHEN
Institut für Klinische Pharmacologie
Inselspital
Murtenstr. 35
CH-3010 Bern
Switzerland

M. RIZZETTO
Institute of Internal Medicine
Molinette
Corso Bramante 88
I-10126 Torino
Italy

J. RODES
Liver Unit
Hospital Clinico y Provincial
Villarroel, 170
E-08036 Barcelona
Spain

LIST OF PRINCIPAL CONTRIBUTORS

R. SCHMID
University of California
School of Medicine, S-224
Box 0410
San Francisco
CA 94143-0410
USA

J. SCHÖLMERICH
Medizinische Klinik und Poliklinik 1
Universitätsklinikum Regensburg
Franz-Josef-Strauss-Allee 11
W-8400 Regensburg
Germany

R. W. SCHRIER
Department of Medicine
University of Colorado Health Sciences Center
4200 East 9th Avenue
Denver
CO 80262
USA

T. E. STARZL
Department of Surgery
University of Pittsburgh
School of Medicine
3601 Fifth Avenue
Pittsburgh
PA 15213
USA

I. STERNLIEB
Liver Research Center
Albert Einstein College of Medicine
1300 Morris Park Avenue, Ullman 517
Bronx
NY 10461
USA

R. W. STREMMEL
Abteilung für Innere Medizin der
Heinrich-Heine Universität
Moorenstr. 5
W-4000 Düsseldorf 1
Germany

J. A SUMMERFIELD
Department of Medicine
QEQM Wing
St Mary's Hospital Medical School
Imperial College of Science and Technology
London
W2 1NY
UK

D. H. VAN THIEL
Oklahoma Transplant Institute
Baptist Medical Center of Oklahoma
3300 Northwest Expressway
Oklahoma City
OK 73112
USA

G. Y. WU
University of Connecticut
Department of Medicine
Division of Gastroenterology
263 Farmington Avenue
Farmington
CT 06030
USA

R. ZIEGLER
Abteilung Innere Medizin 1
Medizinische Klinik der Universität Heidelberg
Bergheimer Str. 58
W-6900 Heidelberg 1
Germany

Preface and Introduction of Professor Thomas E. Starzl

R. SCHMID

Ladies and Gentlemen,
This evening's lecture is the first general event of the Basel Liver Week 1992. As the chairman of the symposium I would like to take this opportunity to welcome you in Basel to this mega-assembly of the world's hepatologists. It is also the ninth International Congress on Liver Disease which Dr Herbert Falk has organized, and the sixth time that it is taking place in Basel. I am certain I speak on behalf of all present when I express to Dr Falk our deep gratitude for his extraordinary and unique contributions to hepatology and his enduring support of the interaction and communication among hepatologists worldwide.

Thank you, Herbert Falk.

Meine Damen und Herren,
Als Vorsitzender des neunten Internationalen Kongresses über Leberkrankheiten entbiete ich Ihnen ein herzliches Willkommen in Basel.

Heute Abend beginnen wir gleich mit einem Höhepunkt der Basler Leberwoche, nämlich Professor Thomas Starzl's 'state-of-the-art' Vorlesung über Lebertransplantation. Beim Ausdruck 'state-of-the-art' hat die Art in diesem Zusammenhang natürlich wenig zu tun mit Kunst, obwohl ja beide, Kunst und Wissenschaft, kreatives Schaffen gemeinsam haben. Aber mit 'state-of-the-art' ist hier gemeint der gegenwärtige Stand der wissenschaftlichen und technischen Entwicklung, in unserem Fall der Entwicklung der Lebertransplantation. Das ungewöhnliche und bemerkenswerte an der heutigen Vorlesung ist, dass es der Vortragende selber war, der diese Entwicklung in Bewegung gesetzt hat und der sie dank seiner aussergewöhnlichen wissenschaftlichen und chirurgischen Leistungen drei Jahrzehnte lang im Brennpunkt des medizinischen Fortschrittes hielt.

Ladies and Gentlemen, it therefore is very appropriate to consider Dr Starzl as *the father* of liver transplantation.

Thomas Earl Starzl was born in Iowa in 1926, and earned his MD together with a PhD degree in 1952 at Northwestern University in Chicago. He then took extended postgraduate surgical and research training at Johns Hopkins Medical School, which provided him with his proverbial surgical skill, judgement and self-control for which he is internationally recognized. In 1962 he was appointed Professor of Surgery at the University of Colorado, and in 1981 he assumed his present position as Distinguished Professor of Surgery at the University of Pittsburgh.

A true visionary, Dr Starzl became fascinated with the possibility of organ transplantation in the late 1950s, at a time when human orthotopic liver transplantation was still a subject of science fiction. But notwithstanding the doubts, if not ridicule, which he initially had to tolerate, he carried on with preparatory studies in animals thought to be of importance for the day when a whole new liver would be implanted in patients with incurable liver failure. These preliminary studies included not only surgical technique, which clearly is unusually demanding, but also investigations of hepatic blood flow, metabolism and regeneration, as well as the immunological problems which one would expect when a foreign organ is grafted onto a living, unrelated body.

The day of reckoning came in 1963 when Starzl and his co-workers for the first time replaced a patient's fatally damaged liver with a healthy human organ. The operation was a technical success, but the recipient unfortunately died during the latter part of the postoperative period. In subsequent transplantations during these early years, Starzl achieved respectable 1-year survival rates of 25–35%, not good enough to silence all vocal critiques, but sufficient to keep up his irrepressible enthusiasm and total commitment. With the refinement of surgical techniques and improvements in liver preservation, perfusion and immunosuppression, survival rates of 85–90% have now become the rule.

In 1983 an international Consensus Conference, held at the National Institutes of Health under my chairmanship, critically reviewed all information then available worldwide. It unanimously concluded that orthotopic liver transplantation had successfully passed the experimental stage and henceforth should be regarded as a promising alternative approach to the treatment of hopeless end-stage liver disease. Based on this recommendation, public and private health care insurance organizations began to accept reimbursement of the operation's costs. As a result, the number of liver transplantations has rapidly increased over the past 8 years, and over 200 hospitals in the US, Europe, and most recently in Japan, are now equipped to perform the operation. The indications for transplantation, which initially were quite restricted, have progressively been broadened and now include fulminant hepatic failure as well as alcoholic and chronic viral liver diseases.

In this dramatic evolution, Starzl has played a central and decisive role of leadership, and his unit at the University of Pittsburgh has accumulated by far the most extensive experience, both in surgical technique as well as in postoperative management, particularly in the handling of immunological rejection and postoperative viral infections of the immune suppressed recipient. He and his co-workers have also made a number of very important observations on the nature of inherited metabolic diseases in which liver transplantation had been performed. These include Wilson's disease, haemochromatosis, alpha-1 antitrypsin deficiency, protoporphyria, Crigler–Najjar disease, type IV glycogen storage disease and homozygous familial hypercholesterolaemia. In some of these conditions, liver transplantation corrected the metabolic defect, and in others substantially improved the patients' survival and quality of life.

Dr Starzl, your life's work represents an exemplary testimony of how unusual imagination, superb skill and complete dedication may produce a quantum leap of progress in science and technology. Ladies and Gentlemen, I am pleased to introduce Professor Thomas Earl Starzl.

State of the Art Lecture
Chimaerism after whole organ transplantation

T. E. STARZL

Throughout the modern history of transplantation, progress with kidney and liver grafting has been interchangeable – and then applicable with very little change to the thoracic organs and most recently the intestine. I will focus today first on why any kind of whole organ allograft and xenograft is accepted, because this not only defines the state of the art for the liver, but predicts the future of transplantation as a whole.

My personal interest in transplantation came via the back door of physiology, during metabolic investigations of the special (so-called hepatotrophic) qualities of portal venous blood. In the course of these inquiries I first developed a new experimental method of total hepatectomy[1] and then the operation of liver replacement[2]. By the end of 1959 we had clarified the surgical secrets of liver transplantation and had also completed a second project in dogs with a multivisceral transplant procedure[3]. Twenty-five years later this latter operation was performed successfully in humans and became the basis for several variations such as the cluster and liver–intestine procedures[4].

However, this research activity in 1958 through early 1960 was in a therapeutic vacuum because there was no such thing as practical immunosuppression. Pharmacological immunosuppression is dated to the classical paper on 6-mercaptopurine by Schwartz and Dameshek[5] in a non-transplant model. Within a few months this drug was shown to prolong survival of skin grafts in rodents[6,7] and kidney allografts in dogs[8,9]. Realizing by now that the road to my primary objective of liver transplantation would have to be through the simpler kidney transplant model, I moved from Northwestern University in Chicago to the University of Colorado in late 1961. There I began a clinical kidney programme.

KIDNEY TRANSPLANTATION AND CHIMAERISM

The programme was based on the simple laboratory discovery that canine kidney rejection under azathioprine could be reversed with prednisone in 88% of dogs[10], an incidence that proved to be the same in humans, as we reported in 1963[11]. The key points were summarized in the title of the 1963 article – the reversal of kidney rejection by steroids and the subsequent ability in successful cases to later reduce the intensity of immunosuppression (referred to as 'tolerance').

The explanation for these two observations was a mystery in 1963, but in retrospect a clue to the mystery was uncovered with exhaustive skin test studies (tuberculin, histoplasmin, coccidiodin, etc.) performed on these early Colorado kidney recipients and their donors. Skin reactions that were positive in the donor but not the recipient were found to cross over to the previously negative recipient along with the transplanted kidney 77% of the time. When this did not occur (the other 23%), it meant that the kidney transplant had failed. Wilson and Kirkpatrick, the immunology fellows who performed these tests, speculated (as it turned out correctly) that the migration of the skin tests was 'caused by adoptive transfer of donor cellular immunity by leukocytes in the renal graft vasculature and hilar lymphoid tissue'[12].

That this actually had occurred was proved 29 years later when some of these original kidney recipients were restudied, proving that there had been an exchange of lymphodendritic leucocytes between the transplanted kidneys and their recipients. These cells still survived nearly three decades later. The presence of the donor cells in the lymph nodes and skin of four recipients of kidneys from HLA mismatched donors was shown with immunocytochemical techniques that stained cells of donor phenotype. These appeared to be dendritic cells. The microchimaerism was confirmed with polymerase chain reaction techniques. In a fifth patient, a female who had received a kidney from her father, male donor cells with the Y chromosome were found in recipient tissues with fluorescent *in situ* hybridization, and confirmed with polymerase chain reaction (PCR) techniques. All of the studied recipients and their grafts were composite structures – no longer the same as at the outset[13].

LIVER TRANSPLANT RECIPIENTS

This was only the beginning of what quickly became a scientific detective story. Between April and July of 1992 evidence was obtained that an even more extensive exchange of tissue leucocytes occurred after liver transplantation, creating a composite graft as well as chimaeric composite host on an even larger scale than after kidney transplantation[14]. For the liver study we began by obtaining follow-ups on all 44 of our first 206 liver recipients who still were alive $10\frac{2}{3}$ to nearly 23 years after transplantation. Six of these patients had stopped their immunosuppressive medications 1–6 years after transplantation and had been drug-free for 5–13 years. The lymphocytes of treated as well as untreated patients reacted vigorously to the lymphocytes of third-party donors. The drug-free patients had achieved lasting immunological tolerance. We also realized that many if not most of those still being treated probably no longer required immunosuppression.

Multiple biopsies were performed on six of the drug-free patients and on 16 more still under maintenance immunosuppression. Specimens were taken of the liver, skin, and a convenient lymph node. Using HLA markers, all 22 were demonstrated to be chimaeras with immunocytochemical and PCR techniques; by PCR, 75% were also blood chimaeras. This could also be documented with sex typing in a subgroup of nine women who had received livers from male donors. Sex chimaerism (the Y chromosome) was detected with fluorescent *in situ* hybridization or with PCR in every case. Using either the HLA alleles of chromosome 6 or the male Y chromosome, the hepatocytes, ducts, and endothelial cells of the allografts remained donor-specific while the Kupffer cells, dendritic cells and other stromal leucocytes were those of the recipients. The systemic chimaerism was usually in more than one site. In one female patient who lost her male graft after 12 years to recurrent viral hepatitis, tissue samples taken at retransplantation (which was successful) showed male cells in blood, skin, lymph nodes, jejunum and the aortic ellipse excised to accommodate a Carrel patch. At the time these samples were collected, this woman had been off medication for 7 years. In the autopsy specimens from another patient who died of B virus hepatitis after 18.4 years, chimaerism was found in essentially all tissues of the body[15].

Aside from their immunological implications the peripheralized chimaeric cells can profoundly alter metabolism[16]. In three additional patients who had undergone liver transplantation 26–91 months previously for metabolic storage diseases, enzyme transport by the seeded peripheral cells explained how amylopectin (in two patients with GSD IV) could be absorbed from the heart as had occurred. Donor cells (thought to be dendritic leucocytes) were detected with monoclonal anti-HLA antibodies and PCR in the myocardium, skin, and lymph nodes. In a patient with Gaucher's disease, donor cells or donor DNA were found in the recipient blood, bone marrow, skin, small bowel, and lymph nodes. In this patient the glucocerebroside deposits (Gaucher's cells) in the lymph nodes had diminished astonishingly over the 26 months post-transplantation.

Thus systemic chimaerism was detected in all 25 liver recipients who were studied from 2 to more than 20 years post-transplantation. The ability to find donor cells wherever they were looked for was striking. Because the same thing was found in the kidney recipients, although less prominently, we concluded that the same thing probably occurred with all kinds of grafts – but so much more extensively with the liver than with other organs, that this accounted for what has been called hepatic tolerogenicity.

WHY PRINCIPLES OF IMMUNOSUPPRESSION ARE NOT DRUG- OR ORGAN-SPECIFIC

These remarkable discoveries in kidney and liver recipients were made only a few months ago. Of course, none of this was known in 1963 when, without knowing why, the observations of rejection reversal and so-called tolerance in kidney recipients led to the empirical therapeutic dogma upon which the transplantation of all whole organ transplantation is based[11,17]. The dogma calls for daily baseline treatment (in those early days with azathioprine) plus intervention with the highly dose-manoeuvrable adrenal cortical steroids (later augmented with antilymphoid agents) to whatever level is required to maintain stable graft function. This creates a trial-and-error situation for every patient as drugs are weaned.

Although the new drugs that have been added through the years have been increasingly potent, they can be viewed as traffic directors, allowing the cell movement to and from all kinds of grafts but preventing the immune destruction that is the natural purpose of the traffic. Apparently, it does not matter exactly how the immune reaction is disrupted, but only that this be achieved without killing all of the migratory cells. The emasculated but living cells that normally cause graft immunogenicity and rejection become instead the missionaries subserving chimaerism, graft acceptance, and ultimately tolerance. Disruption of the function of the lymphocyte can be at the level of antigen processing (claimed for the experimental drug, deoxyspergualin), at an early stage in T-cell activation as occurs with cyclosporin and FK 506, or distal to this with rapamycin which does not inhibit the secretion of cytokines including IL-2 but blocks their action. The so-called antiproliferative drugs (of which azathioprine was the prototype) work even more distally.

RE-EXAMINING TRANSPLANTATION IMMUNOLOGY

With the understanding that cell migration and repopulation is the basis of graft acceptance, no matter what the organ, we now can re-examine some controversies in transplantation immunology that have never been resolved – including why HLA tissue matching to govern the distribution of cadaveric organs has been so imperfect a tool. To understand these controversies we must turn the pages back 50 years, to when Peter Medawar planted the seed of our clinical specialty. If rejection was an immunological response, as Medawar claimed in 1944[18], what could be more logical in preventing it than to weaken the immune system. By 1951, Billingham, Krohn, and Medawar[19] and the American Morgan[20] had taken this crucial step, and had shown that skin graft survival was prolonged with cortisone acetate and ACTH – the first immunosuppressive drugs. The year before, Dempster and co-workers, of Hammersmith, showed mitigation of skin graft rejection with total-body irradiation[21].

Seemingly, these were small steps, but then in 1953 Billingham, Brent, and Medawar[22,23] raised expectations to a new level by showing the possibility of acquiring immunological tolerance, albeit only under the special circumstance of inoculation of immunocompetent adult spleen cells into fetal and perinatal mice. Main and Prehn[24] were able to mimic these developmental conditions in *adult* mice using supralethal total-body irradiation and bone marrow allo-reconstitution. When the reconstituted mice were shown to be tolerant to donor strain skin (the white patch), the clinical possibility of creating radiation bone marrow chimaeras as a means to the end of solid organ transplantation seemed obvious.

These hopes were promptly dashed when the concept of GVHD and runt disease was delineated by Billingham and Brent[25]. However, what was *not* clearly recognized, then or later, was that these whole-animal models, and subsequently the experimental F_1 hybrid model, are almost artifacts in the sense that the interactions of the two-way cell migration and repopulation that I have been discussing were precluded in each case: by the immature state of one party (that was the Billingham, Brent, Medawar model), by the cytoablation used by Main and Prehn (and later bone marrow transplanters), or by genetic manipulation (the F_1 hybrid model). These were whole-animal analogues of the *in vitro* one-way mixed-lymphocyte reaction.

DIVISION OF TRANSPLANTATION INTO TWO FIELDS

Of course, this is hindsight 33 years later. Between 1959 and 1963 – and without really knowing why – the intellectual root that came from Medawar's seed divided into two branches. Although the issue from the roots looked like two separate trees when they surfaced the differences merely reflected different therapeutic dogmas. The bone marrow tree with its precondition of cytoablation mimicked the Billingham, Brent, Medawar model and was the *in vivo* version of a one-way MLR. HLA matching was crucial. Engraftment in a drug-free state (called tolerance) was a realizable objective only with perfect matching. This was not achieved clinically until 1968[26,27], but even with MHC compatibility, GVHD was a constant threat. The reason for the virulence of the GVHD with an HLA mismatch was the complete removal of a counterweight to the transplanted immunocytes.

The whole-organ transplanters who had broken ranks with their bone marrow colleagues, empirically developed the long-term immunosuppression which I discussed earlier with which success (called graft acceptance, not tolerance) did *not* depend on matching and could be accomplished without GVHD – even after the transplantation of lymphoid-rich organs such as the intestine and liver. The explanation for the GVHD resistance with the whole organs is envisioned as the interaction of cells coming out from the allograft with the immunocytes of the recipient (a two-way *in vivo* MLR). The term for the long-term coexistence of two populations of cells is mixed chimaerism.

Of course, the fact that mixed chimaerism interdicts GVHD is only half of the story. The other half is that the midfield cell interaction (which results in what we have called mutual natural immunosuppression) also mitigates rejection (the host versus graft reaction). The details of this donor–recipient rapproachment are not known, but it does seem clear that even organs like the kidney with a poor lymphoreticular constituency have enough dendritic cells (or whatever these leucocytes are) to sometimes induce for themselves donor-specific non-reactivity (tolerance). In the process the donor/recipient interactions are envisioned as occurring on a sliding scale, in which each further level of histo*in*compatibility provokes variable countervailing increases in the mutually cancelling donor versus recipient *and* recipient versus donor cell reactivity.

For renal allografts it becomes possible to understand why Terasaki, Opelz, and others have shown a large advantage only for six-antigen matched cadaver kidney but not for any matching that is less perfect. Most importantly, it becomes possible to understand why the vast majority of unmatched kidneys do well. For liver transplantation the reports from Cambridge and Pittsburgh become comprehensible that have shown an *inverse* relation between the quality of HLA match and survival of liver recipients, but again a difference that is measurable only within a few percentage points.

INDUCTION OF TOLERANCE

It seems obvious that the crucial variable distinguishing one organ from another is the lymphodendritic (not the parenchymal) component – and that these tissue leucocytes can be tolerogenic as well as immunogenic when effective immunosuppression is given. The liver, with its dense constituency of these cells, is high on the favourable list of tolerogenicity, with the lung and intestine following and the heart and kidney bringing up the rear. It is self-evident that the underprivileged kidney and heart could be brought to the same level of tolerogenicity advantage as the liver by the perioperative infusion of lymphoreticular cells obtained from bone marrow of the organ donor, or possibly from the spleen. Now the cycle is complete because this was the starting point for Billingham, Brent, and Medawar, and then Main and Prehn.

THE DRUG REVOLUTION

Of course, what I have said today is our current understanding of transplantation. Rather than limiting a search for better drugs, this insight should encourage their development, as can be illustrated by the different eras of liver transplantation. In July 1967 the first long-surviving liver recipients were produced under azathioprine, prednisone, after an effort which by then had consumed almost 10 years. However, acceptance of the procedure was slow over the next dozen years because of its high mortality. Roy Calne's introduction of cyclosporin[28] and the subsequent combination of this drug with prednisone[29] allowed a doubling or more of survival about a decade ago and brought liver transplantation to centre-stage[30].

Recently, the liver has been the lead organ in the next step of immunosuppression, made possible with the drug, FK 506, whose action is similar to cyclosporin[31]. The patient and graft survival with FK 506 has been improved a further 10–15% compared to the cyclosporin results in the Pittsburgh trials, and in the recent European multicentre randomized trials of FK 506 versus cyclosporin.

These trials suggest that we are at the dawn of another era in transplantation, signalled in addition by an emerging population of recipients of complete cadaveric small bowel, either transplanted alone, with the liver, or as part of a multivisceral graft[32]. Of 23 such patients treated 4 months to more than 2 years ago, all but three are alive. Only one example of GVHD has been seen. The chimaerism I have been discussing has been obvious in every case. In the intestine with epithelial cells of the graft remain those of the donor while the lymphoreticular stromal substrate switches over to predominantly that of the recipient.

XENOTRANSPLANTATION

When organs are transplanted from a significantly disparate species, the first immunological hurdle is that of preformed xenospecific antibodies which quickly devascularize the graft and exclude it from recipient circulation by damaging its blood vessels[33]. If this barrier can be surmounted, the process of xenograft acceptance involves the same bidirectional cell migration and consequent systemic chimaerism as with allotransplantation. After hamster to rat xenotransplantation, the cells displaced from the xenografts can be detected in widespread rat recipient tissues with polyclonal rat absorbed anti-hamster leucocyte antibodies, and confirmed with PCR techniques[14]. As with allotransplantation, the chimaerism is more extensive after liver than after heart transplantation.

Chimaerism was observed recently in a patient who survived for 70 days after receipt of a baboon liver. Death was caused by infectious complications and by complications of biliary stasis rather than rejection or GVHD[34]. This means that successful clinical xenotransplantation must be visualized along the same lines of donor–recipient cellular intimacy which we believe is the fundamental means of xenograft as well as allograft acceptance.

SUMMARY

I have tried to present a unified view of transplantation to which the liver has contributed the central role[35,36]. Thank you for the honour of allowing me to present this to you.

References

1. Starzl TE, Bernhard VM, Benvenuto R, Cortes N. A new method for one-stage hepatectomy in dogs. Surgery. 1959;46:880–6.
2. Starzl, TE, Kaupp HA Jr, Brock DR, Lazarus RE, Johnson RV. Reconstructive problems in canine liver homotransplantation with special reference to the postoperative role of hepatic venous flow. Surg Gynecol Obstet. 1960;111:733–43.
3. Starzl TE, Kaupp HA Jr. Mass homotransplantation of abdominal organs in dogs. Surg Forum. 1960;11:28–30.
4. Starzl TE, Todo S, Tzakis A, Alessiani M, Casavilla A, Abu-Elmagd K, Fung JJ. The many faces of multivisceral transplantation. Surg Gynecol Obstet. 1991;172:335–44.
5. Schwartz R, Dameshek W. Drug-induced immunological tolerance. Nature. 1959;183:1682–3.
6. Schwartz, R, Dameshek W. The effects of 5-mercaptopurine on homograft reactions. J Clin Invest. 1960;39:952–8.

7. Meeker W, Condie R, Weiner D, Varco RL, Good RA. Prolongation of skin homograft survival in rabbits by 6-mercaptopurine. Proc Soc Exp Biol Med. 1959;102:459–61.
8. Calne RY. The rejection of renal homografts: inhibition in dogs by 6-mercaptopurine. Lancet. 1960;1:417–18.
9. Zukoski CF, Lee HM, Hume DM. The prolongation of functional survival of canine renal homografts by 6-mercaptopurine. Surg Forum. 1960;11:470–2.
10. Marchioro TL, Axtell HK, LaVia MF, Waddell WR, Starzl TE. The role of adrenocortical steroids in reversing established homograft rejection. Surgery. 1964;55:412–17.
11. Starzl TE, Marchioro TL, Waddell WR. The reversal of rejection in human renal homografts with subsequent development of homograft tolerance. Surg Gynecol Obstet. 1963;117:385–95.
12. Wilson WEC, Kirkpatrick CH. Immunologic aspects of renal homotransplantation. In: Starzl TE, editor. Experience in renal transplantation. Philadelphia: Saunders; 1964:239–61.
13. Starzl TE, Demetris AJ, Trucco M, Zeevi A, Ramos H, Terasaki P, Rudert WA, Kocova M, Ricordi C, Ildstad S, Murase N. Chimerism and donor specific nonreactivity 27 to 29 years after kidney allotransplantation. Transplantation. 1993: In press.
14. Starzl TE, Murase N, Demetris AJ, Giorda R, Valdivia L, Trucco M. Drug development and testing in relation to cell migration and chimerism. Transplant Proc. 1993;25:469–72.
15. Starzl TE, Demetris AJ, Trucco M, Murase N, Ricordi C, Ildstad S. Cell migration and chimerism after whole organ transplantation: The basis of graft acceptance. Hepatology. 1993;17:issue 5.
16. Starzl TE, Demetris AJ, Trucco M, Ricordi C, Ildstad S, Terasaki P, Murase N, Kendall RS, Kocova N, Rudert WA, Zeevi A, Van Thiel D. Chimerism after liver transplantation for Type IV glycogen storage disease and Type I Gaucher's disease. N Engl J Med. 1993;328:745–9.
17. Starzl TE: Experience in Renal Transplantation. Philadelphia: Saunders; 1964:1–383.
18. Medawar PB. The behaviour and fate of skin autografts and skin homografts in rabbits. J Anat. 1944;78:176–99.
19. Billingham RE, Krohn PL, Medawar PB. Effect of cortisone on survival of skin homografts in rabbits. Br Med J. 1951;1:1157–63.
20. Morgan JA. The influence of cortisone on the survival of homografts of skin in the rabbit. Surgery. 1951;30:506–15.
21. Dempster WJ, Lennox B, Boag JW. Prolongation of survival of skin homotransplants in the rabbit by irradiation of the host. Br J Exp Pathol. 1950;31:670–9.
22. Billingham RE, Brent L, Medawar PB. 'Actively acquired tolerance' of foreign cells. Nature. 1953;172:603–6.
23. Billingham R, Brent L, Medawar P. Quantitative studies on tissue transplantation immunity. III. Activity acquired tolerance. Phil Trans R Soc Lond (Biol). 1956;239:357–412.
24. Main JM, Prehn RT. Successful skin homografts after the administration of high dosage X radiation and homologous bone marrow. J Natl Cancer Inst. 1955;15:1023–9.
25. Billingham R, Brent L. Quantitative studies on transplantation immunity. IV. Induction of tolerance in newborn mice and studies on the phenomenon of runt disease. Phil Trans R Soc Lond (Biol). 1956;242:439–77.
26. Gatti RA, Meuwissen HJ, Allen HD, Hong R, Good RA. Immunological reconstitution of sex-linked lymphopenic immunological deficiency. Lancet. 1968;2:1366–9.
27. Thomas ED. Allogeneic marrow grafting – a story of man and dog: In: Terasaki PI, Cecka JM, editors. Clinical transplants. Los Angeles, CA: UCLA Press, 1991:381–90.
28. Calne RY, Rolles K, White DJG, Thiru S, Evans DB, McMaster P, Dunn DC, Craddock GN, Henderson RG, Aziz S, Lewis P. Cyclosporin A initially as the only immunosuppressant in 34 recipients of cadaveric organs: 32 kidneys, 2 pancreases, and 2 livers. Lancet. 1979;2:1033–6.
29. Starzl TE, Weil R III, Iwatsuki S, Klintmalm G, Schroter GPJ, Koep LJ, Iwasaki Y, Terasaki PI, Porter KA. The use of cyclosporin A and prednisone in cadaver kidney transplantation. Surg Gynecol Obstet. 1980;151:17–26.
30. Starzl TE, Klintmalm GBG, Porter KA, Iwatsuki S, Schroter GPJ. Liver transplantation with use of cyclosporin A and prednisone. N Engl J Med. 1981;305:266–9.
31. Starzl TE, Todo S, Fung J, Demetris AJ, Venkataramanan R, Jain A. FK 506 for human liver, kidney, and pancreas transplantation. Lancet. 1989;2:1000–4.
32. Todo S, Tzakis AG, Abu-Elmagd K, Reyes J, Nakamura K, Casavilla A, Selby R, Nour BM, Wright H, Fung JJ, Demetris AJ, Van Thiel DH, Starzl TE. Intestinal transplantation

in composite visceral grafts or alone. Ann Surg. 1992;216:223–34.
33. Starzl TE. The future of xenotransplantation. Ann Surg. 1992;216(4):October (supplement).
34. Starzl TE, Fung J, Tzakis A, Todo S, Demetris AJ, Marino IR, Doyle H, Zeevi A, Warty V, Michaels M, Kusne S, Rudert WA, Trucco M. Baboon to human liver transplantation. Lancet. 1993;341:65–71.
35. Starzl TE, Demetris AJ, Murase N, Ildstad S, Ricordi C, Trucco M. Cell migration, chimerism, and graft acceptance. Lancet. 1992;339:1579–82.
36. Starzl TE, Demetris AJ, Trucco M, Ramos H, Zeevi A, Rudert WA, Kocoua M, Ricordi C, Ildstad S, Murase N. Systemic chimerism in human female recipients of male livers. Lancet. 1992;340:876–7.

Hans Popper Award 1992: Introduction of Dr Mario Rizzetto

R. SCHMID

Ladies and Gentlemen,
The Hans Popper Award is sponsored by the Falk Foundation to recognize outstanding contributions to clinical and experimental hepatology by scientists under the age of 50. The award is given in memory of Hans Popper, whose charismatic personality and intellectual genius dominated these meetings from their inception to his death. Although Hans passed away in 1988, like an invisible hand, his vision seems to continue hovering over the Basel Liver Week and to spiritually steer and enrich it.

An international committee of distinguished hepatologists was charged with the selection of this year's awardee. This turned out to be a difficult task, because almost a dozen candidates had been nominated, all with impressive qualifications and widely recognized scientific achievements. What led the committee to award the prize to *Dr Mario Rizzetto* of Torino, Italy, was the far-reaching scope and worldwide impact of his work on viral hepatitis, culminating in his discovery of delta hepatitis.

Dr Rizzetto received his medical education at the venerable University of Padova, and subsequently specialized in gastroenterology and hepatology in Torino and Milano. He early on developed a strong interest in the immunopathology of liver disease, particularly of viral hepatitis. In the early 1970s he spent a year of fellowship at the Middlesex Hospital Medical School in London, where he learned from Deborah Doniach the secrets of autoimmunity and, in fact, discovered a few new and important autoantibodies.

But Dr Rizzetto's most important contribution by far was his discovery in 1977 of a new antigen–antibody system in patients with hepatitis B virus infection. This of course turned out to reflect superinfection with a new pathogenic hepatotropic agent, the delta agent, a defective RNA virus that in some ways resembles virions in plants. Perhaps the most curious aspect of this new infective agent was that it required the coexistence of infection with the hepatitis B virus, a feature which seemed to make it difficult to distinguish the two superimposed infections. This may explain the surprise and reservations which initially met Dr Rizzetto's challenging report. But all ambivalence was soon dispersed when, at the invitation of Dr Robert Purcell at NIH and John Gerin at Georgetown University, Dr Rizzetto was able to present his exciting findings to a critical audience of peers in the US Capital. There followed an exceptionally productive year of fellowship at the NIH and Georgetown, during which Dr Rizzetto began to clarify the nature of the hepatitis D agent and its many pathological and immunological features.

After his return to Italy in 1980, Dr Rizzetto established in Torino a powerful unit for hepatitis research which has become very productive, and is attracting international recognition and people from all over the world. Over the past 12 years he and his co-workers have succeeded in characterizing most of the pathogenic, morphological, and epidemiological aspects of delta hepatitis. Indeed, Dr Rizzetto not only *discovered* delta hepatitis, but he made it *his* own disease. Yet, he by no means neglected his interests in other types of viral hepatitis and liver disease. For example, in 1989 he and his co-workers *co*discovered the bizarre hepatitis B variants in which the hepatitis B virus had lost its ability to produce precore hepatitis B-e antigen. This unexpected finding touched off a world-wide flood of investigations which revealed that these variants are by no means infrequent and reflect on-going viral mutations.

In a relatively short period of time Dr Rizzetto has become one of the most productive and admired investigators in hepatology, and one of the world's foremost experts in liver disease. He represents the scientific forefront in the field, and is uniquely deserving of the distinction of the award which honours the founder of scientific hepatology, Dr Hans Popper.

Dr Rizzetto, may I ask you to come forward.

Hans Popper Award
The hepatitis delta virus: a unique human pathogen

M. RIZZETTO

To a person like me, who has committed his working life to the study and treatment of liver disorders, it is the greatest honour to receive the 1992 prize in the name of Dr Hans Popper, the father of modern hepatology, its most fervent apostle and the most important contemporary representative of the new discipline. I wish to thank the International Selection Committee, and in particular its President Professor Leonardo Bianchi, for this honour.

The enthusiasm of Hans, and his endless interest in all aspects of liver diseases, made him a charismatic figure who has inspired generations of hepatologists, and the protagonist of all major advances in liver pathology.

This is true also of hepatitis delta. When Hans first learnt about the delta antigen his intellectual curiosity drove him to verify the claim. To my satisfaction he almost immediately became a vigorous and vocal supporter of the delta novelty at a time when scepticism was still widespread. Hans decided personally to investigate the morphological aspects of the new disease. He produced a number of papers on the peculiar cytopathic aspects of hepatitis D which remain a classic in liver pathology[1,2].

I take further personal pleasure in delivering this lecture, as it was here in Basel that the hepatitis delta virus was baptized as a new infectious agent by my American mentor Dr Robert Purcell, 2 years after its birth in Italy as a novel hepatitis B virus (HBV)-related antigen[3].

In 1979 Dr Purcell was celebrated for his numerous and important achievements in the field of viral hepatitis at Falk Symposium 28 on Viruses and the Liver. Together with my other American mentor, Dr John Gerin, Bob also deserves credit, among his many merits, for having been the first to foresee clearly the unique nature of the delta virus. Although in his lecture on 'Unfinished business in hepatitis'[4] he considered the hypothesis that the newly identified virus might be a genotype of the HBV, he was clearly inclined to believe the assumption that it was instead a defective non-A, non-B agent requiring the presence of the HBV for infection. He was of course right.

By the beginning of the last decade, infectivity studies in chimpanzees[5] had conclusively shown that the delta antigen was the component of a new hepatotropic agent which needed an obligatory helper function for its infection. This could be provided not only by human HBV[6], but also by the woodchuck hepatitis virus[7]. The development of diagnostic assays has made it possible to carry out epidemiological investigations and detailed clinical analysis of the disease[8]. It has emerged that the hepatitis delta virus (HDV) is a major health problem throughout the world, and it is likely that not less than 5% of the 300 million carriers of HBsAg worldwide are also infected by HDV[9].

As HDV needs HBV in order to thrive, this means that HDV infection only strikes people who have also been infected by the HBV[8]. Those who acquire protective antibodies to the HBsAg (anti-HBs) either by HBV infections which have resolved, or by vaccination, seem to be protected from HDV. Those who are long-term carriers of the HBV are susceptible to HDV, as are those who are infected by HBV and HDV at the same time. The first case is called superinfection, where HDV is rescued by the pre-existing HBV infection of the patient. The second case is known as coinfection, where HDV is rescued by the HBV contained in the infectious inoculum which transmits both viruses.

In simultaneous HBV/HDV infection expression of the HDV is dependent on the virulence of the associated HBV infection and it is also limited by it. The expression of HDV is variable because the interactions between the two viruses are variable. Coinfection only rarely progresses to cause chronic HDV infections, because the underlying HBV infection is usually self-limited and HDV cannot survive after its helper virus has been eliminated[9].

Vice-versa, when HDV infects a carrier of HBsAg the pre-existing HBV infection provides fertile ground for the swift activation and spread of HDV. In this instance the HDV does not depend on the virulence of the HBV in the inoculum, but is instead rescued by the pre-existing HBV infection of the carrier[9]. This means that inocula containing HBV/HDV may not be infectious to normal people, as the HBV component is not sufficiently virulent to initiate a 'helper' infection. They may nonetheless transmit HDV to HBV carriers, as the HBsAg state can rapidly rescue even infinitesimal amounts of the defective agent.

Superinfections in humans result most often in chronic HDV infections because the persistence of the HBsAg state provides a long-term biological setting that HDV can flourish in, and reproduce from, continually.

THE UNIQUE NATURE OF THE HDV: RESEMBLANCE TO THE VIROIDS OF PLANTS

Characterization studies using chimpanzees and well-pedigreed human sera showed that the HDV virion is made up of a 36 nm particle which is coated with the envelope protein of the coinfecting hepadnavirus. The particle contains hepatitis delta antigen (HDAg) and a single-stranded circular 1.7 kilobase RNA. Although this chimaeric structure has earned HDV the definition of 'defective' agent, there are no parallels between HDV and the defective interfering particles generated during the infection of many RNA viruses, as there is no significant sequence homology between HDV and the helper hepadnaviruses.

The virion that is infectious in humans is coated by HBsAg, similar to the 22 nm particle of HBsAg[10]. Antibodies other than anti-HBs have not been found to immunoprecipitate the HDV particle. It therefore seems that no epitopes are present on the HDV envelope apart from those of HBsAg.

The HDV is solubilized in detergent. The antigen is a nuclear phosphoprotein with RNA binding activity that is composed of two crossreacting peptides. In different laboratories the molecular weights of these peptides have varied from 24 to 27 kDa and from 27 to 30 kDa.

The dependence of HDV on a genetically unrelated virus resembles the way that subviral pathogens of the vegetable world, called the viroid-like satellite RNAs, establish infection in plants. These are small RNA molecules that are not replication autonomous but need a simultaneous infection with a mature plant virus for progeny production[11]. Based on these analogies it was suggested in 1981 that the nature of HDV was more akin to the pseudoviruses of the vegetable world than to conventional RNA viruses of animals[12], a hypothesis which has received in the past decade confirmation from the molecular characterization of the HDV genome.

When the HDV-RNA was cloned in the mid-1980s by Dr Kos[13] and the American group of Dr Houghton[14], it was found that this genome was distinctly smaller in size than that of all known animal viruses. It had a single-strand circular structure that was also unheard of in conventional RNA viruses. *In-situ* hybridization experiments have shown that the HDV-RNA resides in the nuclear compartment of the hepatocytes[15]; in infections with conventional RNA viruses the genome is located in the cytoplasm of the hepatocytes.

Many nucleotide stretches contained in the HDV-RNA molecule are complementary to one another. These stretches collapse the RNA into an unbranched rod-like structure which under native conditions has left-hand and right-hand terminal loops.

These conformational features are typical of the viroids and related satellite RNAs. Both have minute single-strand RNA genomes, a genome conformation that is often circular and a cellular localization that is predominantly nuclear[16]. True viroids, however, are not capable of coding for any protein. As satellite RNAs have a genome that is larger than viroid RNA, and that codes for their own proteins, HDV would appear to be more closely related to these pseudoviruses.

Further exciting evidence for the relationship between HDV and the viroid-like satellite RNAs of plants stems from the sequence homologies between two regions of HDV-RNA, one in the genomic strand and the other in the antigenomic strand, and regions conserved in the viroids and satellite RNAs throughout their evolution. These homologous regions were identified in the first description of the molecular anatomy of HDV-RNA[13,14], but their functional role has been clarified only recently. Both regions show an ability to self-cleave and self-ligate *in vitro* in the absence of protein catalysts[17]. They therefore qualify as ribozymes; in other words as a unique RNA molecule which contains the genetic information and an enzymatic activity in itself[18]. The cleavage and ligation of HDV-RNA take place through a process of transesterification. This is activated by a stretch of no more than 100 nucleotides[19] arranged in a complex secondary structure. The direction of the reaction is determined by the temperature and by the concentration of magnesium. The HDV ribozyme in the antigenome is unusually stable, and this results in a very efficient self-cleavage even under biologically adverse conditions[19].

Similar autocatalytic activity has been observed in the satellite RNAs in the regions homologous to the ribozymic sites of HDV[20].

Thus the hepatitis delta virus appears to be made up of two conjoined parts, an ancestral viroid-like domain containing the ribozymic site and a protein-coding domain that directs the synthesis of HDAg. The viroid remnant must have gained a distinct evolutionary advantage with the acquisition of the antigen, but the functions of the HDAg are at present still not clear. It is probably important for the regulation of replication[21].

Translation of the HDAg gene can lead to the expression of two proteins, the small HDAg, which is 155 amino acids long, and the large HDAg, which is 214 amino acids long. When a stop codon is converted into a tryptophan codon by a strategic single nucleotide change in the small HDAg sequence, the large HDAg is synthesized[22]. This mutation occurs in the course of the infection and appears to modulate the rate of HDV-RNA replication, the small antigen accelerating the synthesis of the genome, and the large antigen acting as an inhibitor of its synthesis. The large antigen may be involved in the packaging of the viral nucleic acid in the envelope provided by the helper hepadnavirus[23].

REPLICATION OF HDV

The similarity of the HDV-RNA genome to the viroids of plants has suggested that it may replicate according to the rolling circle model of replication which has been proposed for the plant pseudoviruses[24]. In this model[25] a multimeric antigenomic strand is rolled onto the circular HDV genome which serves as the input. A multimeric genomic strand is copied onto the antigenomic intermediate. The genomic intermediate is then cleaved into monomers of genomic length. In the end the linear monomer is ligated into the circular HDV viral progeny. Double-stranded forms of HDV-RNA, some of them twice the size of genomic RNA, have been found in the livers of infected chimpanzees[26], in agreement with the hypothesis of a direct RNA–RNA synthesis.

While the rolling circle model may provide the mechanism by which HDV replicates, the question of the nature of the polymerase involved remains as yet unanswered. The hypothesis that HDV is replicated via the retroviral mechanism by which the helper HBV is replicated has been ruled out, as the HDAg is too small to act as a polymerase and no DNA copy of HDV-RNA has been found in infected livers. HDV is therefore presumably copied by the host replicative machinery. Known host polymerases, however, normally use DNA rather than RNA templates; thus if HDV is replicated by a normal cell polymerase it must be capable of redirecting the host enzyme to copy RNA[19].

In vitro experiments have confirmed that HDV can replicate within infected cells in the absence of coinfection with a hepadnavirus, and that replication does not depend on specific liver functions. Primary cultures of chimpanzees and woodchuck hepatocytes[27] have been successfully infected with HDV alone, and transfection experiments with cDNA clones of HDV have led to the synthesis of HDV not only in liver but also in non-liver cell lines such as mouse fibroblasts and CHO cells[28]. Furthermore, full-blown hepatitis D accompanied by markers of a virulent HDV infection has been induced by injection of a cDNA clone of HDV directly into the liver of a chimpanzee carrying the HBsAg[29].

THE DISEASE

Despite the advances in the virology of HDV, and in the knowledge of its interactions with the HBV, the medical sequelae of HDV infection continue to represent an unresolved clinical problem. All clinical studies conducted in the past decade have shown a significant correlation between HDV expression and the presence of severe liver disease, and hepatitis D has developed in all chimpanzees experimentally infected with HDV. The disease[30] has also developed in animals inoculated with serum containing HDV diluted 10^{-11}.

Replication of HDV during primary infection often leads to the temporary suppression of HBV synthesis, with a decrease or apparent disappearance of HBV-DNA and of HBV gene products from serum. Interestingly, HDV adapts during intraspecies and interspecies transfers with an exchange of the virus envelope. For example woodchucks infected with HDV coated with HBsAg from primates circulate HDV particles coated with surface antigen derived from the woodchuck hepatitis virus; however, progeny virions contain HDAg and RNA with no modification with relation to the parental virus[7]. Although the close association between HDV and liver disease led in the 1980s to the conclusion that HDV is highly pathogenic, and almost invariably creates new disease or aggraves pre-existing HBV disease, it was observed recently that on the Greek island of Rhodes[31] and in American Samoa, Polynesia[32], many HBV carriers also infected with the HDV had no biochemical or histological signs of liver damage. Moreover the long-term follow-up of HBsAg carrier chimpanzees which were superinfected at the National Institutes of Health in Bethesda further supports the theory that HDV infection may run a harmless course[33]. This study revealed that more than 50% of the animals have continued to circulate HDV-RNA in the absence of significant liver lesions.

It thus appears that the clinical expression of HDV infections is disparate, and there may be considerable geographical differences. However, while an unknown proportion of HDV infections run a subclinical course, patients who develop hepatitis D appear nevertheless to suffer from a disease that is more serious than other forms of viral hepatitis[34]. Unequivocal pointers of virulence are the peak prevalence rates of HDV in patients with fulminant HBsAg hepatitis and in patients with HBsAg cirrhosis, i.e. at the two clinical extremes of the spectrum of HBsAg-positive liver disorders.

The rate of spread of HDV may be one factor that influences the severity of HDV infection in a given population. Asymptomatic cases appear to predominate in populations where the circulation of the virus is relatively slow, whereas disease predominates in communities, such as in drug addicts, where circulation of the virus is rapid[35].

Although genetic differences in the infecting HDV strain or in the helper HBV may be important in explaining clinical disparities, at present there is no evidence that genetic variations are relevant in pathogenesis. The pathogenic mechanism of HDV damage remains unknown, but it would appear to be complex, as a spectrum of inflammatory and cytopathic lesions accompanies human hepatitis D. In one study, over time a correlation was found between the presence and extent of inflammation in the portal tracts and the number of HDAg-positive hepatocytes in the lobule[36]. The extent of the inflammatory reaction was determined by the amount of HDAg in the liver; this would imply that the host's immune system plays a role in creating the disease.

There is, however, evidence that HDV may cause cytopathic lesions without inflammation. HDV may exert direct cytotoxity on the liver cells based on the significant sequence homology between conserved regions of HDV-RNA and two regions of human 7SL RNA, which is a small cytoplasmic RNA associated with the signal recognition particle[37]. This structure plays a part in the correct targeting of secretory and membrane proteins to the membrane of the endoplasmic reticulum. The sequence analogies suggest that antigenomic intermediates of HDV-RNA may base pair to the corresponding 7SL RNA regions. This would disturb the metabolic processes promoted by the normal signal recognition particle. An alternative possibility is that 7SL RNA might be the target of a ribozymic cleavage, as the annealing site would involve the ribozymic domain of HDV. This would also lead to the dysfunction of the particle.

A cytotoxic effect might also be caused by expression of the HDAg. HeLA and HepG2 cell lines were transfected with HDV-RNA constructs under the control of the methallothionein promoter[38]. These cell lines were fatally damaged by the expression of the short form of the HDAg. Cells that did not express the HDAg but which expressed non-coding HDV-RNA showed no damage.

CONCLUSIONS

Although many unsuspected properties of the HDV have been elucidated, and the clinical implications of its infections have been established, the aspects of HDV biology and pathobiology that lie ahead for further studies appear to be even more fascinating than the discoveries of the recent past.

For example, the liver transplantation model now provides the clinical counterpart to the *in vitro* observation that HDV can thrive in the absence of HBV. Patients transplanted for terminal HDV cirrhosis often harbour reinfecting HDV without HBV, and yet they remain well and disease-free[39]. Vice-versa, the recent recognition that the product of c-myc, a proto-oncogene involved in transformation of cells, selectively accumulates in hepatocytes infected with HDV[40] may cast some light on the role of HDV in the early development of cirrhosis and hepatocellular carcinoma. It is also exciting to note that molecular biologists are currently exploring the possibility that some of the biological properties of HDV which make it a devastating and elusive pathogen may be converted into useful therapeutic options. One of these potential options is the use of the viral RNA as a suitable vector for the delivery of biologically active RNAs with antiviral and other beneficial effects[41].

This remarkable and rapid progress in the understanding of the HDV biology and pathology was made possible by a joint, integrated effort between the group in Turin, the National Institutes of Health and Georgetown University. This productive association began when I first had the privilege of working with Dr Purcell and Dr Gerin in the US in the late 1970s. Since then our cooperation has been extended and strengthened by Dr Bonino, Dr Ponzetto, Dr Smedile, Dr Rosina and Dr Negro. One after the other they have shared the expertise and friendship of our American colleagues. Back in Italy they have reproduced their American achievements in the medical reality of Turin. Together with Dr Crivelli, who ran our laboratory in the early 1980s, they have all contributed towards the gradual construction of the HDV image. Thus they all share with me the honour of this prize.

I and my younger colleagues, however, have also been able to enjoy a unique opportunity in Turin thanks to the will and far-sighted intelligence of my former chief and long-time friend Professor Giorgio Verme. He created the research group of Turin anew, staking his enthusiasm and the enthusiasm of his colleagues on future success.

I wish to thank Professor Verme for his continuous support and encouragement throughout the many vicissitudes of medical research in Italy. Were it not for him, I have no doubt that I would not be here today to receive the Hans Popper prize.

References

1. Popper H, Thung SN, Gerber MA *et al.* Histologic studies of severe delta infection in Venezuelan indians. Hepatology. 1983;3:906–12.
2. Popper H, Buitrago B, Hadler SC *et al.* Pathology of hepatitis delta infection in the Amazon Basin. In: Rizzetto M, Gerin JL, Purcell RH, editors. The hepatitis delta virus and its infection. Progress in clinical and biological research, vol. 234. New York: Alan R Liss; 1987:121–8.
3. Rizzetto M, Canese MG, Arico S, Crivelli O, Bonino F, Trepo CG, Verme G. Immunofluorescence detection of a new antigen–antibody system (δ-antiδ) associated with the hepatitis B virus in the liver and in the serum of HBsAg carriers. Gut. 1977;18:997–1003.

4. Purcell RH. Viral hepatitis: some unanswered questions and unfinished business. In: Bianchi L, Gerok W, Sickinger K, Stalder GA, editors. Virus and the liver. Falk Symposium 28. Lancaster: MTP Press; 1980:75–82.
5. Rizzetto M, Canese MG, Gerin JL, London WT, Sly LD, Purcell RH. Transmission of the hepatitis B virus-associated delta antigen to chimpanzees. J Infect Dis. 1980;141:590–602.
6. Rizzetto M, Hoyer B, Canese MG, Shih JW-K, Purcell RH, Gerin JL. Delta agent: association of delta antigen with hepatitis B surface antigen and RNA in serum of delta-infected chimpanzees. Proc Natl Acad Sci USA. 1980;77:6124–8.
7. Ponzetto A, Cote PJ, Popper H *et al.* Transmission of the hepatitis B-associated delta agent to the eastern woodchuck. Proc Natl Acad Sci. 1984;81:2208–21.
8. Rizzetto M. The delta agent. Hepatology. 1983;3:729–37.
9. Rizzetto M, Verme G, Gerin JL, Purcell RH. Hepatitis delta virus disease. In: Popper H, Schaffner F, editors. Progress in liver diseases, vol. VIII. New York: Grune & Stratton; 1986:417–31.
10. Bonino F, Heermann KH, Rizzetto M, Gerlich WH. Hepatitis delta virus: protein composition of delta antigen and its hepatitis B virus derived envelope. J Virol. 1986;58:945–50.
11. Diener TO, Prusiner SB. The recognition of subviral pathogens. In: Marmorosch K, McKelvey JJ, editors. Subviral pathogens of plants and animals: viroids and prions. Florida: Academic Press; 1985:3–20.
12. Rizzetto M, Gerin JL, Purcell RH. Delta antigen: evidence for a variant of hepatitis B virus or a defective non-A non-B agent. In: Pollard M, editor. Perspectives in virology, vol. XI. New York: Alan Liss; 1981:195–217.
13. Kos A, Dijkema R, Arnberg AC, Van der Meide PH, Schelleken H. The hepatitis delta virus possesses a circular RNA. Nature. 1986;322:558–60.
14. Wang K-S, Choo Q-L, Weiner AJ *et al.* Structure, sequence and expression of the hepatitis delta virtal genome. Nature. 1986;323:508–13.
15. Gowans EJ, Baroudy BM, Negro F, Ponzetto A, Purcell RH, Gerin JL. Evidence for the replication of hepatitis delta virus RNA in nuclei after *in vivo* infection. Virology. 1988;167:274–8.
16. Diener TO. Autonomous and helper-dependent small pathogenic RNA of plants: viroids and satellites. In: Rizzetto M, Gerin JL, Purcell RH, editors. The hepatitis delta virus (HDV) and its infection. Progress in clinical and biological research, vol. 234. New York: Alan R Liss; 1987:3–18.
17. Branch AD, Levine BJ, Robertson HD. The brotherhood of circular RNA pathogens: viroids, circular satellites and the delta agent. Semin Virol. 1990;1:143–52.
18. Young B, Hicke B. Delta virus as a cleaver. Nature. 1990;343:28.
19. Taylor J, Negro F, Rizzetto M. Hepatitis delta virus: from structure to disease expression. Rev Med Virol. 1992;2:161–7.
20. Prody GA, Balos JT, Buzauan JM. Autolytic processing of dimeric plant virus satellite RNA. Science. 1986;231:1577–80.
21. Kuo MY-P, Chao M, Taylor J. Initiation of replication of the human hepatitis delta virus genome from cloned DNA: role of the delta antigen. J Virol. 63:1945–50.
22. Luo G, Chao M, Hsieh SY *et al.* A specific base transition occurs on replicating hepatitis delta virus RNA. J Virol. 1990;64:1021–7.
23. Lai MMC, Chao YC, Chang MF *et al.* Functional studies of hepatitis delta antigen and delta virus RNA. In: Gerin JL, Purcell RH, editors. The hepatitis delta virus. Progress in clinical and biological research, vol. 364. New York: Wiley/Liss; 1991:283–92.
24. Branch AD, Robertson HD. A replication cycle for viroids and small infectious RNAs. Science. 1984;223:450–5.
25. Taylor JM, Sharmeen L, Kuo M, Dinter-Gottlieb G. The self-cleaving RNAs of human hepatitis delta virus. In: Cech T, editor. Molecular biology of RNA. UCLA Symposia on molecular and cellular biology, new series, vol. 94. New York: Alan R Liss; 1989:99–108.
26. Chen P-J, Kalpana G, Goldberg J, Mason W, Werner B, Gerin J, Taylor JM. The structure and replication of the genome of the hepatitis delta virus. Proc Natl Acad Sci USA. 1986;83:8774–8.
27. Taylor J, Mason W, Summers J *et al.* Replication of human hepatitis delta virus in primary cultures of woodchuck hepatocytes. J Virol. 1987;71:2891–5.
28. Taylor JM. Structure and replication of hepatitis delta virus. Semin Virol. 1990;1:135–41.

29. Sureau C, Taylor JM, Chao M, Eichberg JE, Lanford RE. Cloned hepatitis delta virus complementary DNA is infectious in the chimpanzees. J Virol. 1989;63:4292–7.
30. Ponzetto A, Negro F, Popper H *et al.* Serial passage of hepatitis delta virus in chronic hepatitis B virus carrier chimpanzees. Hepatology. 1988;8:1655–61.
31. Hadziyannis SJ, Hatzakis A, Papaioannou C *et al.* Endemic hepatitis delta virus infection in a Greek community. In: Rizzetto M, Gerin JL, Purcell RH, editors. The hepatitis delta virus and its infection. Progress in clinical and biological research, vol. 234. New York: Alan R Liss; 1987:181–202.
32. Hadler SC, de Monzon MA, Bensabath G, Duran MM, Schatz G, Fields H. Epidemiology of hepatitis delta infection in less developed countries. In: Gerin JL, Purcell RH, Rizzetto M, editors. The hepatitis delta virus. Progress in clinical and biological research, vol. 364. New York: Wiley–Liss; 1991:21–31.
33. Negro F, Bergmann KF, Baroudy BM, Satterfield WC, Popper H, Purcell RH, Gerin JL. Chronic hepatitis D virus (HDV) infection in hepatitis B virus carrier chimpanzees experimentally superinfected with HDV. J Infect Dis. 1988;158:151–9.
34. Rizzetto M, Verme G, Recchia S *et al.* Chronic HBsAg hepatitis with intrahepatic expression of delta antigen. An active and progressive disease unresponsive to immunosuppressive treatment. Ann Intern Med. 1983;98:437–41.
35. Rizzetto M, Hadziyannis S, Hansson BG, Toukan A, Gust I. Hepatitis delta virus infection in the world: epidemiologic patterns and clinical expression. Gastroenterol Int. 1992;5:18–32.
36. Negro F, Baldi M, Bonino F *et al.* Chronic HDV (hepatitis delta virus) hepatitis. Intrahepatic expression of delta antigen, histologic activity and outcome of liver disease. J Hepatol. 1988;6:8–14.
37. Negro F, Gerin JL, Purcell RH, Miller RH. Basis of hepatitis delta virus diseases. Nature. 1989;341:111.
38. Cole S, Gowans EJ, Macnaughton TB, De La Halle PM, Burrell CJ. Direct evidence for cytotoxicity associated with expression of hepatitis delta virus antigen. Hepatology. 1992;13:845–51.
39. Ottobrelli A, Marzano A, Smedile A *et al.* Patterns of hepatitis delta virus reinfection and disease in liver transplantation. Gastroenterology. 1991;101:1649–55.
40. Tappero G, Anfossi G, Rosina F *et al.* Detection of c-myc nuclear oncoprotein in nuclei expressing the hepatitis delta virus antigen (HDAg). J Hepatol. 1991;13:S75.
41. Netter H, Hsieh S-Y, Lazinski D, Taylor J. Modified HDV as a vector for the delivery of biologically-active RNAs. In: Hadzyiannis S, Taylor JM, Bonino F, editors. Hepatitis delta virus, molecular biology, pathogenesis and clinical aspects. New York: Wiley/Liss; 1992: In press.

Section I
Portal hypertension

1

Physiology and pathophysiology of portal hypertension in cirrhotic and non-cirrhotic liver

T. D. BOYER

INTRODUCTION

Portal hypertension is a common sequela of liver disease. The rise in pressure within the portal veins leads to the opening of portal-systemic collaterals and the common clinical problems of gastrointestinal bleeding from varices/gastropathy and hepatic encephalopathy. Increases in pressure within the splanchnic capillaries and hepatic sinusoids increase formation of hepatic and splanchnic lymph, and lead eventually to the appearance of ascites. Thus, portal hypertension is a cause of significant morbidity and mortality in patients with liver disease.

This chapter will review the role of increased resistance versus increased portal venous flow in the pathogenesis of portal hypertension. Techniques used to measure portal vein pressure and flow are reviewed in an accompanying chapter by Dr Bosch (Chapter 2). The potential causes of the increase in portal venous inflow will be reviewed only briefly in this chapter as Dr Reichen reviews the pathogenesis of the hyperdynamic circulation in Chapter 5. The reader is referred to a number of reviews published recently on this topic[1-4].

NORMAL LIVER BLOOD FLOW

Normal hepatic blood flow is approximately 1500 ml/min. Thirty per cent of the flow and 30–60% of the oxygen consumed by the liver are provided by the hepatic artery[5-7]. The intrahepatic circulation has two unique features. The first relates to outflow resistance[8]. In skeletal muscle the ratio of pre-to post-capillary resistance is about 4:1. Arteriolar dilation in skeletal muscle leads to a significant rise in capillary pressure, and the transudation of fluid from the vascular space to the interstitial space. The endothelial lining of most capillaries is quite impermeable to the passage of proteins into the interstitium. Therefore, the rise in capillary pressure is counteracted by rises in intravascular oncotic pressure and increases in hydrostatic pressure in the interstitial space (Starling forces) limiting vascular fluid losses. In contrast, the pre- to post-capillary resistance in the liver is high, 49:1. The high ratio is due to a low outflow resistance from the liver. The site of the outflow resistance appears, in cats, to be in the small veins just beyond the sinusoids[9]. Whether similar sites are present in humans is unknown. Because of the low outflow resistance from the sinusoids, increases in flow cause a minimal rise in sinusoidal pressure. High flow states therefore uncommonly cause portal hypertension. Maintenance of a low sinusoidal pressure is important because of the permeability characteristic of the sinusoids. The endothelial linings of the hepatic sinusoids contain fenestrae. In the space of Disse there is a permeability barrier to the passage of proteins at low sinusoidal pressures. However, this barrier is lost in the normal liver when the sinusoidal pressure exceeds 10 mmHg, and Starling forces do not apply to the liver when the pressure in the hepatic sinusoids rises significantly[10]. A rise in sinusoidal pressure causes the rapid movement of large amounts of fluid and protein from the vascular to the interstitial space. Maintaining a low pressure in the sinusoids is therefore critical to normal hepatic function.

The second unique feature of the hepatic circulation is the interrelationship between hepatic artery and portal vein blood flow[11,12]. In both animals and humans a decrease in portal venous flow or sinusoidal pressure causes a reflex increase in hepatic arterial flow. Conversely, an increase in sinusoidal pressure or flow causes a reflex decrease in hepatic arterial flow. This reflex change in hepatic arterial flow appears to be intrinsic to the liver as transplanted livers which are denervated still demonstrate this response[13]. This 'buffer' response may be mediated by adenosine, and it maintains a constant hepatic blood flow despite changes in portal venous flow[12]. Changes in hepatic arterial flow, however, do not cause alterations in portal venous blood flow. The latter is controlled by splanchnic haemodynamics which appear to be independent of metabolic events in the liver. The one exception to this may be that a fall in portal flow will cause splanchnic vasodilation[14]. As discussed below, however, changes in splanchnic flow can have a significant impact on portal pressure when there is increased resistance within the portal venous system.

PORTAL HYPERTENSION

The pressure within a vessel is determined by the flow and resistance within that vessel. This relationship is expressed by Ohm's law: $\Delta P = Q \times R$, where P is pressure, and Q and R are flow and resistance, respectively. Resistance depends on a number of factors as defined by Poiseuille's law: $R = 8nL/\pi r^4$ where n is the coefficient of viscosity, L the length of the vessel and r the radius. The length of the vessel and viscosity are usually constant, although the latter may change during resuscitation of a patient who has recently bled. Radius appears to be the most important factor, as small changes in radius are associated with large changes in resistance.

The normal portal venous pressure is 5–10 mmHg (7–14 cmH_2O). Intra-abdominal pressure can vary, and therefore the portal pressure gradient (wedged hepatic vein pressure (WHVP) or portal vein pressure (PVP) – free hepatic vein pressure or IVC pressure) is used to identify individuals with portal hypertension. A gradient that exceeds 5 mmHg is considered to be abnormal[15,16]. Levels of pressure that exceed 12 mmHg are associated with large varices and bleeding[17,18] (Fig. 1); however, ascites and encephalopathy can develop in patients with gradients of less than 12 mmHg.

The term 'portal hypertension' was first used in 1906[19]. In the late 1800s Guido Banti concluded that an enlarged spleen caused an increase in portal vein blood flow which led to an increase in portal pressure[20]. In the middle of the 20th century investigators concluded that increased resistance, not flow, was the principal event in causing portal hypertension in cirrhosis. This argument was strengthened when portal vein blood flow in patients with cirrhosis measured at the time of surgery was found to be normal or low[21]. Measurements at surgery, however, failed to account for flow in portosystemic collaterals. Subsequently, when total portal venous inflow was measured in animals with portal hypertension caused by partial ligation of the portal vein, CCl_4-induced cirrhosis or schistosomiasis, portal venous inflow was

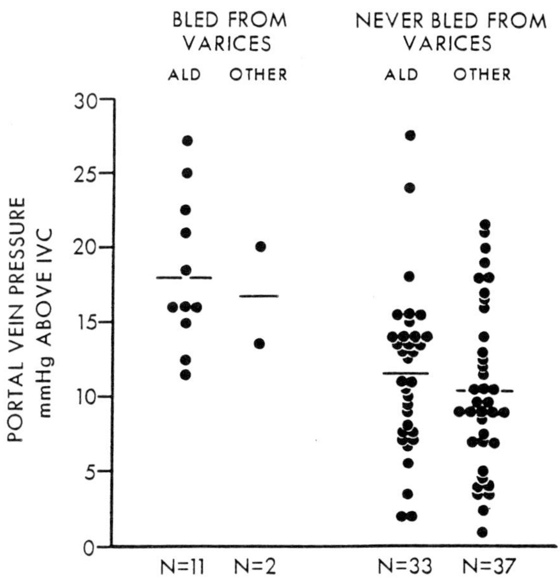

Fig. 1 Portal vein pressures in patients with alcoholic liver disease (ALD) and other causes of liver disease (non-ALD). Pressures were corrected for intra-abdominal pressure. Taken from Boyer, T. D. Portal hypertension and bleeding esophageal varices in hepatology. In: *A textbook of liver disease*, 2nd edn, W. B. Saunders, Philadelphia, PA, 1990, pp. 572–615. Reproduced with permission

increased[1,3]. These observations have reopened the debate as to the relative importance of resistance (backward) versus flow (forward) in the pathogenesis of portal hypertension in patients with cirrhosis[22].

HEPATIC RESISTANCE IN CIRRHOSIS AND NON-CIRRHOTIC PORTAL HYPERTENSION

The site of the increased resistance in cirrhosis has been the subject of much study and controversy. Studies of alcoholic cirrhotics have shown that the WHVP and PVP are equal (Fig. 2), suggesting that the site of the increase in resistance includes the entire sinusoid. Others, however, believe that the major site of resistance is in the hepatic veins immediately beyond the sinusoid[12]. The sphincters thought to exist in animals in these small veins[12], however, have never been identified in humans. In contrast, some patients with non-alcoholic cirrhosis have a significantly lower WHVP as compared to the PVP, suggesting an uneven resistance across the sinusoids[23] (Fig. 2). The anatomical differences in the alcoholic and non-alcoholic patients that account for these haemodynamic differences have not been defined. Studies in animals suggest that periportal fibrosis is associated with alterations in the portal venules that could lead to an increase in resistance in the peripheral branches of the portal vein[24], and perhaps a similar situation exists in humans with non-alcoholic cirrhosis. Alternatively, preservation of collaterals between sinusoids in the non-alcoholic cirrhotic liver may cause the WHVP to underestimate PVP[16].

Studies of cirrhotic livers have shown distortion and reduction of the hepatic microcirculation. These vascular changes, in concert with compression of portal and less likely hepatic veins by regenerative nodules, were thought to account for the increase in vascular resistance seen in cirrhosis[25–27]. Portal hypertension may, however, be present without cirrhosis, especially in the alcoholic[28]. Collagen deposition in the space of Disse may be an early finding in alcoholic liver injury (Fig. 3). The relationship between collagen deposition and portal pressure was examined in a group of patients with alcoholic liver disease. A positive correlation ($r = 0.85$) was found between intrahepatic pressure and the amount of collagen in the liver[29]. The correlation between collagen deposition and pressure was observed in patients with fatty liver, alcoholic hepatitis and cirrhosis. A similar relationship was found in alcohol-fed baboons[30]. Involvement of the entire lobule is again consistent with the haemodynamic findings in alcoholic liver disease.

Portal pressure may fall in patients with alcoholic liver disease if their liver disease improves[23,31]. One possible explanation for the improvement in pressure is a decrease in the size of the hepatocytes. In a series of studies, Orrego, Blendis, and their colleagues estimated the size of hepatocytes and sinusoidal volume in patients with alcoholic and non-alcoholic liver disease[32–36]. They correlated these measurements with intrahepatic parenchymal pressure (not corrected for intra-abdominal pressure). Cell size correlated directly with parenchymal pressure, whereas sinusoidal area correlated inversely with pressure in alcoholic liver disease. This relationship was

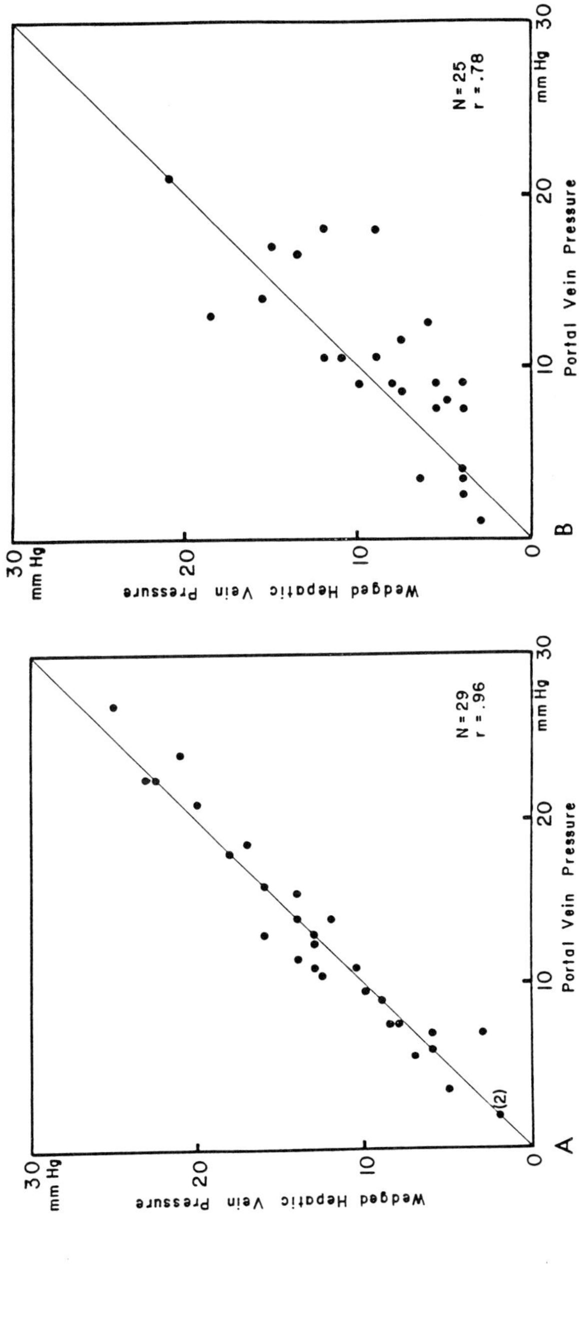

Fig. 2 Relationship between portal vein pressure and wedge hepatic vein pressure in cirrhotic (**A**) and non-alcoholic (**B**) liver disease. From ref. 23. Reproduced with permission

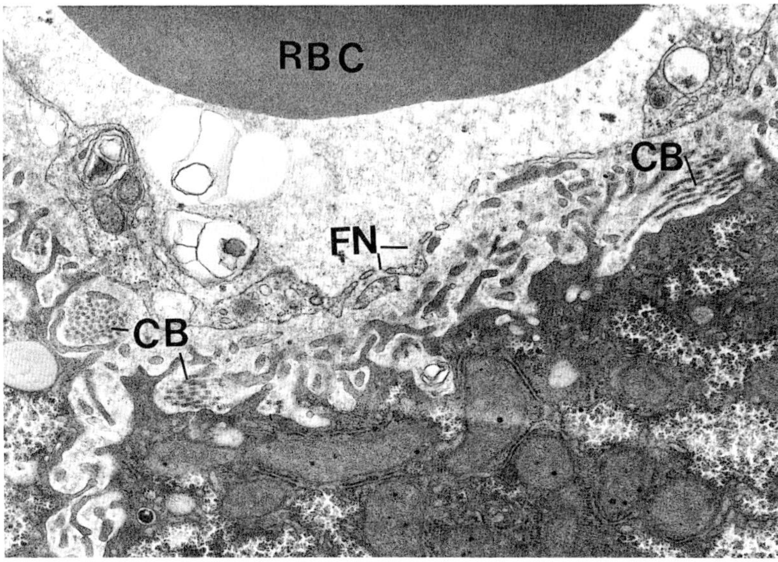

Fig. 3 Transmission electronic micrograph of a hepatic sinusoid. Tissue obtained from a patient with alcoholic liver disease. FN = Fenestrae. CB = Collagen bundles. Taken from Boyer, T. D., Portal hypertension and bleeding esophageal varices in hepatology. In: *A Textbook of Liver Disease*, 2nd edn. W. B. Saunders, Philadelphia, PA, 1990, pp. 572–615. Reproduced with permission

observed only up to 20 mmHg. There was no relationship between pressure and cell size. There was no relationship between cell size and sinusoidal area in non-alcoholic patients with liver disease. Studies by other investigators in humans and alcohol-fed rats and baboons have not found a relationship between pressure and cell size[30,37,38]. There are a number of differences between the various studies which may explain the lack of consistent findings[36]. Perhaps the most important variable is the fact that hepatocyte size appears to have a significant influence only at relatively low levels of pressure. If the pressure measurements are corrected for intra-abdominal pressure using a value of 7 mmHg[23], then with pressure gradients greater than 13 mmHg hepatocyte size does not influence portal pressure. As bleeding from varices is seen only in patients with a portal pressure gradient greater than 12 mmHg[17,18] (Fig. 1), hepatocyte enlargement would not be expected to be a major factor in these patients.

All of the changes in resistance that have been considered are largely passive, i.e. reflect changes in cell size or are secondary to scarring. Recent work suggests that intrahepatic resistance may also change in an active manner. Present in perivenous and perisinusoidal areas of cirrhotic but not normal livers are contractile cells termed myofibroblasts[39]. These cells appear to develop from activated lipocytes[40]. The infusion of vasodilators into a normal rat liver is not associated with a change in vascular tone, whereas similar infusions into a perfused cirrhotic liver caused significant falls in resistance[41]. Also, exposure of these myofibroblasts to endothelin caused contraction of the cells[42]. Whether similar events occur *in vivo* is unclear, but the findings suggest that the use of pharmacological agents in an attempt to reduce portal pressure may affect the myofibroblasts and therefore influence the response to therapy.

The site of resistance in non-cirrhotic portal hypertension is better understood. In alcoholic liver disease cell size and collagen deposition in the space of Disse may be important factors (see above). In schistosomiasis there is obstruction of the portal venules by the inflammatory and fibrotic reaction to the eggs, leading to an increase in hepatic resistance[43]. The situation in idiopathic portal hypertension (IPH) is somewhat less clear as the relative roles of increased flow versus increased resistance have not been resolved. It is clear that many patients with IPH have an increase in intrahepatic resistance because of phlebosclerosis of the portal veins and hepatic fibrosis[44,45–48]. Based on studies using Doppler ultrasound these patients also appear to have increased portal vein flow because of increased flow from the splenic artery[45,46]. What is unclear is the temporal relationship between the development of increased resistance and flow in the portal vein as measured by Doppler ultrasound. In one study increased flow appeared to precede increased resistance[47], but this conclusion was not based on prospective observations. Given the low outflow resistance from the liver, increased portal flow, in the absence an increase in resistance, is unlikely to cause a significant rise in portal pressure.

EFFECT OF CIRRHOSIS ON HEPATIC ARTERIAL FLOW

Most research has focused on portal venous flow as a determinant of portal pressure. Hepatic arterial flow also contributes to intrasinusoidal pressure. As discussed above, changes in portal flow/pressure influence hepatic artery flow. Portal venous flow is known to be low in cirrhosis but sinusoidal pressure is high. The primacy of flow over pressure can be determined by measuring hepatic artery resistance in humans or animals with cirrhosis. Hepatic haemodynamics were measured in patients pre- and post-liver transplant with electromagnetic flow meters[49]. In the cirrhotic liver hepatic artery flow was low and resistance high despite low portal vein flow. Following transplant hepatic artery resistance was low despite increased portal vein flow. These findings suggest that sinusoidal pressure, not flow, is the principal determinant of arterial resistance in cirrhosis. This conclusion is not consistent with the adenosine model[12]. In an animal model of schistosomiasis[50], a fall in portal venous flow was accompanied by increases in hepatic arterial flow despite a rise in portal pressure. The change in hepatic arterial flow, however, only partially compensated for the decrease in portal venous flow. Similarly, diversion of portal venous flow in some patients with cirrhosis is associated with an increase in hepatic arterial flow[51]. Hence, the normal 'buffer' response of the hepatic artery is maintained in cirrhosis, albeit probably at a reduced level compared to the normal liver.

EFFECT OF PORTAL HYPERTENSION ON PORTAL VENOUS INFLOW

As mentioned previously, increased flow in the portal vein is an uncommon cause of portal hypertension because of the low outflow resistance from the liver. However, in cirrhosis and non-cirrhotic forms of portal hypertension with increased hepatic outflow resistance, portal venous inflow will have a significant impact on pressure. Portal-systemic collaterals that develop in cirrhosis will tend to reduce the portal vein pressure. However, large portal-systemic collaterals are seen in patients with high portal pressures, and in fact the higher the pressure the more extensive the collateral circulation[52]. These observations suggest that either the resistance in these vessels is very high, or portal venous inflow increases as the collaterals develop maintaining a high portal pressure. Although resistance in the collaterals may be higher than in normal animals[22] it seems unlikely that resistance in the collateral vessels is unusually high, as they persist after pressure in the portal vein is normalized either by removing the portal vein obstruction[53], performing a portal-systemic shunt or following liver transplantation[54]. Therefore, portal-venous inflow appears to increase as the portal-systemic collateral system develops, which encourages further development of the collateral system and keeps portal pressure high.

Studies by Dr Groszman and his colleagues in partial portal vein-ligated and cirrhotic rats have shown that total portal inflow (portal system plus collaterals) increases as the collateral system develops[55–59]. The increased portal venous inflow results from a fall in splanchnic arterial resistance. In humans high flows are present in the collateral circulation[60], and the hyperdynamic circulation that develops in animals with portal hypertension is also present in cirrhotic patients (refs 1–3 and Chapter 5 of this volume). Hence, it seems reasonable to conclude that increased portal venous inflow is an important factor in maintaining a high portal pressure in patients with liver disease.

In the portal vein-ligated rat model about 40% of the increase in pressure is accounted for by the increase in flow[22]. However, in the latter model flow returns to normal if the animals are followed for a prolonged period of time[58]. Additionally, relief of the obstruction is associated with a fall in portal pressure to normal, despite persistence of the hyperdynamic circulation[53]. Therefore even in this experimental situation the rise in vascular resistance in the portal system is the principal factor in increasing portal pressure. Also, in humans, only 2% of the increase in pressure present with cirrhosis can be accounted for by increased portal venous inflow[22]. Based on studies in animals and humans the following sequence of events appears to occur both in cirrhotic and non-cirrhotic causes of portal hypertension (Fig. 4). Pressure in the portal vein is increased either because of hepatic fibrosis or partial or complete occlusion of the portal vein. Total portal flow initially decreases, and hepatic blood flow is partially maintained by an increase in hepatic arterial flow. In response to the rise in portal pressure portal-systemic collaterals develop, vascular resistance falls in the splanchnic and systemic arterial bed leading to the development of a hyperdynamic circulation. Splanchnic and portal inflow increase, and portal pressure continues to be elevated despite the

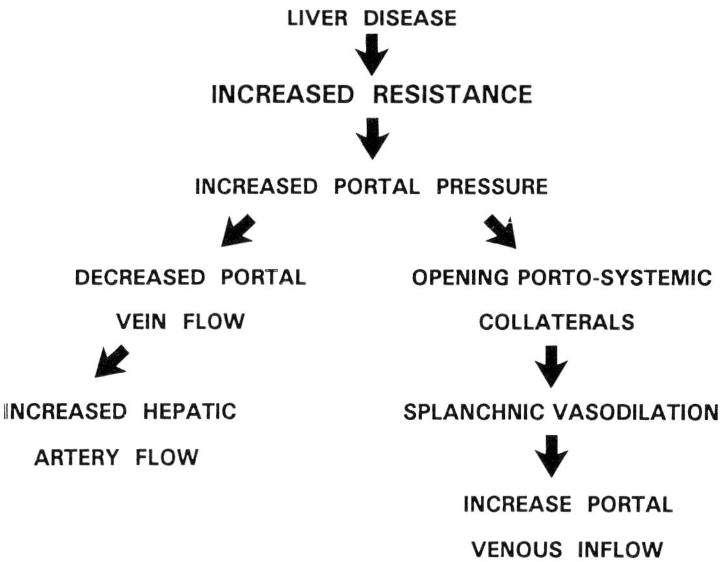

Fig. 4 Proposed sequence of events in the development of portal hypertension in both cirrhotic and non-cirrhotic forms of liver disease

opening of the collateral circulation. As resistance in the liver continues to increase, there is a rise in portal pressure, a fall in portal flow to the liver, and an increasing percentage of portal blood is shunted through the collateral bed. The increase in portal inflow therefore helps support the high pressure and keeps the collaterals open.

The relative importance of resistance versus flow in IPH is less clear. Clearly, there is an increase in intrahepatic resistance in patients with this disorder[48]. In addition, they tend to have marked splenomegaly with increased splenic artery flow. When haemodynamic measurements are made in patients with IPH and compared to patients with cirrhosis $\pm$ splenomegaly, the IPH patients have the highest portal vein flows. However, these high flows are not significantly greater than measured flows in patients with cirrhosis and splenomegaly[46]. Attempts to reduce PVP in patients with cirrhosis and splenomegaly by ligating the splenic artery had little effect on pressure[61]. Therefore, as resistance is also increased in IPH, the high portal vein flow appears to be a secondary factor in the development of portal hypertension.

OTHER FACTORS INFLUENCING PORTAL PRESSURE

Changes in portal-collatoral or portal-venous resistance could have an effect on portal pressure. For example, administration of propanolol to portal hypertensive rats was found to increase resistance in the collateral circulation which limited the effect of propranolol on portal pressure despite reductions in flow[59]. Splanchnic veins have receptors for 5-hydroxytryptamine (5-HT). When exposed to 5-HT superior mesenteric veins from portal hypertensive animals were found to be more sensitive to this agent than were normal vessels[62]. Administration of 5-HT antagonist to portal hypertensive rats caused a fall in portal pressure[63]. Systemic haemodynamics were unaffected in the latter study, so the effect appeared to be on collateral resistance and portal venous inflow. As mentioned earlier, myofibroblasts contract when exposed to endothelin[42]. Levels of endothelin-1 have been measured in patients with cirrhosis, and levels were lower that controls[64]. The physiological significance of the low levels is unclear, but with increased numbers of myofibroblasts present in cirrhotic livers and an increase in the number of endothelin receptors on activated lipocytes[65] small changes in blood endothelin levels could alter portal pressure.

There is increasing interest in nitric oxide as a vasodilator in a number of pathological states. Vallance and Moncada suggested that nitric oxide may contribute to the hyperdynamic circulation seen in cirrhosis[66]. In one study superior mesenteric arteries from normal and portal hypertensive rats were perfused and their response to vasoconstrictors determined. The vessels from portal hypertensive animals were hyporesponsive to vasoconstrictors and this hyporesponsiveness could be overcome by an inhibitor of nitric oxide synthesis[67]. In a second study[68] nitric oxide synthesis was inhibited in rats with portal hypertension. Inhibition of synthesis was associated with an increase in porto-collateral resistance as well as splanchnic and peripheral resistance. Both studies support a role for nitric oxide in regulating resistance and blood flow in the splanchnic bed and collaterals of portal hypertensive animals. Nitroglycerine also is thought to exert its effects by being metabolized to nitric oxide in vascular smooth muscle cells. Studies have suggested that the first step in activation is the release of NO_2 from nitroglycerine by the glutathione S-transferases. The NO_2 is then converted to NO by an undefined reaction[69]. We examined the metabolism of nitroglycerine by dog vascular smooth muscle cells to define the role of the glutathione S-transferases[70]. Both NO and NO_2 were produced by the vascular homogenate. Increasing the activity of the transferases by adding GSH led to an increase in NO_2 production but a fall in NO release. Conversely, inhibition of the transferases was associated with a fall in NO_2 production and no change in NO release. These and additional studies suggest that the glutathione S-transferases are a degradative, not an activating, pathway for nitroglycerine. Therefore, changes in cellular levels of GSH or the transferases in vascular tissue may affect the response of the splanchnic circulation to nitroglycerine.

Patients with bleeding varices commonly are admitted to the hospital and are found not to be bleeding at the time of endoscopy. The risk of rebleeding is greatest immediately following the index bleed, which is when patients are transfused[71]. Diuretic- and phlebotomy-induced falls in plasma blood volume were associated with a fall in portal pressure, whereas expansion of the plasma volume was associated with a rise in portal pressure and enlargement of varices[72,73]. Therefore, the temporal relationship between transfusion and rebleeding may be significant. The mechanism behind the transfusion-induced rise in pressure has been investigated in animals. Following a phlebotomy, portal pressure falls in both normal and portal hypertensive animals. With correction of the anaemia portal pressure rises to prehaemorrhage levels in the normal rats, but pressure actually goes above the baseline value in the portal hypertensive animals. The increase in pressure in the portal hypertensive rats was secondary to a rise in collateral resistance[73,74]. Hence, preventing rapid increases in blood/plasma volume may be an important factor in minimizing the risk of rebleeding from varices.

CONCLUSIONS

Our understanding of the basic mechanism behind the increase in portal pressure seen in patients with liver disease has increased greatly in recent years. The realization that both flow and resistance are important factors has stimulated interest in the basic mechanisms behind regulation of hepatic blood flow. Additionally, realizing the importance of flow has led to new forms of therapy, which are having a significant impact on our management of patients with portal hypertension.

References

1. Mahl TC, Groszmann RJ. Pathophysiology of portal hypertension and variceal bleeding. Surg Clin N Am. 1990;70:251–66.
2. Okumura H, Aramaki T, Katsuta Y. Pathophysiology and epidemiology of portal hypertension. Drugs. 1989;37:2–12.
3. Bosch J, Pizcueta P, Feu F, Fernandez M, Garcia-Pagan JC. Pathophysiology of portal hypertension. Gastroenterol Clin N Am. 1992;21:1–14.
4. Groszmann RJ, Atterbury CE. The pathophysiology of portal hypertension: a basis for classification. Semin Liv Dis. 1982;2:177–86.
5. Bradley SE, Ingelfinger FJ, Bradley GP *et al.* The estimation of hepatic blood flow in man. J Clin Invest. 1945;24:890–7.
6. Brandt JL, Castleman L, Greenwald J *et al.* The effect of oral protein and glucose feeding on splanchnic blood flow and oxygen utilization in normals and cirrhotic subjects. J Clin Invest. 1955;34:1017–25.
7. Greenway CV, Stark RD. Hepatic vascular bed. Physiol Rev. 1971;51:23–65.
8. Lautt WW. Hepatic vasculature: a conceptual review. Hepatology. 1977;73:1163–9.
9. Lautt WW, Greenway CV, Legare DJ, Weisman H. Localization of intrahepatic portal vascular resistance. Am J Physiol. 1986;14:G375–81.
10. Granger D, Miller T, Allen R *et al.* Permselectivity of cat liver blood lymph barrier to endogenous macromolecules. Gastroenterology. 1979;77:103–9.
11. Richardson PDI, Withrington PG. Physiological regulation of the hepatic circulation. Ann Rev Physiol. 1982;44:57–69.
12. Lautt WW, Greenway CV. Conceptual review of the hepatic vascular bed. Hepatology. 1987;7:952–63.
13. Henderson JM, Gilmore GT, Mackay GJ, Galloway JR, Dodson TF, Kutner MH. Hemodynamics during liver transplantation: the interactions between cardiac output and portal venous and hepatic arterial flows. Hepatology. 1992;16:715–18.
14. Henderson JM, Mackay GJ, Lumsden AB *et al.* The effect of liver denervation on hepatic hemodynamics during hypovolemic shock in swine. Hepatology. 1992;15:130–3.
15. Reynolds TB, Redeker AG, Geller HM. Wedged hepatic vein pressure. Am J Med. 1957;22:341–50.
16. Reynolds T, Ito S, Iwatsuki S. Measurement of portal pressure and its clinical application. Am J Med. 1970;49:649–57.

17. Viallet A, Marleau D, Huet M *et al*. Hemodynamic evaluation of patients with intrahepatic portal hypertension: relationship between bleeding varices and the portohepatic gradient. Gastroenterology. 1975;69:1297–1300.
18. Garcia-Tsao G, Groszmann RJ, Fisher RL *et al*. Portal pressure, presence of gastroesophageal varices and variceal bleeding. Hepatology. 1985;5:419–24.
19. Thompson WP. The pathogenesis of Banti's disease. Ann Intern Med. 1941;14:255–62.
20. Grannis F. Guido Banti's hypothesis and its impact on the understanding and treatment of portal hypertension. Mayo Clin Proc. 1975;50:41–8.
21. Moreno A, Burchell A, Reddy R *et al*. The hemodynamics of portal hypertension revisited: determinants and significance of occluded portal pressures. Surgery. 1975;77:167–79.
22. Benoit JN, Granger DN. Splanchnic hemodynamics in chronic portal hypertension. Semin Liver Dis. 1986;6:287–98.
23. Boyer TD, Triger D, Horisawa M *et al*. Direct transhepatic measurement of portal vein pressure using a thin needle: comparison with wedged hepatic vein pressure. Gastroenterology. 1977;72:584–9.
24. Shibayama Y, Nakata K. The relation of periportal fibrosis to portal hypertension. J Hepatol. 1990;11:313–17.
25. Kelty RH, Baggenstoss AH, Butt HR. The relation of the regenerated liver nodule to the vascular bed in cirrhosis. Gastroenterology. 1950;15:285–95.
26. Baldus WP, Hoffbauer FW. Vascular changes in the cirrhotic liver as studied by the injection technic. Am J Dig Dis. 1963;8:689–700.
27. Shibayama Y, Nakata K. Localization of increased hepatic vascular resistance in liver cirrhosis. Hepatology. 1985;5:643–8.
28. Edmondson H, Peters R, Reynolds T *et al*. Sclerosing hyaline necrosis of the liver in the chronic alcoholic. Ann Intern Med. 1973;59:646–73.
29. Orrego H, Blendis LM, Crossley IR, Medline A, MacDonald A, Ritchie S, Israel Y. Correlation of intrahepatic pressure with collagen in Disse space and hepatomegaly in humans and the rat. Gastroenterology. 1981;80:546–56.
30. Miyakawa H, Iida S, Leo MA, Greenstein RJ, Zimmon DS, Lieber CS. Pathogenesis of precirrhotic portal hypertension in alcohol-fed baboons. Gastroenterology. 1985;88:143–50.
31. Reynolds TB, Geller H, Kuzma O *et al*. Spontaneous decrease in portal pressure with clinical improvement in cirrhosis. N Engl J Med. 1960;263:734–9.
32. Blendis LM, Orrego H, Crossley IR, Blake JE, Medline A, Israel Y. The role of hepatocyte enlargement in hepatic pressure in cirrhotic and non-cirrhotic alcoholic liver disease. Hepatology. 1982;2:539–46.
33. Colman JC, Britton RS, Orrego H, Saldivia V, Medline A, Israel Y. Relation between osmotically induced hepatocytes enlargement and portal hypertension. Am J Physiol. 1983;245:G382–7.
34. Vidins EI, Britton RS, Medline A, Blendis LM, Israel Y, Orrego H. Sinusoidal caliber in alcoholic and non-alcoholic liver disease: diagnostic and pathogenic implications. Hepatology. 1985;5:408–14.
35. Orrego H, Israel Y, Blake JE *et al*. Relationships between liver histologic lesions and portal hypertension in patients with alcoholic cirrhosis. Hepatology. 1985;5:703–5.
36. Blendis LM. Hepatocyte swelling and portal hypertension. J Hepatol. 1992;15:4–5.
37. Krogsgaard K, Gludd C, Henriksen JH, Christoffersen P. Correlation between liver morphology and portal pressure in alcoholic liver disease. Hepatology. 1984;4:699–703.
38. Dagenais M, Giroux L, Belgiorno J, Huet PM. The effect of alcohol-induced hepatomegaly on portal hypertension in cirrhotic rats. J Hepatol. 1992;15:88–93.
39. Rudolph R, McClure WJ, Woodward M. Contractile fibroblasts in chronic alcoholic cirrhosis. Gastroenterology. 1979;76:704–9.
40. Rockey DC, Boyles JK, Gabbiani G *et al*. Rat hepatic lipocytes express smooth muscle actin upon activation *in vivo* and in culture. J Submicrosc Cytol Pathol. 1992;24:193–203.
41. Bhathal PS, Grossman HJ. Reduction of the increased portal vascular resistance of the isolated perfused cirrhotic rat liver by vasodilators. J Hepatol. 1985;1:325–37.
42. Rockey DC, Housset CN, Friedman SL. Contractility of hepatic lipocytes: implications for the pathogenesis of portal hypertension. Hepatology. 1992;16:123A.
43. Da Silva LC, Carrilho FJ. Hepatosplenic schistosomiasis. Pathophysiology and treatment. Gastroenterol Clin N Am. 1992;21:163–77.

44. Okuda K, Kono K, Ohnishi K *et al.* Clinical study of eighty-six cases of idiopathic portal hypertension and comparison with cirrhosis and splenomegaly. Gastroenterology. 1984;86:600–10.
45. Ohnishi K, Sato S, Nomura F, Iida S. Splanchnic hemodynamics in idiopathic portal hypertension: comparison with chronic persistent hepatitis. Am J Gastroenterol. 1989;84:403–8.
46. Ohnishi K, Chin N, Tanaka H, Iida S, Sato S, Terabayashi H, Nomura F. Differences in portal hemodynamics in cirrhosis and idiopathic portal hypertension. Am J Gastroenterol. 1989;84:409–12.
47. Ohnishi K, Saito M, Sato S *et al.* Portal hemodynamics in idiopathic portal hypertension (Banti's syndrome): comparison with chronic persistent hepatitis and normal subjects. Gastroenterology. 1987;92:751–8.
48. Moriyasu F, Nishida O, Ban N, Nakamura T, Miura K, Sakai M, Miyake T, Uchino H. Measurement of portal vascular resistance in patients with portal hypertension. Gastroenterology. 1986;90:710–17.
49. Paulsen AW, Klintmalm BG. Direct measurement of hepatic blood flow in native and transplanted organs, with accompanying systemic hemodynamics. Hepatology. 1992;16:100–11.
50. Morgan JS, Groszmann RJ, Rojkind M, Enriquez, R. Hemodynamic mechanisms of emerging portal hypertension caused by schistosomiasis in the hamster. Hepatology. 1990;11:98–104.
51. Zimmon D, Kessler R. Effect of portal venous blood flow diversion on portal pressure. J Clin Invest. 1980;65:1388–98.
52. Rousselot L, Moreno A, Panke W. Studies on portal hypertension. IV. The clinical and physiopathologic significance of self-establishment (non-surgical) portal venous shunts. Ann Surg. 1959;150:384–410.
53. Sikuler E, Groszmann RJ. Interaction of flow and resistance in maintenance of portal hypertension in a rat model. Am J Physiol. 1986;250:6205–12.
54. Chezmar JL, Redvanly RD, Nelson RC, Henderson JM. Persistence of portal systemic collaterals and splenomegaly on CT after orthotopic liver transplantation. Am J Roentgenol. 1992;159:317–20.
55. Groszmann RJ, Vorobioff J, Riley E. Splanchnic hemodynamics in portal-hypertensive rats: measurement with y-labeled microspheres. Am J Physiol 1982;242:G146–60.
56. Vorobioff J, Bredfeldt JE, Groszmann RJ. Increased blood flow through the portal system in cirrhotic rats. Gastroenterology. 1984;87:1120–26.
57. Sikuler E, Kravetz D, Groszmann RJ. Evolution of portal hypertension and mechanisms involved in its maintenance in a rat model. Am J Physiol. 1985;248:G618–25.
58. Sikuler E, Groszmann RJ. Hemodynamic studies in long- and short-term portal hypertensive rats: the relation to systemic glucagon levels. Hepatology. 1986;6:414–18.
59. Kroeger RJ, Groszmann RJ. Increased portal venous resistance hinders portal pressure reduction during the administration of β-adrenergic blocking agents in a portal hypertensive model. Hepatology. 1985;5:97–101.
60. Bosch J, Groszmann RJ. Measurement of azygous venous blood flow by a continuous thermal dilution technique: an index of blood flow through gastroesophageal collaterals in cirrhosis. Hepatology. 1984;4:424–9.
61. Witte C, Witte M, Renert W *et al.* Splenic artery ligation in selected patients with hepatic cirrhosis and in Sprague-Dawley rats. Surg Gynecol Obstet. 1976;142:1–12.
62. Cummings SA, Groszmann RJ, Kaumann AJ. Hypersensitivity of mesenteric veins to 5-hydroxytryptamine- and ketanserin-induced reduction of portal pressure in portal hypertensive rats. Br J Pharmacol. 1986;89:501–13.
63. Kaumann AJ, Morgan JS, Groszmann RJ. ICI 169,369 selectively blocks 5-hydroxytryptamine$_2$ receptors and lowers portal pressure in portal hypertensive rats. Gastroenterology. 1988;95:1601–6.
64. Veglio F, Pinna G, Melchio R, Rabbia F, Panarelli M, Gagliardi B, Chiandussi L. Plasma endothelin levels in cirrhotic subjects. J Hepatol. 1992;15:85–7.
65. Housset CN, Rockey DC, Bissell DM. Endothelin (ET) in liver: expression receptor distribution and contractile effect on activated lipocytes. Hepatology. 1992;16:90A.
66. Vallance P, Moncada S. Hyperdynamic circulation in cirrhosis: a role for nitric oxide? Lancet. 1991;337:776–8.
67. Sieber CC, Groszmann RJ. Nitric oxide mediates hyporeactivity to vasodepressors in

mesenteric vessels of portal hypertensive rats. Gastroenterology. 1992;103:235–9.
68. Pizcueta MP, Pique JM, Bosch J, Whittle BJ, Moncada S. Effects of inhibiting nitric oxide biosynthesis on the systemic and splanchnic circulation of rats with portal hypertension. Br J Pharmacol. 1992;105(1):184–90.
69. Hill KE, Hunt RW, Jones R *et al.* Metabolism of nitroglycerin by smooth muscle cells. Involvement of glutathione and glutathione S-transferase. Biochem Pharmacol. 1992;43:561–6.
70. Kurz MA, Boyer TD, Whalen R, Peterson TE, Harrison DG. Nitroglycerin metabolism in vascular tissue: role of glutathione-*S*-transferases and the relationship between NO^o and NO_2^- formation. Biochem J. 1993 (in press).
71. Smith JH, Graham DY. Variceal hemorrhage: a critical evaluation of survival analysis. Gastroenterology. 1982;82:968–73.
72. Okumura H, Aramaki T, Katsuta Y *et al.* Reduction in hepatic venous pressure gradient as a consequence of volume contraction due to chronic administration of spironolactone in patients with cirrhosis and no ascites. Am J Gastroenterol. 1991;86:46–52.
73. Kravetz D, Sikuler E, Groszmann RJ. Splanchnic and systemic hemodynamics in portal hypertensive rats during hemorrhage and blood volume restitution. Gastroenterology. 1986;90:1232–40.
74. Kravetz D, Bosch J, Arderiu M, Pizcueta MP, Rodes J. Hemodynamic effects of blood volume restitution following hemorrhage in rats with portal hypertension due to cirrhosis of the liver: influence of the extent of portal-systemic shunting. Hepatology. 1989;9:808–14.

2

Diagnostic tools in portal hypertension

J. BOSCH

Portal hypertension is a common complication in liver diseases. It should be suspected in every patient with cirrhosis, as well as in other chronic liver diseases, especially if there is a history of past bleeding, ascites or encephalopathy, or if there are clinical signs such as splenomegaly, visible collateral vessels on the abdominal wall, decreased platelets and WBC counts and fluid retention.

Evaluation of the portal hypertensive patient is based on visualization of varices at endoscopy, on the definition of the portocollateral anatomy by ultrasonography and/or angiography, and on the measurement of portal pressure. Recently, techniques that allow assessment of changes in pressure and blood flow at the collateral circulation have been introduced. These have allowed a better understanding of the haemodynamic changes associated with portal hypertension, of the mechanism of bleeding, and of the effects of new forms of pharmacological therapy[1,2].

NON-INVASIVE DIAGNOSTIC METHODS

Imagining techniques: ultrasonography, pulsed-Doppler measurements of portal blood flow, CT scans and nuclear magnetic resonance

Imaging techniques are very useful in the initial evaluation of the portal hypertensive patient. Frequently, portal hypertension is detected by the finding of a dilated portal vein, of portosystemic collaterals or splenomegaly using either of these diagnostic techniques. Moreover, ultrasonography, CT scans and nuclear magnetic resonance imaging are almost as accurate as angiography in detecting the patency of the portal vein or the presence of portal vein thrombosis[2], which should be investigated in every patient suspected of having portal hypertension. Ultrasonography, because of its low cost and high accuracy, is the preferred initial investigation.

The accuracy of ultasonography in detecting portal vein thrombosis is increased by the concomitant use of pulsed-Doppler flowmetry (the so-called 'duplex' technique). This allows determination of the presence, direction and velocity of portal blood flow. This latter measurement can be used to estimate portal blood flow. This is done by multiplying portal flow velocity by the cross-sectional area of the portal vein, estimated by planimetry on ultrasound imaging. This method is subject to many errors, and should thus be used with caution[3]. A recent study showed a large variability in these estimations of portal blood flow, especially when comparing measurements by different observers[4]. Variation is reduced with skill and by careful selection of patients, but is still considerable, which makes a critical evaluation and double-blind design of studies mandatory. Despite its limitations the fact of being totally non-invasive makes it attractive and it is being increasingly used. It is hoped that rapid technological improvement may increase its accuracy, making it suitable for physiological and pharmacological research. Ultrasonography and Doppler flow measurements are also useful in the assessment of the patency of surgical portacaval or splenorenal shunts, and in the evaluation of patency of arterial and venous anastomosis after orthotopic liver transplantation[2,3].

Endoscopy

Oesophagoscopy is the best method of evaluating the presence of varices, and should be performed in every patient suspected of having portal hypertension. Endoscopy provides important prognostic information: variceal bleeding will not occur if there are no varices, which is not unusual even in the presence of other complications of portal hypertension such as ascites. Actually, it has been shown that varices are present in only 60% of cirrhotics at diagnosis, although this percentage increases to up to 90% on long-term follow-up. In addition to demonstrating the presence of varices, it is possible at endoscopy to grade variceal size on a I to IV scale. This is important because bleeding is directly related to the size of the varices[1]. For that reason, endoscopy should be performed routinely in all patients with cirrhosis at the time of diagnosis. If no varices are present a follow-up endoscopy should be scheduled 2 years later[5]. Patients with small varices usually evolve to have large varices, which makes it convenient to plan follow-up endoscopies at yearly intervals. At endoscopy it is important to pay attention to the presence on the wall of the varices of 'red signs' (telangiectasias, red 'wale markings', cherry-red spots), since these are markers of increased bleeding risk[6]. A recent multicentre prospective study has shown that the risk of variceal haemorrhage in patients with cirrhosis and oesophageal varices is significantly related to the size of varices, to the presence of red colour signs and to liver function, evaluated by Child–Pugh's classification. On the basis of these three variables a prognostic index (the so-called NIEC index) was derived and validated prospectively[6]. This index allows identification of groups of patients with high or low risk of variceal haemorrhage; however, its value in individual subjects has been questioned.

Endoscopy may also disclose the presence of *portal hypertensive gastropathy*, a recently described complication of portal hypertension which is responsible for many of the non-variceal bleeding episodes in patients with cirrhosis[7,8]. These lesions are characterized histologically by enlarged mucosal capillaries. Endoscopically, the condition is characterized by the presence of the 'mosaic pattern' or by a diffuse reddening of the gastric mucosa ('scarlatina pattern') in mild cases, or by cherry-red spots on a finely granular mucosa, sometimes oozing blood or showing intramucosal bleeding (black spots) in severe cases[9].

INVASIVE PROCEDURES

Measurement of portal pressure (Table 1)

This is still the single most important haemodynamic measurement in portal hypertension. Other methods provide additional information but are no substitute for measurements of portal pressure. Portal pressure should be expressed in terms of the *pressure gradient* with the inferior vena cava (IVC), since this gradient is not modified by changes in intra-abdominal pressure[1]. Clinically significant portal hypertension, with formation of oesophageal varices, requires this gradient to increase above 10 mmHg. Variceal bleeding is rarely – if ever – observed[10] if this gradient is less than 12 mmHg. Conversely, patients with a high portal pressure gradient become completely protected[11] against the risk of variceal bleeding when the portal pressure gradient is decreased to values equal to or lower than 12 mmHg.

Direct measurements of portal pressure are invasive investigations based on the surgical, percutaneous transhepatic, or transvenous (transjugular) catheterization of the portal vein. In these techniques, except for the transjugular approach, measurement of IVC pressure will require a separate simultaneous procedure[1].

Because of these inconveniences, the indirect approach of hepatic vein catheterization, with measurements of wedged and free hepatic venous

Table 1 Methods for the measurement of portal pressure

A. *Direct method*
1. Transvenous portal catheterization using transjugular liver biopsy needle
2. Transhepatic percutaneous puncture[a]
3. Catheterization of a mesenteric vein during abdominal surgery[a]
4. Surgical repermeabilization of umbilical vein[a,b]

B. *Indirect methods*
1. Measurement of WHVP, PHVP and HVPG at hepatic vein catherization
2. Splenic pulp puncture[a,c]

[a] Requires separate procedure to measure the inferior vena cava pressure in order to calculate the portal pressure gradient
[b] Difficult and invasive procedure
[c] Abandoned because of its dangers

pressure (WHVP and FHVP) is the preferred technique to determine portal pressure. WHVP is measured by occluding the hepatic vein, either by inflating a balloon at the tip of the catheter, or by advancing the catheter until it becomes 'wedged' into a small branch of an hepatic vein[1,2,12]. When blood flow in a hepatic vein is stopped by a 'wedged' catheter, the static column of blood transmits the pressure existing in the preceding communicated vascular territory (the hepatic sinusoids). Thus, WHVP is a measurement of the hepatic sinusoidal pressure and not of portal pressure itself[1]. When portal hypertension is due to increased sinusoidal resistance (as happens in alcoholic liver disease) WHVP is equal to portal pressure (*sinusoidal portal hypertension*). However, when increased resistance is located at presinusoidal sites, WHVP underestimates portal pressure (*presinusoidal portal hypertension*). This happens in prehepatic diseases causing portal hypertension. In addition, some liver diseases affecting predominantly the portal tracts also cause a presinusoidal portal hypertension[13-15]. The more frequent examples are schistosomiasis, initial stages of primary biliary cirrhosis, and idiopathic portal hypertension. Also, in non-alcoholic cirrhosis there may be such a presinusoidal component to the portal hypertension. In these cases direct measurement of portal pressure may be preferable[15]. We recommend percutaneous transhepatic puncture with thin needles under ultrasonographic and radiological guidance because this method is easier to perform and more acceptable to the patient than other ways of obtaining a direct measurement. Diseases causing hepatic outflow block, such as the Budd–Chiari syndrome, are classified as *postsinusoidal, posthepatic portal hypertension*.

Hepatic vein catheterization is a simple and safe technique. The complications of the procedure in a series of 2500 consecutive studies performed in our laboratory have been limited to one femoral arteriovenous fistula, one leakage requiring blood transfusion, and rupture of a venous introducer requiring phlebotomy and surgical reconstruction of the femoral vein under local anaesthesia. There were no fatalities. An additional advantage of the technique is that it allows in the same procedure the measurement of portal pressure in absolute values, as WHVP, and as the pressure gradient WHVP–FHVP (the so-called hepatic vein pressure gradient, HVPG). With hepatic vein catheterization it is also possible to measure the hepatic blood flow using indocyanine green as the indicator[1,16], as well as the intrinsic clearance of ICG, a valuable quantitative liver function test assessing overall liver metabolic activity. Finally, measurement of HVPG has been found to be closely related with prognosis in patients with cirrhosis, suggesting that these can be used to monitor the course of the disease.

Measurement of azygos blood flow

Measurement of azygos blood flow represents an index of blood flow through the gastro-oesophageal collaterals and oesophageal varices in portal hypertension[17-19]. This technique is based in the well-known fact that most gastro-oesophageal collaterals drain into the azygos venous system; therefore an increased azygos blood flow in patients with portal hypertension reflects the collateral blood flow emptying in the azygos vein. Obviously, the technique does not allow differentiation of how much of the increase in azygos blood flow is contributed by oesophageal varices and how much by peri-oesophageal collaterals also draining into the azygos vein. It should be noted that in up to 25% of the cases these cephalad collaterals drain in other thoracic veins (subclavian, innominate, and pulmonary) instead of the azygos vein. Therefore, the absence of an increased azygos blood flow does not indicate the absence of oesophageal varices[18].

Measurement of azygos flow requires the retrograde catheterization of the azygos vein using a continuous thermal dilution catheter. This is a very simple procedure in the course of routine haemodynamic investigations using the femoral vein approach, but much more difficult from the jugular vein. Measurement of blood flow is performed by indicator dilution during a constant infusion of isotonic glucose solution at room temperature, while simultaneously recording the temperature of the indicator and of azygos blood. The whole procedure, including repeated measurements of blood flow, does not take more than 15 min. The technique is accurate and reproducible: the variation of repeated measurements is less than 10%. Technical aspects of measurements of azygos blood flow have been recently reviewed[19].

Azygos blood flow is usually markedly increased in portal hypertension. Values in normal subjects range between 0.15 and 0.25 l/min, whereas in patients with cirrhosis and portal hypertension[19] these are increased on average to 0.65 l/min. Patients with non-cirrhotic portal hypertension also have increased azygos flow (Table 2). These increased values are markedly reduced following surgical portacaval shunt or oesophageal tamponade with a Sengstaken–Blakemore tube[18]. Azygos blood flow shows a direct, significant correlation with portal pressure and, in patients with varices, there is a parallelism between azygos blood flow and the size and extent of the oesophageal varices. However, as already mentioned, these correlations are not helpful in assessing the risk of bleeding in individual patients.

The main application of measurements of azygos blood flow is the monitoring of the effects of pharmacological therapy in portal hypertension.

Table 2 Azygos blood flow and hepatic venous pressure gradient (HVPG) in diseases causing portal hypertension

Aetiology	*Azygos blood flow (ml/min)*	*HVPG (mmHg)*
Alcoholic cirrhosis ($n = 54$)	722 ± 41	19.3 ± 0.7
Non-alcoholic cirrhosis ($n = 35$)	646 ± 42	19.3 ± 0.8
Primary biliary cirrhosis:		
with portal hypertension ($n = 7$)	647 ± 321	14.1 ± 6.2[b]
without portal hypertension ($n = 9$)	319 ± 121[a]	5.1 ± 2.3[c]
Idiopathic portal hypertension ($n = 4$)	480 ± 256	6.1 ± 2.8[c]
Portal vein thrombosis ($n = 7$)	519 ± 192	3.1 ± 1.7[c]

[a] Significantly lower than in patients with portal hypertension of any cause ($p < 0.01$)
[b] Significantly lower than in alcoholic and non-alcoholic cirrhosis ($p < 0.05$)
[c] Significantly lower than in diseases causing intrahepatic portal hypertension ($p < 0.001$)
Reproduced from ref. 19, with permission

The ability of the technique to sense changes in portal-collateral blood flow has allowed a better understanding of the beneficial effects of vasoactive drugs currently used in the medical treatment of portal hypertension[19]. In addition, it has been demonstrated that some of these drugs, such as propranolol, cause greater decreases in azygos blood flow than in portal pressure, and that with equal falls in portal pressure there can be different effects in azygos blood flow[20,21]. These findings have introduced the important concept that vasoactive agents may have specific effects at the collaterals, which cannot be assessed adequately by measurements of portal pressure.

Measurement of variceal pressure

The pressure of the oesophageal varices can be measured at endoscopy using two different approaches: direct variceal puncture, which has been increasingly used since the popularization of sclerotherapy, and by the use of endoscopic pressure-sensitive gauges, that allow measurement of variceal pressure without puncturing the varices, and therefore without the risk of precipitating variceal haemorrhage[22-25]. The endoscopic gauge technique is based on the assumption that, because of their thin walls and lack of external tissue support, the varices behave as an elastic structure; thus, the pressure needed to compress a varix equals the pressure inside the varix. We have demonstrated an excellent agreement between measurements by both methods both in *in vitro* studies using artificial varices and *in vivo*, in patients with cirrhosis who had measurements of both methods in the course of the first session of sclerotherapy[24].

Measurements of variceal pressure are, at the moment, research procedures. The results may be difficult to interpret because of artifacts caused by oesophageal peristalsis. In addition, there are limitations inherent to any of the proposed techniques. Thus, the real risk of measurements involving the puncture of the varices (bleeding, bacteraemia, etc.) is still unknown. Probably this technique is justified only in patients undergoing therapeutic sclerotherapy. Endoscopic pressure-sensitive ('capsule') measurements can be influenced by construction of the capsule and by the skill of the physician performing the measurements. Recent studies from our laboratory using an improved, miniaturized, pressure-sensitive capsule evaluated under double-blind conditions have shown that this technique is highly reproducible when adopting strict criteria to define a satisfactory measurement[25].

The main findings of studies measuring variceal pressure in patients with cirrhosis are: (a) variceal pressure is significantly lower than portal pressure; this is due to the resistance offered by the collaterals feeding the varices, and indicates that measurements of variceal pressure cannot be used to estimate portal pressure[22-24]; (b) variceal pressure is greater in patients who have bled from the varices than in those who have not[23], suggesting that increased variceal pressure plays a key role in the mechanism of bleeding and that measurement of variceal pressure may have a prognostic value to assess the risk of bleeding, although this has still not been proved by prospective longitudinal studies; and (c) the technique may be useful to assess the effects of pharmacological agents; however, due to the technical limitations outlined above, these investigations should be performed under strict double-blind conditions by critical investigators. It should be emphasized in that regard that these measurements are done in conditions far from physiological, and that they complement, but are no substitute for, the information obtained by conventional haemodynamic studies[25].

SUMMARY: DIAGNOSTIC APPROACH TO THE PORTAL HYPERTENSIVE PATIENT

Patients suspected of having portal hypertension should undergo ultrasonography and upper gastrointestinal endoscopy. At endoscopy particular attention should be paid to the presence, extent, size and appearance of the wall of the varices. Ultrasonography, preferably combined with Doppler flowmetry, will show if the portal vein is patent or not, and may disclose additional useful information on liver, biliary or pancreatic diseases that may be the cause of portal hypertension. Portal hypertensive patients with a patent portal vein should have hepatic vein catheterization. If the patient has varices and the hepatic venous pressure gradient is less than 12 mmHg, presinusoidal intrahepatic portal hypertension is likely; this should be investigated by liver biopsy and percutaneous transhepatic measurement of portal pressure. If the hepatic vein pressure gradient is above 12 mmHg and the patient has oesophageal varices, the possibility of instituting prophylactic medical therapy should be considered[26–28]. Finally, if the gradient is increased but endoscopy shows no varices, it is wise to re-evaluate the patient at 12-month periods because of the risk of developing varices and bleeding if portal pressure remains elevated. It should be emphasized that portal pressure does not remain steady during the evolution of cirrhosis. Actually, it usually varies in parallel with the severity of the disease. Many abstinent patients may exhibit a spontaneous reduction in portal pressure, while alcoholic hepatitis or development of hepatocellular carcinoma are associated with marked aggravations of the portal hypertension.

ACKNOWLEDGEMENTS

Research reported in this paper has been supported by grants from the Fondo de Investigaciones Sanitarias (FIS 91-0374) and Fundació Catalana per l'Estudi de les Malalties del Fetge. The author is indebted to Drs J. C. Garcia-Pagán, F. Feu, A. Luca and J. M. Bordas for their enthusiastic cooperation, to Ms M. A. Baringo for expert technical assistance and to Ms E. Gutierrez for secretarial help.

References

1. Bosch J, Mastai R, Kravetz D *et al.* Hemodynamic evaluation of the patients with portal hypertension. Semin Liver Dis. 1986;6:309–17.
2. Bosch J, Navasa M, Garcia-Pagán JC *et al.* Portal hypertension. Med Clin N Am. 1989;73:931–53.
3. Consensus Conference Committee. The value of Doppler US in the study of hepatic hemodynamics. Consensus conference (Bologna, Italy, 12 September 1989). J Hepatol. 1990;10:353–5.
4. Sabbá C, Weltin GG, Cicchetti DV *et al.* Observer variability in echo-doppler measurements of portal flow in cirrhotic patients and normal volunteers. Gastroenterology. 1990;98:1603–11.
5. Calés P, Pascal JP. Histoire naturelle des varices oesophagiennes au cours de la cirrhose (de la naisance a la rupture). Gastroeneterol Clin Biol. 1988;12:245–54.
6. North Italian Endoscopic Club for the Study and Treatment of Esophageal Varices. Prediction of the first variceal hemorrhage in patients with cirrhosis of the liver and esophageal varices. N Engl J Med. 1988;13:983–9.
7. Quintero E, Piqué JM, Bombi JA *et al.* Gastric mucosal vascular ectasias causing bleeding in cirrhosis. A distinct entity associated with hypergastrinemia and low serum levels of pepsinogen I. Gastroenterology. 1987;93:1054–61.
8. Pérez-Ayuso RM, Piqué JM, Bosch J *et al.* Propranolol in prevention of recurrent bleeding from severe portal hypertensive gastropathy in cirrhosis. Lancet. 1991;337:1431–4.
9. Papazian A, Braillon A, Dupas JL *et al.* Portal hypertensive gastric mucosa: an endoscopic study. Gut. 1986;27:1199–202.
10. Garcia-Tsao G, Groszmann RJ, Fisher RL *et al.* Portal pressure, presence of gastroesophageal varices and variceal bleeding. Hepatology. 1985;5:419–24.
11. Groszmann RJ, Bosch J, Grace ND *et al.* Hemodynamic events in a prospective randomized trial of propranolol versus placebo in the prevention of a first variceal hemorrhage. Gastroenterology. 1990;99:1401–7.
12. Groszmann RJ. Reassessing portal venous pressure measurements. Gastroenterology. 1984;80:1611–17.
13. Lebrec D, Benhamou JP. Noncirrhotic intahepatic portal hypertension. Sem Liver Dis. 1986;6:332–40.
14. Navasa M, Parés A, Bruguera M *et al.* Portal hypertension in primary biliary cirrhosis. Relationship with histological feature. J Hepatol. 1987;5:292–8.
15. Pomier-Layrargues G, Kusielewicz D *et al.* Presinusoidal portal hypertension in non-alcoholic cirrhosis. Hepatology. 1985;5:415–18.
16. Navasa M, Bosch J, Mastai R *et al.* Measurement of hepatic blood flow, hepatic extraction and intrinsic clearance of indocyanine green in patients with cirrhosis. Comparison of a non-invasive pharmacokinetic method with measurements using hepatic vein catheterization. Eur J Gastroenterol Hepatol. 1991;3:305–12.
17. Bosch J, Groszmann RJ. Measurement of the azygos venous blood flow by a continuous thermal dilution technique. An index of blood flow through gastroesophageal collaterals in cirrhosis. Hepatology. 1984;4:424–9.
18. Bosch J, Mastai R, Kravetz D *et al.* Measurement of azygos venous blood flow in the evaluation of portal hypertension in patients with cirrhosis. Clinical and haemodynamic correlations in 100 patients. J Hepatol. 1985;1:125–39.
19. Bosch J, Feu F, García-Pagán JC. Measurement of azygos blood flow. In: Okuda K, Benhamou JP, editors. Portal hypertension – clinical and physiological aspects. Tokyo: Springer-Verlag; 1991:139–150.
20. Bosch J, Mastai R, Kravetz D *et al.* Effects of propranolol on azygos blood flow and hepatic and systemic hemodynamics in cirrhosis. Hepatology. 1984;4:1200–5.
21. Mastai R, Bosch J, Nevasa M *et al.* Effects of alpha-adrenergic stimulation and beta-adrenergic blockade on azygos blood flow and splanchnic haemodynamics in patients with cirrhosis. J Hepatol. 1987;4:71–9.
22. Bosch J, Bordas JM, Mastai R *et al.* Effects of vasopressin on the intravariceal pressure in patients with cirrhosis: comparison with the effects on portal pressure. Hepatology. 1988;8:861–5.

23. Rigau J, Bosch J, Bordas JM, Navasa M *et al.* Endoscopic measurement of variceal pressure in cirrhosis: correlation with portal pressure and variceal haemorrhage. Gastroenterology. 1989;96:873–80.
24. Bosch J, Bordas JM, Rigau J *et al.* Non-invasive measurement of the pressure of esophageal varices using an endoscopic gauge. Comparison with measurements by variceal puncture in patients undergoing sclerotherapy. Hepatology. 1986;6:667–72.
25. Feu F, Bordas JM, García-Pagán JC *et al.* Double-blind investigation of the effects of propranolol and placebo on the pressure of the esophageal varices in patients with portal hypertension. Hepatology. 1991;13:917–22.
26. Pagliaro L, Burroughs AK, Sorensen TIA *et al.* Therapeutic controversies and randomised controlled trials (RCTs): prevention of bleeding and rebleeding in cirrhosis. Gastroenterol Int. 1989;2:71–84.
27. Poynard T, Calés JP, Pasta L *et al.* Beta-adrenergic-antagonist drugs in the prevention of gastrointestinal bleeding in patients with cirrhosis and esophageal varices. An analysis of data and prognostic factors in 589 patients from four randomized clinical trials. N Engl J Med. 1991;324:1532–8.
28. De Franchis R, Pascal JP, Ancona E *et al.* Definitions, methodology and therapeutic strategies in portal hypertension. A Consensus Development Workshop, Baveno, Lake Maggiore, Italy, 5 and 6 April 1990. J Hepatol. 1992;15:256–61.

3

Drugs for prevention and therapy of portal hypertension

D. LEBREC

The pharmacological treatment of portal hypertension consists of reducing portal pressure to prevent oesophageal variceal bleeding or treating active variceal bleeding. Since portal pressure depends on both elevated portal tributary blood flow and intrahepatic or collateral vascular resistance, drugs should induce a reduction in either portal blood flow or vascular resistance or both.

Many vasoactive drugs have been tested in patients and animals with portal hypertension (Table 1). A certain number of vasoactive agents which are only effective for a short period are used for the treatment of acute variceal bleeding. Others may be used over a long period and are therefore potentially useful in preventing gastrointestinal bleeding. In this chapter the main findings of the haemodynamic effects and the results of clinical studies for the prevention of bleeding are reported.

β-Adrenergic antagonists

In patients with portal hypertension, acute and chronic administration of β-blockers reduces portal pressure, hepatic venous pressure and variceal pressure, but these effects differ from one patient to another and the decrease ranges from 0% to 40%[1–18]. In contrast, azygos blood flow decreases with remarkable consistency, and ranges from 30% to 35%. In some patients, β-blockers have a minor effect (a decrease of less than 10%) or no effect on the hepatic venous pressure gradient. The lack of response of the hepatic venous pressure gradient may be due to a reflex increase in hepatic and collateral vascular resistances since azygos blood flow significantly decreases in these 'non-responders'. The portal hypotensive effect of β-blockers has been found in different types of cirrhosis and in patients with extrahepatic

Table 1 Drugs which decrease portal hypertension

Category	*Drug*
β-adrenergic antagonists	
Non-selective	Propranolol
	Long-acting propranolol
	Nadolol
	Mepindolol
	Sotalol
	Penbutolol
	Tertatolol
Cardioselective	Atenolol
	Metoprolol
	Betaxolol
	Levomoprolol
α-β-antagonists	Labetalol
β_2-antagonists	ICI 118551
β-antagonists with nitroxy base	Nipradilol
β_2-adrenergic agonist	Terbutaline
α-adrenergic antagonists	Phenoxybenzamine
	Prazosin
	Regitine
α_1-adrenergic agonist	Methoxamine
α_2-adrenergic agonist	Clonidine
5-hydroxytryptamine-receptor antagonists	Ketanserin
	Ritanserin
Growth hormone inhibiting factors	Somatostatin
	SMS 201-995
Vasoconstrictors	Vasopressin
	Triglycyl-vasopressin
	Octapressin
	Angiotensin
Nitrovasodilators	Sodium nitroprusside
	Nitroglycerine
	Isosorbide dinitrate
	Isosorbide mononitrate
Vasodilators	Molsidomine
	Pentoxifylline
	Parathyroid hormone
	Atrial natriuretic factor
Diuretics	Furosemide
	Spironolactone
	Mersalyl
	Chlorothiazide
Platelet-activating factor antagonist	BN 52021
Antiglucagon	Antiglucagon
Inhibitor of nitric oxide release	N^Gmonomethyl-L-arginine
Blocker of ATP-sensitive K^+ channels	Glibenclamide

portal hypertension[19]. The severity of liver disease does not influence the haemodynamic effects of β-blockers[5,20]. At present neither clinical, laboratory, nor haemodynamic criteria can predict which patient will respond, nor can other tests, such as plasma propanolol measurement[21] or isoproterenol infusion[22]. Moreover, in conscious portal hypertensive rats it has been demonstrated that systemic β-blockade differed from β-blockade of the splanchnic circulation[23]. This suggests that decreases in heart rate do not directly reflect the splanchnic effect of propranolol.

The hepatic blood flow was not affected by propranolol[24]. However, following propranolol administration, portal blood flow, which is a fraction of total hepatic blood flow, significantly decreased both in patients with cirrhosis[12,25] and in rats with portal hypertension[23]. Renal blood flow and cerebral blood flow were not altered in patients receiving propranolol[26,27].

A few studies using other non-selective β-blockers show haemodynamic effects similar to propranolol[28,29]. In contrast, selective β_1- or β_2-blockers reduce portal pressure less than non-selective β-blockers[30–32].

The combinations of portal hypotensive substances and propranolol have been tested. One experimental study showed that nitroglycerine combined with propranolol reduced portal pressure and portal tributary blood flow more than nitroglycerine or propranolol alone in anaesthetized rats with portal vein stenosis[33]. The long-term administration of propranolol and isosorbide-5-mononitrate in cirrhotic patients also had a greater beneficial effect on the hepatic venous pressure gradient than either drug alone[34]. Similarly, the combination of propranolol and molsidomine, a venous dilator, caused a greater reduction in portal blood flow measured by pulsed Doppler flowmetry than propranolol or molsidomine alone[35]. In these three haemodynamic studies, however, the combination of propranolol with a vasodilator significantly decreased arterial pressure, whereas propranolol alone did not affect it.

The association of propranolol and clonidine induced a significant decrease in portal pressure and portal tributary blood flow in conscious cirrhotic rats[36]. These changes were significantly more marked following the combined administration of these substances than following either clonidine or propranolol alone. No change in arterial pressure was observed, but cardiac output significantly decreased. The additive effect of these two drugs verifies the action of clonidine and propranolol at central and peripheral levels and on α- and β-receptors.

The combination of propranolol and 5-hydroxytryptamine (5-HT_2) receptor antagonist has also been tested. In cirrhotic patients receiving propranolol, the addition of ketanserin induced a further significant reduction in wedged hepatic venous pressure, the hepatic venous pressure gradient, and azygos blood flow[37]. Moreover, among non-responders to propranolol, certain patients had a reduced wedged hepatic venous pressure after ketanserin was added. In conscious cirrhotic rats, ritanserin significantly reduced portal pressure, which was further reduced by the addition of propranolol[38]. Arterial pressure was not affected in these two last studies.

β-Adrenergic agonist

Results of one study showed that administration of terbutaline, a β_2-adrenergic agonist, significantly reduced portal pressure despite an increased portal tributary blood flow in cirrhotic rats[39]. These results may be explained by a decrease in hepatic and collateral vascular resistance. Clinical studies are needed, however, to confirm the portal hypotensive effect of this drug.

α-Adrenergic antagonists

The α-blockers have been used to reduce portal pressure in patients with portal hypertension. In one study, phenoxybenzamine was used in anaesthetized patients[40], and a second study demonstrated that continuous administration of prazosin induced a decrease in the hepatic venous pressure gradient in cirrhotic patients[11]. It is possible that the systemic arteriodilating and venodilating effects of these agents might influence the splanchnic circulation and thereby portal hypertension.

α_1-Adrenergic agonist

In one study performed in patients with cirrhosis, methoxamine, a powerful vasoconstrictor, induced a decrease in the hepatic venous pressure gradient[9]. This effect was associated with a marked increase in arterial pressure and a decrease in cardiac output.

α_2-Adrenergic agonist

Clonidine, a centrally acting α_2-agonist, decreases sympathetic nervous activity which is elevated in cirrhotic patients. In two clinical investigations, acute administration of clonidine significantly reduced portal pressure or the hepatic venous pressure gradient, arterial pressure and cardiac output[41,42]. In one of these studies, decreased intrahepatic resistance was considered the cause of this portal hypotensive effect[41]. In the other, splanchnic vasoconstriction mediated by baroreflexes and triggered by the fall in arterial presure was hypothesized[42]. In three studies, long-term clonidine administration in patients with cirrhosis continued to improve splanchnic haemodynamics and did not induce deleterious systemic effects[43–45]. Long-term effects of clonidine administration on renal haemodynamics are controversial[43,44]. In cirrhotic rats, clonidine reduced portal pressure but did not affect systemic haemodynamics. Accordingly, clonidine probably reduced portal pressure by inducing an increase in portal tributary vascular resistance.

5-Hydroxytryptamine (5-HT_2) receptor antagonists

Different experimental studies have shown that 5-HT_2 is a mediator for intestinal vasodilation and may help to maintain portal hypertension. Moreover, the isolated superior mesenteric veins from portal hypertensive rats appear to be more sensitive to 5-HT_2 than veins from normal rats[46]. Several clinical studies have shown that 5-HT_2 receptor antagonists such as ketanserin or ritanserin significantly decrease portal pressure or the hepatic venous pressure gradient in patients with cirrhosis[47-49] and in animals with portal hypertension[50,51]. In one study, acute administration of ketanserin also decreased azygos blood flow while hepatic blood flow was not affected[47]. The long-term administration of ketanserin produced a sustained decrease in the hepatic venous pressure gradient[49]. In this last study, however, large doses of ketanserin in patients in poor condition also induced reversible hepatic encephalopathy.

Growth hormone release inhibitory factors

The haemodynamic effects of somatostatin on portal hypertension are not clear. Somatostatin may decrease portal, hepatic venous or variceal pressure and azygos blood flow in patients with cirrhosis[52-58]. The extent of change differs greatly from one patient to another and ranges from 0% to 50%. The effects of a bolus injection on portal pressure seem to be more pronounced than intravenous infusion. These results indicate that the splanchnic response depends on the dose of somatostatin. This correlation has recently been demonstrated in cirrhotic rats with a somatostatin analogue (SMS 201-995)[59].

The mechanisms responsible for the haemodynamic effects of somatostatin are not clearly understood. Somatostatin decreases gastric mucosal blood flow in normal subjects but not in patients with cirrhosis[57]. In anaesthetized subjects, somatostatin decreased splanchnic blood flow and in conscious cirrhotic patients, total hepatic blood flow was decreased[58]. These results indicate that decreased portal pressure is caused by a reduction in portal tributary blood flow. Similar effects have been demonstrated in cirrhotic rats[59]. In most studies, somatostatin had no or minor systemic haemodynamic effects. In one investigation, however, decreased cardiac output was observed[55]. This cardiac output reduction lasted less than 5 min, and could explain the decrease in splanchnic blood flow. Finally, in a study with portal hypertensive rats, it was suggested that the reduction of glucagon by somatostatin may explain the haemodynamic effects of this substance[60].

Vasoconstrictors

The haemodynamic effects of vasopressin have been extensively studied[61]. Several studies have demonstrated that the intravenous or intra-arterial administration of vasopressin or vasopressin analogues such as Glypressin decreases portal pressure or the hepatic venous pressure gradient and azygos blood flow in patients with cirrhosis. These portal hypotensive effects have also been demonstrated in animals. Portal hypotensive responses to vasopressin range from 0% to 60% of basal values.

Vasopressin decreases portal pressure by reducing portal tributary blood flow through vasoconstriction of splanchnic arterioles. It has been well established that the vasoconstrictive effects of vasopressin increase arterial pressure, pulmonary wedged pressure, and systemic vascular resistance, and decrease cardiac output. Since severe side-effects may occur, nitrovasodilators have been used to counteract the effects of vasopressin in cirrhotic patients[62]. The effects of vasodilators on vasopressin-induced systemic vasoconstrictors, however, have not yet been firmly established.

Finally, one study has shown that the effects of vasopressin on the splanchnic circulation in bleeding portal hypertensive rats differ from the effects observed when blood volume is normal[63]. In this case, in fact, both haemorrhage and vasopressin alone decreased portal pressure.

Nitrovasodilators

The portal hypotensive effects of nitroglycerine, isosorbide mononitrate and dinitrate are still being debated[64]. These agents may decrease portal pressure, have no effect or even increase portal hypertension (see ref. 64). Even if nitrovasodilators decrease portal pressure, the underlying mechanisms have not yet been clarified. At low doses, nitroglycerine induces venous pooling and thus decreases venous return, while arterial pressure remains unchanged. The decreased venous return causes splanchnic arterial constriction. On the other hand, low doses of nitrovasodilators have no effect on portal pressure, which suggests an anomaly in the cardiopulmonary baroreflexes of cirrhosis. At high doses, nitrovasodilators reduce both venous return and arterial pressure, and arterial hypotension induces splanchnic vasoconstriction. Thus, in cirrhotic patients, arterial baroreceptor unloading could reduce both portal inflow and portal pressure.

Overall, the use of nitrovasodilators in patients with portal hypertension seems hazardous, since a drop in arterial pressure associated with a decrease in systemic oxygen consumption has been observed in patients with cirrhosis receiving nitroglycerine. The correct combination of a nitrovasodilator with a vasoconstrictor for portal hypertension must still be established.

Other vasodilators

Molsidomine[65], parathyroid hormone[66], and pentoxifylline[67,68] have been shown to reduce portal hypertension in patients or animals with cirrhosis. In these studies the reduction in arterial pressure probably induced splanchnic vasoconstriction or nitrovasodilation and caused a decrease in portal pressure.

Diuretics

Since cirrhotic patients have augmented blood volume which correlates with the degree of portal hypertension, diuretics have been suggested to reduce portal pressure through a reduction of blood volume. Different types of diuretics have been used, and all show that acute or chronic administration of these substances significantly reduces blood volume and portal pressure[69–72]. One study using furosemide also showed decreased cardiac output and azygos blood flow[70].

Platelet-activating factor (PAF) antagonist

PAF, a potent hepatic vasoconstrictor, has been suggested as one of the substances involved in the systemic hyperdynamics of portal hypertension. In this case, PAF antagonist should correct the hyperkinetic syndrome observed in portal hypertension. This hypothesis has been investigated in cirrhotic rats[73]. In these animals BN 52021, a PAF receptor antagonist, significantly decreased cardiac output and portal pressure. Further clinical studies are, however, needed to determine the role of PAF in patients with portal hypertension.

Other drugs

N^G-monomethyl-L-argine (L-NMMA) has recently been shown to decrease portal pressure in conscious rats with cirrhosis[74]. L-NMMA, a competitive inhibitor of nitric oxide synthesis, has been used to reduce nitric oxide since this substance is considered to be a potential vasodilator in cirrhosis[75].

Finally, glibenclamide, a blocker of ATP-sensitive K^+ channels, has also been found to significantly decrease portal pressure and hyperkinetic circulation in portal hypertensive rats[76].

TREATMENT

Acute treatment of variceal bleeding

The management of acute gastrointestinal bleeding due to portal hypertension is still controversial[77]. Although many studies have been performed, only a few of them were controlled. As a result no firm conclusions can be drawn. Two points must still be clarified. First, survival rate depends mainly on the severity of liver disease, and not on gastrointestinal bleeding. Second, criteria for the efficacy of treatment have not yet been clearly established, and differ among studies. Finally, it should be emphasized that most patients stop bleeding spontaneously without any treatment.

Although endoscopic sclerotherapy is an effective treatment for variceal bleeding, pharmacological therapy may also be used before this procedure, i.e. while waiting for sclerotherapy.

Vasopressin and its analogues, alone or combined with vasodilators, have been suggested for the management of acute variceal bleeding. Vasopressin or Glypressin controls variceal bleeding in 9–90% of patients. Among the five trials that compared vasopressin or Glypressin with a placebo, three showed a significant difference between the two groups (see ref. 77). The association of nitroglycerin with vasopressin or Glypressin does not markedly increase the efficacity of the vasoconstrictors[78,79].

Two trials that compared placebo and somatostatin in acute variceal bleeding showed discrepant results[80,81]. In one study, somatostatin was effective in controlling acute variceal bleeding[80] but these results were not found in the second study[81]. Somatostatin has been shown to be as effective as vasopressin or balloon tamponade. Finally, somatostatin has fewer side-effects than vasopressin.

Prevention of the first episode of gastrointestinal bleeding

The results of nine controlled studies for the prevention of the first gastrointestinal bleeding in cirrhotic patients with oesophageal varices have been published (Table 2)[82-90]. Moreover, another controlled trial, performed in 95 patients with portal hypertension with or without oesophageal varices, has shown that among the 48 patients receiving a placebo, three developed gastrointestinal bleeding over a 1-year period, while of the 47 patients receiving long-acting propranolol, none bled[91]. Among the nine controlled studies performed with cirrhotic patients, seven used propranolol or long-acting propranolol administered at doses which decreased heart rate by approximately 25%. In two studies, nadolol – a non-selective β-adrenergic blocker – was used. Four studies showed that β-blockers significantly decrease the risk of gastrointestinal bleeding. One study showed that this difference was observed only among compliant patients and another only when patients without or with mild ascites were considered. Only one study showed a significant difference in survival rate between treated and non-treated patients. Three studies did not find any significant difference between the two groups of patients.

Three meta-analyses have recently been published[92-94]. All concur that β-blockers significantly decrease the risk of the first episode of gastrointestinal bleeding in patients with cirrhosis. Death from bleeding was also significantly different between patients receiving β-blockers and patients receiving a placebo. One meta-analysis, which used individual data, showed that the severity of liver failure and ascites were strong independent prognostic factors

Table 2 Results of the controlled studies for the prevention of the first episode of gastrointestinal bleeding in patients with cirrhosis

	Bleeding (%)				*Survival rate (%)*			
	Control		*β-Blocker*		*Control*		*β-Blocker*	
First author	*1 year*	*2 years*	*1 year*	*2 years*	*1 year*	*2 years*	*1 year*	*2 years*
Andreani[82]	30	39	6*	6*	66	54	79	66
Colman[83]	—	5	—	31	—	69	—	80
Conn[84]	22	—	4*	—	78	—	84	—
Idéo[85]	19	30	0*	6*	84	78	95	94
Lebrec[86]	21(23)	26	17(3†)	21	80	74	78	72
Pascal[87]	25	61	15	26*	66	51	76	72*
PROVA[88]	18	—	18	—	89	—	93	—
Strauss[89]	—	25	—	20	—	56	—	65
The Italian multicenter[90]	12	31	8**	22**	87	59	94	74

* Significantly different from the control group
† Significantly different from the control group only in compliant patients
** Significantly different from the control group only in patients without ascites

for bleeding and death in all patients[93]. Moreover, this study showed that β-blockers significantly decreased the risk of the first episode of bleeding and death from bleeding among patients with or without ascites, with or without severe liver failure, with small or large varices and in patients receiving nadolol or propranolol.

Side-effects occurred in 3–40% of patients receiving β-blockers; β-blockers were interrupted in only 5% of the patients. Dizziness occurred in approximately 6% of the treated patients and was the main complication. Raynaud's syndrome and pulmonary or cardiac complications occurred in less than 2% of the patients. Except for hepatic encephalopathy, these side-effects were similar to those observed in patients without liver disease receiving β-blockers. Encephalopathy occurred in less than 1% of the cases. This complication was mild and transient. In all the studies the resuscitation of patients receiving β-blockers who bled, was not more difficult than in untreated patients.

Finally preliminary results have showed that isosorbide-5-mononitrate was as effective as propranolol in the prevention of the first gastrointestinal bleeding in patients with cirrhosis[95].

Prevention of recurrent gastrointestinal bleeding

β-Blockers

The results of 13 controlled studies of the prevention of rebleeding in patients with cirrhosis have been published (Table 3)[3,84,96–106]. Two other trials have been performed in patients with non-cirrhotic portal hypertension. Among these 13 studies there are discrepant results. Eight trials show a significant

Table 3 Results of the controlled studies of the prevention of recurrent gastrointestinal bleeding in patients with portal hypertension

	Rebleeding (%)				*Survival rate (%)*			
	Control		*β-Blocker*		*Control*		*β-Blocker*	
First author	*1 year*	*2 years*	*1 year*	*2 years*	*1 year*	*2 years*	*1 year*	*2 years*
Burroughs[3]	44	70	46	72	77	—	85	—
Cerbelaud[96]	—	87	—	49*	—	71	—	88
Colman[84]	—	50	—	31	—	95	—	95
Colombo[97]	—	51	—	24*	—	68	—	90
Garden[98]	—	77	—	47*	—	44	—	49
Gatta[99]	33	74	10*	30*	90	65	100	89
Kiire[100]	80	—	20*	—	80	—	96	—
Lebrec[101]	58	68	13*	21*	84	57	94	90*
Queuniet[102]	52	—	50	—	79	—	76	—
Qureshi[103]	—	63	—	40*	—	94	—	91
Rossi[104]	46	61	19	47	81	66	92	80
Sheen[105]	41	85	13*	43*	—	89	—	100
Villeneuve[106]	76	—	71	—	62	—	64	—

* Significantly different from the control group

difference between the risk of rebleeding in patients receiving β-blockers and those receiving a placebo, whereas in the five other studies significant differences were not found between the two groups. Finally, a recent study showed that propranolol significantly reduced the risk of rebleeding from portal hypertensive gastropathy and improved survival rate in patients with cirrhosis for a period of 2 years[108]. Although none of these studies explains the discrepancies certain points should be considered. First, time intervals between episodes of gastrointestinal bleeding and inclusion in the study might explain the percentage of rebleeding, since it has been demonstrated that the risk of rebleeding decreases over time. In fact, the time intervals differ greatly from one study to the other. Moreover, a controlled study performed in cirrhotic patients showed that propranolol significantly prevented early recurrent gastrointestinal bleeding[107]. It has also been suggested that the severity and cause of cirrhosis might play a role in the risk of rebleeding. In the studies where β-blockers reduced the risk of rebleeding, or where β-blockers had no beneficial effect, most of the selected patients were in good condition. In most studies, patients had cirrhosis due to alcohol intoxication: accordingly, a comparison between alcoholic and non-alcoholic cirrhosis could not be performed. Two meta-analyses showed that β-blockers significantly reduced the risk of recurrent gastrointestinal bleeding in patients with portal hypertension[92,109]. A significant difference in mortality between treated and untreated patients was found in one meta-analysis[92] but not in the other.

Certain factors have been found to be associated with recurrent gastrointestinal bleeding in patients treated with β-blockers[110]. All patients who developed hepatocellular carcinoma rebled. Non-compliant patients and patients whose heart rate did not significantly decrease, rebled more than compliant patients. The risk of rebleeding was higher in patients with previous bleeding than in those who bled for the first time. In this study the cause and severity of cirrhosis was not associated with rebleeding. Moreover, haemodynamic studies showed that the risk of recurrent gastrointestinal bleeding in patients receiving propranolol could not be predicted using either basal splanchnic and systemic haemodynamic values or the acute response to propranolol.

β-Blockers vs endoscopic sclerotherapy

Ten randomized studies comparing the efficacy of propranolol and sclerotherapy in the prevention of rebleeding have been reported (Table 4)[103,111–119]. In two studies the risk of rebleeding in patients receiving propranolol was higher than in patients treated by sclerotherapy. In one study the risk of rebleeding was higher in patients treated with endoscopic sclerotherapy than in patients receiving propranolol. There were no significant differences in survival rate in any of the studies.

Finally, the results of the association of propranolol with sclerotherapy showed that the risk of rebleeding was lower than in patients treated with sclerotherapy alone[120–124].

Table 4 Comparison between β-blockers and endoscopic sclerotherapy for the prevention of recurrent gastrointestinal bleeding in patients with portal hypertension

First author	*Period of follow-up (months)*	*Rebleeding (%)*		*Survival rate (%)*	
		β-Blocker	*Sclerotherapy*	*β-Blocker*	*Sclerotherapy*
Alexandrino[111]	17–57	58	27*	54	69
Andreani[112]	12	34	42*	74	58
Dasarathy[113]	24	67	42*	59	78
Dollet[114]	13–53	52	63	65	68
Fleig[115]	12	28	29	92	93
Martin[116]	24	53	55	77	59
Qureshi[103]	24	40	47	91	86
Rossi[117]	27/26	24	47	50	80
Terès[118]	33/39	12	24	20	79
Westaby[119]	48/52	12–64	54	45	55

* Significantly different from β-blocker group

CONCLUSION

Pharmacological treatment for the prevention of the first episode of gastrointestinal bleeding or for the prevention of recurrent gastrointestinal bleeding in compliant and abstinent patients should be administered. If this treatment fails, other procedures such as encoscopic sclerotherapy, intrahepatic shunts, or surgery can be proposed. At the same time, new experimental and clinical studies are needed to evaluate the most appropriate pharmacological treatment of portal hypertension.

References

1. Bendtsen F, Henriksen JH, Becker U, Sorensen TIA. Effect of oral propranolol on splanchnic oxygen uptake and haemodynamics in patients with cirrhosis. J Hepatol. 1987;5:137–43.
2. Bosch J, Masti R, Kravetz D, Bruix J, Gaya J, Rigau J, Rodes J. Effects of propranolol on azygos venous blood flow and hepatic and systemic hemodynamics in cirrhosis. Hepatology. 1984;4:1200–5.
3. Burroughs AK, Jenkins WJ, Sherlock S, Dunk A, Walt RP, Osuafor TOK, Mackie S, Dick R. Controlled trial of propranolol for the prevention of recurrent variceal hemorrhage in patients with cirrhosis. N Engl J Med. 1983;309:1539–42.
4. Calès P, Braillon A, Jiron MI, Lebrec D. Superior portosystemic collateral circulation estimated by azygos blood flow in patients with cirrhosis. Lack of correlation with oesophageal varices and gastrointestinal bleeding. Effect of propranolol. J Hepatol. 1984;1:37–46.
5. Garcia-Tsao G, Grace ND, Groszmann RJ, Conn HO, Bermann MM, Patrick MJC, Morse SS, Alberts JL. Short-term effects of propranolol on portal venous pressure. Hepatology. 1986;6:101–6.
6. Kanazawa H, Matsusaka S, Tada N, Kuroda H, Kobayashi M. Measurement of azygos blood flow by a continuous thermodilution method in liver disease. Acta Hepatol Jpn. 1986;27:1132–40.
7. Kong CW, Lay CS, Tsai YT, Lee SD, Lai KH, Lo KJ, Chiang BN. Hemodynamic effect of propranolol on portal hypertension in patients with HBsAg-positive cirrhosis. Dig Dis Sci. 1986;31:1303–6.

8. Lebrec D, Hillon P, Munoz C, Goldfarb G, Nouel O, Benhamou JP. The effect of propranolol on portal hypertension in patients with cirrhosis: a hemodynamic study. Hepatology. 1982;2:523–7.
9. Mastai R, Bosch J, Navasa M, Kravetz D, Bruix J, Viola C, Rodès J. Effects of alpha-adrenergic stimulation and beta-adrenergic blockade on azygos blood flow and splanchnic haemodynamics in patients with cirrhosis. J Hepatol. 1987;4:71–9.
10. Meacci E, La Villa G, Laffi G, Cominelle F, Di Donato M, Dabizz P, Alban F, Gentilini P. Systemic haemodynamics, renal and platelet function during chronic propranolol administration in patients with compensated cirrhosis. Liver. 1987;7:110–15.
11. Mills PR, Rae AP, Farah DA, Russell RI, Lorimer AR, Carter DC. Comparison of three adrenoreceptor blocking agents in patients with cirrhosis and portal hypertension. Gut. 1984;25:73–8.
12. Onishi K, Nakayama T, Saito M, Hatano H, Tsukamoto T, Terabayashi H, Sugita S, Wada K, Nomura F, Koen H, Okuda K. Effects of propranolol on portal hemodynamics in patients with chronic liver disease. Am J Gastroenterol. 1985;80:132–4.
13. Okumura H, Sekiyama T, Katsuta Y, Aramaki T, Satomura K, Akaike M, Terada H, Sekino M. Effect of propranolol on portal venous pressure in patients with chronic liver disease: comparison with vasopressin. Acta Hepatol Jpn. 1984;25:1534–40.
14. Pomier-Layrargues G, Villeneuve JP, Willems B, Huet PM, Marleau D. Systemic and hepatic hemodynamics after variceal hemorrhage: effects of propranolol and placebo. Gastroenterology. 1987;93:1218–24.
15. Rector WG. Propranolol for portal hypertension. Evaluation of therapeutic response by direct measurement of portal vein pressure. Arch Intern Med. 1985;145:648–50.
16. Valla D, Bercoff E, Menu Y, Bataille C, Lebrec D. Discrepancy between wedged hepatic venous pressure and portal venous pressure after acute propranolol administration in patients with alcoholic cirrhosis. Gastroenterology. 1984;86:1400–3.
17. Vorobioff J, Picabea E, Villavicencio R, Puccini V, Rossi O, Bordato J, Audano M. Acute and chronic hemodynamic effects of propranolol in unselected cirrhotic patients. Hepatology. 1987;7:648–53.
18. Westaby D, Bihari DJ, Gimson AES, Crossley IR, Williams R. Selective and nonselective beta receptor blockade in the reduction of portal pressure in patients with cirrhosis and portal hypertension. Gut. 1984;25:121–4.
19. Braillon A, Moreau R, Hadengue A, Roulot D, Sayegh R, Lebrec D. Hyperkinetic circulatory syndrome in patients with presinusoidal portal hypertension. Effect of propranolol. J Hepatol. 1989;9:312–18.
20. Braillon A, Calès P, Valla D, Gaudy D, Geoffroy P, Lebrec D. Influence of the degree of liver failure on systemic and splanchnic haemodynamics and on response to propranolol in patients with cirrhosis. Gut. 1986;27:1204–9.
21. Jiron MI, Delhotal B, Lebrec D. Relationship between dose, blood level and haemodynamic response in patients with cirrhosis receiving propranolol. Eur J Clin Pharmacol. 1985;28:353–5.
22. Bercoff E, Bataille C, Pariente AE, Valla D, Delhotal B, Lebrec D. Assessment of β-adrenergic blockade with propranolol in patients with cirrhosis. Hepatology. 1984;4:451–3.
23. Koshy A, Girod C, Lee SS, Hadengue A, Cerini R, Lebrec D. Discrepancy between portal pressure and systemic hemodynamic changes after incremental doses of propranolol in awake portal hypertensive rats. Hepatology. 1989;9:269–73.
24. Braillon A, Jiron MI, Valla D, Calès P, Lebrec D. Effect of propranolol on hepatic blood flow in patients with cirrhosis. Clin Pharmacol Ther. 1985;37:376–80.
25. Zoli M, Marchesini G, Brunori A, Cordiani RM, Pisi E. Portal venous flow in response to acute β-blocker and vasodilatory treatment in patients with liver cirrhosis. Hepatology. 1986;6:1248–51.
26. Bataille C, Bercoff E, Pariente EA, Valla D, Lebrec D. Effects of propranolol on renal blood flow and renal function in patients with cirrhosis. Gastroenterology. 1984;86:129–33.
27. Calès P, Pierre-Nicolas M, Guell A, Mauroux JL, Franco-Sempe A, Vinel JP, Gerauc G, Pascal JP. Propranolol does not alter cerebral blood flow and functions in cirrhotic patients without previous hepatic encephalopathy. Hepatology. 1989;9:439–42.
28. Braillon A, Calès P, Lebrec D. Comparison of the short-term effects of mepindolol and propranolol on splanchnic and systemic haemodynamics in patients with cirrhosis. Int J Clin Pharmacol Res. 1985;5:223–8.

29. Gatta A, Sarcerdoti D, Merkel C, Caregaro L, Borsato M, Bolognesi M, Ruol A. Renal effects of nadolol in cirrhosis. Eur J Clin Pharmacol. 1987;37:22–8.
30. Bihari D, Westaby D, Gimson A, Crossley I, Harry J, Williams R. Reductions in portal pressure by selective β_2-adrenoceptor blockade in patients with cirrhosis and portal hypertension. Br J Clin Pharmacol. 1984;17:753–7.
31. Butzow GH, Remmecke J, Brauer A. Metoprolol in portal hypertension. A controlled study. Klin Wochenschr. 1982;60:311–14.
32. Hillon P, Lebrec D, Munoz C, Jungers M, Goldfarb G, Benhamou JP. Comparison of the effects of a cardioselective and a nonselective β-blocker on portal hypertension in patients with cirrhosis. Hepatology. 1982;2:528–31.
33. Kroeger RJ, Groszmann RJ. The effects of the combination of nitroglycerin and propranolol on splanchnic and systemic hemodynamics in a portal hypertensive rat model. Hepatology. 1985;5:425–30.
34. Garcia-Pagan JC, Navasa M, Bosch J, Bru C, Pizcueta P, Rodès J. Enhancement of portal pressure reduction by the association of isosorbide-5-mononitrate to propranolol administration in patients with cirrhosis. Hepatology. 1990;11:230–8.
35. Monnin JL, Vinel JP, Pascal JP, Dauzat M, Bruel JM, Blanc F, Michel H, Le Quellec A, Ciurana AJ. Pulsed Doppler flowmetry assessment of molsodomine and molsidonine + propranolol effects portal hemodynamic in patients with cirrhosis (abstract). J Hepatol. 1989;9(suppl 1):S192.
36. Roulot D, Gaudin C, Braillon A, Sekiyama T, Bacq Y, Lebrec D. Hemodynamic effects of combination of clonidine and propranolol in conscious cirrhotic rats. Can J Physiol Pharmacol. 1989;67:1369–72.
37. Hadengue A, Moreau R, Cerini R, Koshy A, Lee SS, Lebrec D. Combination of ketanserin and verapamil or propranolol in patients with alcoholic cirrhosis. Research for an additive effect. Hepatology. 1989;9:183–7.
38. Pomier-Layrargues G, Biroux L, Rocheleau B, Huet PM. Combined treatment of portal hypertension with ritanserin and propranolol in conscious and unrestrained cirrhotic rats. Hepatology. 1992;15:878–82.
39. Poo JL, Braillon A, Hadengue A, Gaudin C, Lebrec D. Hemodynamic effects of terbutaline, a β_2-adrenoceptor agonist in conscious rats with secondary biliary cirrhosis. Hepatology. 1992;15:459–63.
40. Ikeda M. Effect of phenoxybenzamine (POB) on portal venous pressure in patients with portal hypertension. Am J Gastroenterol. 1979;71:389–94.
41. Willett IR, Esler M, Jennings G, Dudley FJ. Sympathetic tone modulates portal venous pressure in alcoholic cirrhosis. Lancet. 1986;1:773–5.
42. Moreau R, Lee SS, Hadengue A, Braillon A, Lebrec D. Hemodynamic effects of a clonidine-induced decrease in sympathetic tone in patients with cirrhosis. Hepatology. 1987;7:149–54.
43. Roulot D, Moreau R, Gaudin C, Bacq Y, Braillon A, Hadengue A, Frohly P, Lebrec D. Long-term sympathetic and hemodynamic responses to clonidine in patients with cirrhosis and ascites. Gastroenterology. 1992;102:1309–18.
44. Esler M, Dudley F, Jennings G, Debinski H, Lambert G, Jones P, Crotty B, Colman J, Willett I. Increased sympathetic nervous activity and the effects of its inhibition with clonidine in alcoholic cirrhosis. Ann Intern Med. 1992;116:446–55.
45. Albillos A, Banares R, Barrios C, Clemente G, Rossi I, Escartin P, Bosch J. Oral administration of clonidine in patients with alcoholic cirrhosis. Hemodynamic and liver function effects. Gastroenterology. 1992;102:248–54.
46. Cummings SA, Groszmann RJ, Kaumann AJ. Hypersensitivity of mesenteric veins to 5-hydroxytryptamine- and ketanserin-induced reduction of portal pressure in portal hypertensive rats. Br J Pharmacol. 1978;64:851–8.
47. Hadengue A, Lee SS, Moreau R, Braillon A, Lebrec D. Beneficial hemodynamic effects of ketanserin in patients with cirrhosis: possible role of serotonergic mechanisms in portal hypertension. Hepatology. 1987;7:644–7.
48. Huet PM, Pomier-Layrargues G, Semret M. Effects of ritanserin, a serotonin antagonist, in cirrhotic patients with portal hypertension. (abstract). Hepatology. 1988;8:1422.
49. Vorobioff J, Garcia-Tsao G, Groszmann R, Aceves G, Picabea E, Villavicencio R, Hernandez-Ortiz J. Long-term hemodynamic effects of ketanserin a 5-hydroxytryptamine

bloocker, in portal hypertensive patients. Hepatology 1989;9:88–91.
50. Mastai R, Rocheleau B, Huet PM. Serotonin blockade in conscious, unrestrained cirrhotic dogs with portal hypertension. Hepatology. 1989;9:265–8.
51. Mastai R, Giroux L, Semret M, Huet PM. Ritanserin decreases portal pressure in conscious and unrestrained cirrhotic rats. Gastroenterology. 1990;98:141–5.
52. Bosch J, Kravetz D, Rodes J. Effects of somatostatin on hepatic and systemic hemodynamics in patients with cirrhosis of the liver; comparison with vasopressin. Gastroenterology. 1981;80:518–25.
53. Eriksson LS, Brundin T, Söderlund C, Wahren J. Haemodynamic effect of a long-acting somatostatin analogue in patients with liver cirrhosis. Scand J Gastroenterol. 1987;22:919–25.
54. Kleber G, Sauerbruch T, Fischer G, Paumgartner G. Somatostatin does not reduce oesophageal variceal pressure in liver cirrhotics. Gut. 1988;29:153–6.
55. Lebrec D, Nouel O. Comment la somatostatine diminue-t-elle la pression portale chez le cirrhotique? Gastroenterol Clin Biol. 1980;4:498–9.
56. Merkel C, Gatta A, Zuin R, Finucci GF, Nosadinin R, Ruol A. Effect of somatostatin on splanchnic hemodynamics in patients with liver cirrhosis and portal hypertension. Digestion. 1985;32:92–8.
57. Sonnenberg A, West C. Somatostatin reduces gastric mucosal blood flow in normal subjects but not in patients with cirrhosis of the liver. Gut. 1983;24:148–53.
58. Tydén G, Samnegard H, Thulin L, Muhrbeck O, Efendié S. Circulatory effects of somatostatin in anesthetized man. Acta Chir Scand. 1979;145:443–6.
59. Cerini R, Lee SS, Hadengue A, Koshy A, Girod C, Lebrec D. Circulatory effects of somatostatin analogue in two conscious rat models of portal hypertension. Gastroenterology. 1988;94:703–8.
60. Kravetz D, Bosch J, Arderiu MT, Pizcueta MP, Casamitjana R, Rivera F, Rodés J. Effects of somatostatin on splanchnic hemodynamics and plasma glucagon in portal hypertensive rats. Am J Physiol. 1988;254:G322–8.
61. Lebrec D, Blei AT. Vasopressin analogs and portal hypertension. London: John Libbey Eurotext; 1987.
62. Groszmann RJ, Kravetz D, Bosch J, Glickman M, Bruix J, Bredfeldt J, Conn HO, Rodes J, Storer EH. Nitroglycerin improves the hemodynamic response to vasopressin in portal hypertension. Hepatology. 1982;2:757–62.
63. Valla D, Girod C, Lee SS, Braillon A, Lebrec D. Lack of vasopressin action on splanchnic hemodynamics during bleeding: a study in conscious, portal hypertensive rats. Hepatology. 1988;8:10–15.
64. Moreau R, Lebrec D. Nitrovasodilators and portal hypertension. J Hepatol. 1990;10:263–7.
65. Vinel JP, Monnin JL, Combis JM, Calès P, Desmorat H, Pascal JP. Hemodynamic evaluation of molsidomine: a vasodilator with antianginal properties in patients with alcoholic cirrhosis. Hepatology. 1990;11:239–42.
66. Yand MCM, Pang PKT, Lays CS, Wu SL, Jan KM, Tsai YT, Kuo JS. Effect of parathyroid hormone on portal pressure in portal hypertensive rats. Liver. 1990;10:11–16.
67. Grangé JD, Jaillon P, Noblinski B, Faucherre V, Ballet F, Vasmant D, Poupon R. La pentoxifylline: un traitement potentiel des cirrhoses avec hypertension portale? (abstract) Gastroenterol Clin Biol. 1987;11:161A.
68. Dagenais M, Pomier-Layrargues G, Rocheleau B, Giroux L, Huet PM. Systemic and splanchnic haemodynamic effects of pentifylline in rats with portal hypertension. Clin Sci. 1992;83:41–5.
69. Atkinson M. The effect of diuretic on portal venous pressure. Lancet. 1959;2:819–23.
70. Cereda JM, Roulot D, Braillon A, Moreau R, Koshy A, Lebrec D. Reduction of portal pressure by acute administration of furosemide in patients with alcoholic cirrhosis. J Hepatol. 1989;9:246–51.
71. Klein CP. Spironolacton in der Behandlung der portalen Hypertonie bei Leberzirrhose. Dtsch Med Wochenschr. 1985;110:1774–6.
72. Weisberg H, Rosenthal WS, Jerzy Glass GB. The effect of diuretic therapy on portal pressure in cirrhotic patients with and without ascites. Am J Dig Dis. 1965;10:293–9.
73. Sekiyama T, Gaudin C, Roulot D, Lebrec D, Braquet P, Braillon A. Evidence for platelet-activating factor as a mediator for hyperdynamic circulation in conscious cirrhotic rats. In: Braquet P, editor. Ginkgolides – chemistry, biology, pharmacology and clinical

perspectives. Barcelona, Spain: Prous Science Publishers; 1989;2:313–19.
74. Sogni P, Moreau R, Ohsuga M, Cailmail S, Oberti F, Hadengue A, Pussard E, Lebrec D. Evidence of a normal nitric oxide-mediated vasodilator tone in conscious rats with cirrhosis. Hepatology. 1992;16:980–3.
75. Vallance P, Moncada S. Hyperdynamic circulation in cirrhosis: a role for nitric oxide? Lancet. 1991;237:776–8.
76. Moreau R, Komeichi H, Cailmail S, Lebrec D. Blockade of ATP-sensitive K^+ channels by glibenclamide reduces portal pressure and hyperkinetic circulation in portal hypertensive rats. Hemodynamic responses to glibenclamide in portal hypertension. J Hepatol. 1992;16:215–8.
77. Bernuau J, Rueff B. Treatment of acute variceal bleeding. Clin Gastroenterol. 1985;14:185–207.
78. Gimson AES, Westaby D, Hegarty J, Watson A, Williams R. A randomized trial of vasopressin and vasopressin plus nitroglycerin in the control of acute variceal hemorrhage. Hepatology. 1986;6:410–13.
79. Lee FY, Tsai YT, Lai KH, Lay CS, Chang TT, Malik U, Lin Cy, Lee SD. A randomized controlled study of triglycyl-vasopressin and vasopressin plus nitroglycerin in the control of acute esophageal variceal hemorrhage. Chin J Gastroenterol. 1988;5:131–8.
80. Burroughs AK, McCormick PA, Hughes M, Sprengers D, D'Heygere F, McIntyre N. Randomized, double-blind placebo-controlled trial of variceal bleeding. Emergency control and prevention of early variceal rebleeding. Gastroenterology. 1990;99:1388–95.
81. Valenzuuela JE, Schubert T, Fogel MR, Strong RM, Levine J, Mills PR, Fabry TL, Taylor LW, Conn HO, Posillico JT, and a Multicenter Study Group. A multicenter randomized, double-blind trial of somatostatin in the management of acute hemorrhage from esophageal varices. Hepatology. 1989;10:958–61.
82. Andréani T, Poupon RE, Balkau BJ, Trinchet JC, Grangé JD, Peigney N, Beaugrand M, Poupon R. Preventive therapy of first gastrointestinal bleeding in patients with cirrhosis: results of a controlled trial comparing propranolol, endoscopic sclerotherapy and placebo. Hepatology. 1990;12:1413–19.
83. Colman J, Jones P, Finch C, Dudley F. Propranolol in the prevention of variceal hemorrhage in alcoholic cirrhotic patients (abstract). Hepatology. 1990;12:851.
84. Conn HO, Grace ND, Bosch J, Groszmann RJ, Rodès J, Wright SC, Matloff DS, Garcia-Tsao G, Fisher RL, Navasa M, Drewniak SJ, Atterbury CE, Bordas JM, Lerner E, Bramante C, and Members of the Boston–New Haven–Barcelona Portal Hypertension Study Group. Propranolol in the prevention of the first hemorrhage from esophagogastric varices: a multicenter, randomized clinical trial. Hepatology. 1991;13:902–12.
85. Idéo G, Bellati G, Fesce E, Grimoldi D. Nadolol can prevent the first gastrointestinal bleeding in cirrhotics: a prospective randomized study. Hepatology. 1988;8:6–9.
86. Lebrec D, Poynard T, Capron JP, Hillon P, Geoffroy P, Roulot D, Chaput JC, Rueff B, Benhamou JP. Nadolol for prophylaxis of gastrointestinal bleeding in patients with cirrhosis. A randomized trial. J Hepatol. 1988;7:118–25.
87. Pascal JP, Calès P, and a Multicenter Study Group. Propranolol in the prevention of first upper gastrointestinal and esophageal varices. N Engl J Med. 1987;317:856–61.
88. The Prova Study Group. Prophylaxis of first hemorrhage from esophageal varices by sclerotherapy, propranolol or both in cirrhotic patients: a randomized multicenter trial. Hepatology. 1991;14:1016–24.
89. Strauss E, de Sa MFG, Albano A, Lacet CMC, Leite MO, Maffei RA. A randomized controlled trial for the prevention of the first upper gastrointestinal bleeding due to portal hypertension in cirrhosis sclerotherapy or propranolol versus control groups (abstract). Hepatology. 1988;8:1395.
90. The Italian Multicenter Project for Propranolol in Prevention of Bleeding. Propranolol prevents first gastrointestinal bleeding in non-ascitic cirrhotic patients. Final report of a multicenter randomized trial. J Hepatol. 1989;9:75–83.
91. Hayes PC, Crichton S, Sherpherd AN, Bouchier IAD. Propranolol in chronic liver disease: a controlled trial of its effect and safety over twelve months. Q J Med. 1987;65:823–34.
92. Hayes PC, Davis IM, Lewis JA, Bouchier IA. Meta-analysis of value of propranolol in prevention of variceal haemorrhage. Lancet. 1990;336:153–6.
93. Poynard T, Calès P, Pasta L, Idéo G, Pascal JP, Pagliaro L, Lebrec D. Beta-adrenergic-antagonist drugs in the prevention of gastrointestinal bleeding in patients with

cirrhosis and esophageal varices. An analysis of data and prognostic factors in 589 patients from four randomized clinical trials. N Engl J Med. 1991;324:1532–8.

94. Pagliaro L, D'Amico G, Sörensen TIA, Lebrec D, Burroughs AK, Morabito A, Tiné F, Politi F, Traina M. Prevention of first bleeding in cirrhosis. A meta-analysis of randomized trials of nonsurgical treatment. Ann Intern Med. 1992;77:59–70.
95. Angelico M, Carli L, Piat C, Gentile S, Di Maurizio P, Moscatelli B, Rinaldi V, Bologna E, Capocaccia L. Long-term evaluation of isosorbide-5-mononitrate vs propranolol in the prevention of bleeding in cirrhosis. (abstract). Gastroenterology. 1991;100:A25.
96. Cerbelaud P, Lavignolle A, Perrin D, Jutel P, Beaujard E, Colomb P, Le Bodic L. Propranolol et prévention des récidives de rupture de varice oesophagienne du cirrhotique. (Abstract). Gastroenterol Clin Biol. 1986;10:18A.
97. Colombo M, De Franchis R, Tommasini M, Sangiovanni A, Dioguardi N. β-blockade prevents recurrent gastrointestinal bleeding in well-compensated patients with alcoholic cirrhosis: a multicenter randomized controlled trial. Hepatology. 1989;9:433–8.
98. Garden OJ, Mills PE, Birnie GG, Murray GD, Carter DC. Propranolol in the prevention of recurrent variceal hemorrhage in cirrhotic patients. A controlled trial. Gastroenterology. 1989;98:185–90.
99. Gatta A, Merkel C, Sacerdoti D, Bolognesi M, Caregaro L, Zuin R, Angeli P, Ruol A. Nadolol for prevention of variceal rebleeding in cirrhosis: a controlled clinical trial. Digestion. 1987;37:22–8.
100. Kiire CF. Controlled trial of propranolol to prevent recurrent variceal bleeding in patients with non-cirrhotic portal fibrosis. Br Med J. 1989;298:1363–5.
101. Lebrec D, Poynard T, Bernuau J, Bercoff E, Nouel O, Capron JP, Poupon R, Bouvry M, Rueff B, Benhamou JP. A randomized controlled study of propranolol for prevention of recurrent gastrointestinal bleeding in patients with cirrhosis: a final report. Hepatology. 1984;4:355–8.
102. Queuniet AM, Czemichow P, Lerebours E, Ducrotte P, Tranvouez IL, Colin R. Etude contrôle du propranolol dans la prévention des récidives hémorragiques chez les patients cirrhotiques. Gastroenterol Clin Biol. 1987;11:41–7.
103. Qureshi H, Zuben SJ, Alam E. Efficacy of oral propranolol and injection sclerotherapy in the long-term management of variceal bleeding. Digestion. 1990;46:193–8.
104. Rossi V, Calès P, Burtin P, Charneau J, Person B, Pulol P, Valentin S, D'Aubigny N, Joubaud F, Boyer J. Prevention of recurrent variceal bleeding in alcoholic cirrhotic patients: prospective controlled trial of propranolol and sclerotherapy. J Hepatol. 1991;12:283–9.
105. Sheen IS, Chen TY, Liaw YF. Randomized controlled study of propranolol for prevention of recurrent esophageal varices bleeding in patients with cirrhosis. Liver. 1989;9:1–5.
106. Villeneuve JP, Pomier-Layrargues G, Infante-Rivard C, Willems B, Huet PM, Marleau D, Viallet A. Propranolol for the prevention of recurrent variceal hemorrhage: a controlled trial. Hepatology. 1986;6:1239–43.
107. Marbet UA, Strauman A, Gyr KE, Beglinger C, Schaub N, Vögtlin J, Loosli J, Kiowski W, Ritz R, Stalder GA. Reduction of early recurrence of variceal bleeding by propranolol. Scand J Gastroenterol. 1988;23:369–74.
108. Pérez-Ayuso RM, Piqué JM, Bosch J, Panés J, Gonzales A, Pérez R, Rigau J, Quintero E, Valderrama R, Viver J, Esteban R, Rodrigo L, Bordas JM, Rodés, J. Propranolol in prevention of recurrent bleeding from severe portal hypertensive gastropathy in cirrhosis. Lancet. 1991;337:1431–4.
109. Pagliaro L, Burroughs AK, Sorensen TIA, Lebrec D, Morabito A, D'Amico G, Tinè F. Therapeutic controversies and randomised controlled trials (RCTs): prevention of bleeding and rebleeding in cirrhosis. Gastroenterol Int. 1989;2:71–84.
110. Poynard T, Lebrec D, Hillon P, Sayegh R, Bernuau J, Naveau S, Chaput JC, Klepping C, Rueff B, Benhamou JP. Propranolol for prevention of recurrent gastrointestinal bleeding in patients with cirrhosis: a prospective study of factors associated with rebleeding. Hepatology. 1987;7:447–51.
111. Alexandrino PT, Alves MM, Correia JP. Propranolol or endoscopic sclerotherapy in the prevention of recurrence of variceal bleeding. A prospective, randomized controlled trial. J Hepatol. 1988;7:175–85.
112. Andréani T, Poupon RE, Balkau B, Capron D, Desaint B, Barbare JC, Lagneau M, Grangé JD, Opolon P, Lévy VG, Poupon R. Efficacité comparée du propranolol et des

scléroses endoscopiques de varices oesophagiennes dans la prévention des récidives d'hémorragies digestives au cours des cirrhoses. Etude contrôlée. Gastroenterol Clin Biol. 1991;15(Suppl. 2):A215.

113. Desarathy S, Dwivedi M, Bhargava DK, Sundaram KR, Ramachandran K. A prospective randomized trial comparing repeated endoscopic sclerotherapy and propranolol in decompensated (Child class B and C) cirrhotic patients. Hepatology. 1992;16:89–94.
114. Dollet JM, Chamigneulle B, Patris A, Bigard MA, Gaucher P. Sclérothérapie endoscopique contre propranolol après hémorragie par rupture de varices oesophagiennes chez le cirrhotique. Résultats à 4 ans d'une étude randomisée. Gastroenterol Clin Biol. 1988;12:234–9.
115. Fleig WE, Stange EF, Hunecke R, Schönborn W, Huzler U, Rainer K, Gaus W, Ditschuneit H. Prevention of recurrent bleeding in cirrhotics with recent variceal hemorrhage prospective, randomized comparison of propranolol and sclerotherapy. Hepatology. 1987;7:355–61.
116. Martin T, Taupignon A, Lavignolle A, Perrin D, Le Bodic L. Prévention des récidives hémorragiques chez des malades atteints de cirrhose. Résultats d'une étude contrôlée comparant propranolol et sclérose endoscopique. Gastroenterol Clin Biol. 1991;15:833–7.
117. Rossi V, Calès P, Burtin P, Charneau J, Person B, Pujol P, Valentin S, D'Aubigny N, Joubaud F, Boyer J. Prevention of recurrent variceal bleeding in alcoholic cirrhotic patients: prospective controlled trial of propanolol and sclerotherapy. J Hepatol. 1991;12:283–9.
118. Terès J, Bosch J, Bordas JM, Garcia-Pagan JC, Feu F, Cirera I, Rodès J. Endoscopic sclerotherapy (ES) vs propranolol (PR) in the elective treatment of variceal bleeding. Preliminary results of a randomized controlled clinical trial (abstract). J Hepatol. 1987;5(suppl. 1):S210.
119. Westaby D, Polson RJ, Gimson AES, Hayes PC, Hayllar K, Williams R. A controlled trial of oral propranolol compared with injection sclerotherapy for the long-term management of variceal bleeding. Hepatology. 1990;11:353–9.
120. Ink O, Martin T, Poynard T, Réville M, Anciaux ML, Lenoir C, Marill JL, Labadie H, Masliah C, Perrin D, Chaput JC, Doffoel L, Eugène C, Le Bodic L, Licht H, Etienne JP. Does chronic sclerotherapy improve the efficacy of longterm propranolol for prevention of recurrent bleeding in patients with severe cirrhosis? A prospective, multicenter, randomized trial. J Hepatol. 1991;12(Suppl. 2):S37.
121. Jensen LS, Krarup N. Propranolol may prevent recurrence of oesophageal varices after obliteration by endoscopy sclerotherapy. Scand J Gastroenterol. 1990;25:352–6.
122. O'Connor KW, Lehman G, Yune H, Brunelle R, Christiansen P, Hast J, Compton M, McHenry R, Klatte E, Cockerill E, Holden R, Becker G, Kopecky K, Hawes R, Pound D, Rex D, Lui A, Snodgrass P, Weddle R, Crabb D, Lumeng L. Comparison of three nonsurgical treatments for bleeding esophageal varices. Gastroenterology. 1989;96:899–906.
123. Vinel JP, Lamouliatte H, Calès P, Combis JM, Desmorat H, Roux D, Quinton A, Pascal JP. Comparaison de la sclérose endoscopique (SE) et de l'association sclérose propranolol dans la prévention des récidives hémorragiques (RH) par rupture de varices oesophagiennes (VO) (abstract). Gastroenterol Clin Biol. 1990;14(suppl. 2):195.
124. Westaby D, Melia W, Hegarty J, Gimson AES, Stellon AJ, Williams R. Use of propranolol to reduce the rebleeding rate during injection sclerotherapy prior to variceal obliteration. Hepatology. 1986;6:673–5.

4

Prophylactic and therapeutic surgical intervention in portal hypertension (stents, shunts)

B. LAUNOIS, F. SIRISER and B. MEUNIER

Prophylactic and therapeutic surgical interventions in portal hypertension are end-to-side portacaval shunts, side-to-side portacaval shunts and the more recently described H graft variants, mesocaval shunts and distal and proximal splenorenal shunts. The results of non-surgical portacaval shunts, the percutaneous transjugular intrahepatic portal systemic stent shunt (TIPSS), have recently been described and published.

Surgical treatment should be considered in three circumstances[1]:

1. primary prophylaxis to prevent bleeding from varices which have not bled
2. emergency treatment to stem haemorrhage
3. secondary prophylaxis to prevent later rebleeding.

The aim of surgery is to bring portal pressure back within the normal range, and this depends on the location of obstruction: to the portal vein (extrahepatic obstruction), within the liver (intrahepatic obstruction) and to the hepatic veins (suprahepatic obstruction).

SUPRAHEPATIC OBSTRUCTION: BUDD–CHIARI SYNDROME

Portal hypertension by suprahepatic obstruction is usually due to extensive thrombosis of the hepatic veins. The outcome depends on the underlying cause of the hepatic vein block as well as the acuteness of presentation[2]. Any cause such as a myeloproliferative disorder[3] should be treated.

The surgical possibilities are: side-to-side portacaval shunt, mesoatrial shunt and liver transplantation. The ideal treatment is portacaval shunt in primary or secondary prophylaxis and emergency. Side-to-side portacaval shunt[4–6] or prosthetic[7,8] or venous[9] H graft or mesocaval C graft[10] is indicated in cases of early diagnosis, good liver function tests[11] and the absence of complete or partial obstruction of the vena cava. Ascites always clears when the shunt is functioning. It significantly improves liver blood outflow, as demonstrated by the return to normal values of transaminases and the disappearance of necrosis and sinusoidal dilation on liver biopsies. It dramatically reverses the acute downhill course of the patient with rapidly progressing liver failure[9]. Thrombosis of the shunt has occurred in two circumstances: preoperative thrombosis of the mesenteric or portal vein or vena cava and the use of small-calibre prosthetic material. Therefore an autologous vein should be used whenever possible[9].

Mesoatrial shunt[12–14] can be proposed for patients with complete obstruction of the vena cava, no pressure gradient between the mesenteric vein and the vena cava or an inaccessible vena cava[9].

Liver transplantation[11,15,16] is indicated after acute or progressive shunt failure or the presence of encephalopathy, hypoalbuminaemia $<3\,mg\%$, hyperbilirubinaemia $>3\,mg\%$ or both, and severe fibrosis or cirrhosis at liver biopsy[11].

EXTRAHEPATIC PORTAL VEIN OBSTRUCTION

Portal hypertension by extrahepatic obstruction is due mainly to a thrombosis in the portal system, whatever the cause. The liver is normal. Any underlying cause must be identified and treated. The ideal treatment is sclerotherapy in secondary prophylaxis or emergency.

Indications should be based on three facts:

1. the prognosis for patients with primary extrahepatic obstruction is usually excellent with long-term survival regardless of the form of therapy used[2];
2. definitive surgery for reduction of portal pressure is often difficult;
3. repeated sclerotherapy is very successful in adults[17] and children[18,19].

There is almost no place for surgery. In cases of failure the type of portal shunt depends on the location of the obstruction.

In cases of mesenteric and portal obstruction a splenorenal shunt is indicated, and with splenic and portal obstruction a mesocaval shunt is an ideal procedure.

If the obstruction is diffuse, a makeshift shunt can be performed on epiploic or pancreatic vein if the vein has a diameter greater than 7 mm and if it is not dissected. Use of the autologous jugular vein diminishes the risk of thrombosis. Mortality is nil and the success rate 60%. However, the indication should not be questioned and should be discussed after angiography[20].

INTRAHEPATIC OBSTRUCTION

In intrahepatic obstruction the primary event is obstruction to portal blood flow, due to liver disease, especially cirrhosis. The ideal procedure is liver transplantation.

Primary prophylaxis in surgical treatment of portal hypertension

Four controlled studies[21–24] show the following facts:

1. the risk of rupture of oesophageal varices is significantly less (0–2.7%) than in the control group (19–26%);
2. hepatic encephalopathy is more frequent after portacaval shunt (38–52%) than after medical treatment;
3. long-term survival rates are worst in the shunted group.

Prophylactic shunts (or any other form of major surgery for prophylaxis) are unjustified on current evidence because the first variceal bleed can be successfully treated in most patients when it occurs. In addition, the low incidence of variceal bleeding in the control patients in the prophylactic trials, as well as the impossibility of identifying patients who are vulnerable to a first bleed, make prophylactic shunts unacceptable[2].

Emergency treatment

In three controlled studies[25–27] sclerotherapy stemmed acute variceal bleeding in 90–95% of patients. Portacaval shunts were more effective than injection therapy in preventing early recurrence of bleeding[28]. Six patients out of 32 bled again after shunt, compared to 16 out of 32 in the sclerotherapy group. In that group 12 patients were readmitted for bleeding compared with none in the shunt group (Table 1).

However, portacaval shunt is discouraging for liver transplantation. It is associated with the development of a phlebosclerotic portal vein which becomes difficult to use for subsequent anastomoses. It has been implicated in the development of portal vein thrombosis, or at least of insufficient portal

Table 1 Endoscopic sclerotherapy versus portacaval shunts in acute variceal haemorrhage

	Sclerotherapy ($n = 32$)	*Shunt* ($n = 32$)	p
Duration of procedure	1.0 ± 0.04	4.4 ± 0.30	0.0001
Units transfused	0.3 ± 0.1	7.2 ± 1.1	0.0001
Gastrointestinal haemorrhage after procedure	16	6	0.009
Death ≤ 30 days	17	18	NS
Rehospitalization for haemorrhage	12	0	0.0001
Hospitalized days for encephalopathy	1.6 ± 1.0	1.4 ± 1.08	NS

From ref. 28

flow after mesocaval or splenorenal shunt. Portacaval shunt must be avoided if the patient is a potential candidate for liver transplantation (Table 2).

In emergency, the only indications are: (a) immediate failure of sclerotherapy, (b) recurrent bleeding, (c) gastric varices. However, the choice of portacaval shunt is difficult. Mesocaval shunt is the best alternative, followed by distal splenorenal shunt and proximal splenorenal shunt. The use of a venous jump graft in liver transplantation may make portacaval shunts possible again.

This problem may be solved by a new technique: the percutaneous transjugular intrahepatic portal systemic stent shunt (TIPSS)[29–31].

Routine simultaneous superior mesenteric arterial portography and hepatic venography, with measurement of free and wedged hepatic pressures, is performed pre-TIPSS. A catheter is passed into the hepatic vein via the jugular vein and a tract is opened into a major portal branch with a rigid needle followed by a guide-wire. The tract is dilated with a 8 mm or 10 mm angioplasty balloon catheter and patency is maintained by an expandable metal stent.

Freedman *et al.*[32] at the latest Congress on Transplantation in Paris gave the results for this technique. The mean portal pressure decreased from 33 mmHg to 22 mmHg. Initial technical success was 92% with demonstration angiographically of the newly estblished conduit post-TIPSS in all patients. Patients were followed from 3 to 6 months clinically, biochemically and by doppler examinations. Endoscopy performed 1 month post-TIPSS has shown a dramatic shrinkage, or even the disappearance, of oesophageal varices. One patient died from the procedure (3.8%); six patients out of 22 developed encephalopathy. Four stents thrombosed and hyperbilirubinaemia developed in two patients. There were no significant bleeding complications, whether intrahepatic or intraperitoneal, despite the presence of coagulopathy and thrombocytopenia.

These preliminary results suggest that TIPSS is safe and effective in controlling variceal haemorrhage and in reducing portal venous pressure in patients with end-stage liver disease without altering the extravascular anatomy, thus allowing more 'elective' and technically less arduous, subsequent liver transplantation to be performed.

Therefore the recent advent of percutaneous TIPSS accomplishes the same result in terms of control of variceal haemorrhage in patients who would otherwise require emergency surgery.

Table 2 The best procedure of portacaval shunting before liver transplantation

	PCS ES	*PCS SS*	*PSR*	*DSR*	*MC H*
Dissection of the hepatic pedicle	+	+			
Supramesocolic adhesions	+	+	+		
Risk of portal thrombosis				+	+
Decreased portal flow			+	+	+

PCS: portacaval shunt; ES: end to side; SS: side to side; PSR: proximal splenorenal; DSR: distal splenorenal; MC: mesocaval; H :H-graft

Secondary prophylaxis

The aim of secondary prophylaxis is to prevent recurrent bleeding.

Medical treatment vs portacaval shunts

Four completed controlled studies[33–36] comparing therapeutic portacaval shunts with conventional medical management failed to provide a clear-cut survival advantage.

Sclerotherapy vs medical treatment

In only one[37] out of five controlled clinical trials[37–41] sclerotherapy demonstrated a clear-cut improvement in survival compared to conservative medical treatment. However, in sclerotherapy for long-term management there is increasing evidence to suggest that those patients in whom varices are difficult to eradicate, or those patients who have repeated bleeds during the course of eradication, should be seriously considered for one of the alternative major forms of surgery at an early stage.

Sclerotherapy versus portal systemic shunt

Four controlled studies[42–45] comparing sclerotherapy versus surgery (Warren procedure) showed the following results:

1. surgery prevents bleeding more efficiently than sclerotherapy;
2. long-term survival is similar in the sclerotherapy group and the shunt group;
3. severe recurrent bleeding happened in 20–31% after sclerotherapy, even if the oesophageal varices were totally eradicated;
4. in one study[43] the risk of encephalopathy is identical in both groups and the cost similar.

Surgery and endoscopic treatment should not be regarded as competing approaches; indeed their roles may be complementary. Shunt operations should be considered earlier rather than later in the treatment protocol, in those patients in whom endoscopic sclerotherapy has failed[1]. Warren *et al.*[45] and Paquet *et al.*[46] have claimed better results with such a strategy compared to sclerotherapy alone.

Selective shunts vs non-selective shunts

Total shunts (e.g. end-to-side portacaval, mesocaval) can prevent haemorrhage but, presumably because they reduce liver blood flow, they are followed by portal systemic encephalopathy in about 20% of patients. Of the selective shunts the best-known is the distal splenorenal shunt (Warren), which selectively decompresses the oesophagogastric varices through the splenic renal vein anastomosis but maintains liver perfusion in the hope that hepatoportal encephalopathy can be avoided. The results are mixed[47–52] (Table 3).

Table 3 Randomized and controlled trials of total shunts (TS) versus distal splenorenal shunt (DSR)

First author/ ref.	Control group shunt	*No of patients*		*Mortality 30 days*		*Encephalo-pathy*			*Late mortality*	
		TS	*DSR*	*TS*	*DSR*	*TS*	*DSR*	*Follow-up*	*TS*	*DSR*
Fischer 1981[48]	PSR	19	23	0	4	1	5	2	0	17
Reichle 1979[47]	MC	14	13	7	8			<3	29	33
Millikan 1985[50]	MC(H)	29	26	10	12	76	27	11	72	58
Langer 1985[49]	PCS	40	38	0	13	48	36	5.5	48	58
Harley 1986[52]	PCS	27	26	7	12	32	39	2.5	63	50
Grace 1988[51]	PCS	38	43	13	9	45	51	3.5	68	47

PSR: proximal splenorenal shunt; MC: mesocaval; MC(H): H graft mesocaval; PCS: portacaval shunt

Although Warren's group reported low mortality (9%) and a low incidence of postoperative encephalopathy, larger randomized trials comparing total and selective shunts have shown rates of mortality and long-term encephalopathy which are remarkably similar[1]. Moreover total shunt is a relative contraindication to liver transplantation.

Sarfeh *et al.*[53] and Adam *et al.*[54] claimed the value of narrow-bore portacaval H-graft function, because the advantage of maintaining hepatoportal flow may be an improvement in long-term survival by prevention of impairing hepatocellular function as has previously been suggested in alcoholics after DSRS or small-diameter portacaval shunt. The incidence of post-shunt encephalopathy is smaller.

We need some good randomized controlled trials. In our experience there is a risk of thrombosis which can be prevented by anticoagulation therapy. It seems contraindicated in ascitis.

However, all these types of shunts can be replaced in the future by TIPSS which have the same diameter as a reduced H-graft portacaval shunt.

Portal systemic shunts vs transplantation (Tables 4 and 5)

Portacaval shunt does not reverse the underlying liver disease whose inexorable progress acounts for its failure to influence long-term survival[1]. Moreover the inescapable conclusion from all the work on this subject is that portal systemic diversion is so inherently harmful to the liver that it should be considered only for life-threatening disease conditions or complications[55]. After portacaval shunt the liver parenchyma can be complicated by a slow deterioration in liver functions and hepatocarcinoma.

However, there is no randomized study comparing portacaval shunt and liver transplantation. The 5-year survival after portacaval shunt is between 35% and 55%. In our own series 5-year survival is 45% and 10-year survival 18%. On the other hand, in our group after transplantation survival is 85% at 3 years. It is 100% in Child's class A and B and 67.5% in Child's class C.

Table 4 Survival for shunt versus transplantation

First author/ref.	Type of shunt	No. of patients	Survival rate (%) 1 year	3 years	5 years
Jackson 1971[33]	Non-selective	67	80	62	55
Resnick 1974[34]	Non-selective	54	70	50	48
Reynolds 1981[36]	Non-selective	41	64	44	
Conn 1981[56]	Non-selective	24	76		
	Selective	29	70		
Langer 1985[49]	Selective	38	80	63	51
	Non-selective	40	90	70	56
Millikan 1985[50]	Selective	26	85	65	55
	Non-selective	29	80	70	60
Rikkers 1987[43]	Selective	27	75	60	45
Launois 1992[57]	Non-selective	172	87	65	45
Iwatsuki 1988[58]	Transplantation	302	79	71	71
Launois 1992[59]	Transplantation	20	85	85	

Table 5 Survival for shunt versus transplantation in Child's class C patients

First author/ref.	Type of shunt	No. of patients	Survival rate (%) 1 year	3 years	5 years
Turcotte 1973[60]	Non-selective	50	36	22	17
Warren 1986[45]	Selective	49	60	45	35
	Non-selective	92	50	37	15
Chandler 1985[61]	Both	30	36	30	13
Bismuth 1990[62]	Both	135	88	46	31
Iwatsuki 1988[58]	Transplantation	302	79	71	71

Should all patients have transplants?

The ideal treatment is liver transplantation. PSS (or TIPSS) is indicated: (a) in cases of general contraindications (e.g. age), or (b) in patients who do not opt for transplantation, (c) in patients with alcoholic cirrhosis who cannot cope with the physical and psychological constraints of transplantation. It can be discussed in Child's class A patients.

CONCLUSION

The surgical management of portal hypertension depends on the location of the obstruction:

1. in Budd–Chiari the ideal treatment is surgical portacaval (or mesocaval) shunt;
2. in extrahepatic obstruction the ideal treatment is sclerotherapy;
3. in intrahepatic obstruction the ideal treatment is liver transplantation; but:

(a) primary prophylaxis should never be surgical;
(b) in emergency, sclerotherapy is the first choice, PSS (or TIPSS) the second choice;
(c) elsewhere, liver transplantation should if possible be preferred to portal diversion.

References

1. Shields R. Bleeding oesophageal varices and the surgeon. Br J Surg. 1991;78:513–15.
2. Terblanche J. The surgeon''s role in the management of portal hypertension. Ann Surg. 1989;209:381–95.
3. Valla D, Casadevall N, Lacombe L *et al.* Primary myeloproliferative disorder and hepatic vein thrombosis: a prospective study of erythroid colony formation *in vitro* in 20 patients with Budd–Chiari syndrome. Ann Intern Med. 1985;103:329–34.
4. Prandi D, Rueff B, Benhamou JP. Side to side portacaval shunt in the treatment of Budd–Chiari syndrome. Gastroenterology. 1975;68:137–41.
5. Malt RA, Dalton JC, Johnson RE, Gurewich V. Side to side portacaval shunt versus non-surgical treatment of Budd–Chiari syndrome. Am J Surg. 1978;136:387–9.
6. Orloff MJ, Girard B. Long term results of treatment of Budd–Chiari syndrome by side to side portacaval shunt. Surg Gynecol Obstet. 1989;168:33–41.
7. Huguet C, Liegeois A, Levy VG, Caroli J. Interposition mesocaval shunt for chronic primary occlusion of the hepatic veins. Surg Gynecol Obstet. 1979;148:691–8.
8. Cameron JL, Herlong HF, Sanfey H *et al.* The Budd–Chiari syndrome: treatment by mesenteric systemic venous shunts. Ann Surg. 1983;198:335–44.
9. Vons C, Smadja C, Bourstyn E *et al.* Results of portal systemic shunts in Budd–Chiari syndrome. Ann Chir. 1986;203:366–70.
10. Cameron JL, Harrington DP, Maddrey WL. The mesocaval C shunt. Surg Gynecol Obstet. 1980;150:401–3.
11. Shaked A, Goldstein RM, Klintmalm GB *et al.* Portosystemic shunt versus orthotopic liver transplantation for the Budd–Chiari syndrome. Surg Gynecol Obstet. 1992;174:453–9.
12. Cameron JL, Maddrey WL. Mesoatrial shunts: a new treatment for the Budd–Chiari syndrome. Ann Surg. 1978;187:402–6.
13. Beattie C, Sitzmann JV, Cameron JL. Mesoatrial shunt hemodynamics. Surgery. 1988;104:1–9.
14. Stringer MD, Howard ER, Green DW *et al.* Mesoatrial shunt: a surgical option in the management of the Budd–Chiari syndrome. Br J Surg. 1989;76:474–8.
15. Campbell DA, Rolles K, Jamieson N *et al.* Hepatic transplantation with perioperative and long term anticoagulant as treatment for Budd–Chiari syndrome. Surg Obstet Gynecol. 1988;166:511–18.
16. Halff G, Satoru T, Tzakis AG *et al.* Liver transplantation for Budd–Chiari syndrome. Am J Surg. 1989;211:43–9.
17. Kahn D, Terblanche J, Kitanos S, Bornmann PC. Injection sclerotherapy in adult patients with extrahepatic portal venous shunts. Br J Surg. 1987;74:600–2.
18. Howard ER, Stringer MD, Mowat AP. Assessment of injection sclerotherapy in the management of 152 children with esophageal varices. Br J Surg. 1988;75:404–8.
19. Lilly JR. Endoscopic sclerosis of esophageal varices in children. Surg Gynecol Obstet. 1981;152:513–4.
20. Flamant Y, Branche D, Maillard JM. Les thromboses spléno-portales. In: Mouiel, editor. Actualités Médico-Chirurgicales. Paris: Masson; 1985:170–9.
21. Conn HO, Lindenmuth WW. Prophylactic portacaval anastomosis in cirrhotic patients with esophageal varices. Interim results with suggestions for subsequent investigations. N Engl J Med. 1968;279:725–32.
22. Jackson FC, Perrin EB, Smith AG *et al.* A clinical investigation of the portacaval shunt. II. Survival analysis of the prophylactic operation. Am J Surg. 1968;115:22–41.
23. Resnick RH, Chalmers TC, Ishihara AM *et al.* A controlled study of the prophylactic portacaval shunt: a final report. Ann Intern Med. 1969;70:675–88.
24. Conn HO, Lindenmuth WW, May CJ, Ramsby GR. Prophylactic portacaval anastomosis:

a tale of two studies. Medicine. 1972;51:27–40.
25. Barsoum MS, Bolous FI, El Rooby AA *et al.* Tamponade and injection sclerotherapy in the management of bleeding esophageal varices. Br J Surg. 1982;69:76–8.
26. Paquet KJ, Feussner H. Endoscopic sclerosis and esophageal balloon tamponade in acute hemorrhage from esophagogastric varices: a prospective controlled randomized trial. Hepatology. 1985;5:580–3.
27. Larson AW, Cohen H, Zweinban B *et al.* Acute esophageal variceal sclerotherapy. Results of a prospective randomized controlled trial. J Am Med Assoc. 1986;255:497–500.
28. Cello JP, Grendell JH, Crass RA *et al.* Endoscopic sclerotherapy versus portacaval shunt in patients with severe cirrhosis and acute variceal hemorrhage. Long term follow-up. N Engl J Med. 1987;316:11–15.
29. Colapinto RF, Stronell RD, Gildiner M *et al.* Formation of intrahepatic portosystemic shunts using a balloon dilatation catheter: preliminary clinical experience. Am J Radiol. 1983;140:709–14.
30. Rosch J, Uchida BT, Putnam JS *et al.* Experimental intrahepatic portacaval anastomosis: use of expandable Gianturco stents. Radiology. 1987;162:482–5.
31. Rossle M, Richter GM, Noeldge *et al.* Der intrahepatische porto systemische shunt: Erste klinische erfahrungen bei patienten mit leberzirrhose. Dtsch Med Wochenschr. 1989;114:1511–16.
32. Freedman AM, Sanyal AJ, Tisnado J *et al.* Results with percutaneous transjugular intra-hepatic portal systemic stent shunts (TIPSS) for control of variceal hemorrhage in patients awaiting liver transplantation (OLT). Transplant Proc. 1993 (to be published).
33. Jackson EC, Perrin EB, Felix WR *et al.* A clinical investigation of the portacaval shunt. V. Survival analysis of the therapeutic operation. Ann Surg. 1971;174:672–701.
34. Resnick RN, Iber FL, Ishihara AM *et al.* A controlled study of the therapeutic portacaval shunt. Gastroenterology. 1974;67:843–57.
35. Rueff B, Prandi D, Degos F *et al.* A controlled study of therapeutic portacaval shunt in alcoholic cirrhosis. Lancet. 1976;1:655–9.
36. Reynolds TB, Donovan AJ, Mikkelsen WP *et al.* Results of a 12 year randomized trial of portacaval shunt in patients with alcoholic liver disease and bleeding varices. Gastroenterology. 1981;80:1005–11.
37. Westaby D, MacDougall BRD, Williams R. Improvcd survival following injection sclerotherapy for esophageal varices. Final analysis of a controlled trial. Hepatology. 1985;5:827–30.
38. Terblanche J, Bornman PC, Kahn D *et al.* Failure of repeated injection sclerotherapy to improve long term survival after esophageal variceal bleeding. A five year prospective controlled clinical trial. Hepatology. 1985;5:827–30.
39. Copenhagen Esophageal Varices and Sclerotherapy Project. Sclerotherapy after first variceal hemorrhage in cirrhosis. A randomized multicenter trial. N Engl J Med. 1984;311:1594–600.
40. Korula J, Balart LA, Radvan G *et al.* A prospective randomized controlled trial of chronic esophageal variceal sclerotherapy. Hepatology. 1985;5:584–9.
41. Soderlund C, Ihre C. Endoscopic sclerotherapy versus conservative management of bleeding esophageal varices. A 5 year prospective controlled trial of emergency and long term treatment. Acta Chir Scand. 1985;151:449–56.
42. Korula J, Yellin A, Yamada S *et al.* A prospective randomized controlled comparison of chronic endoscopic variceal sclerotherapy and portal systemic shunt for variceal hemorrhage in Child's class A cirrhotics: a preliminary report. Gastroenterology. 1987;92:1745.
43. Rikkers LF, Burnett DA, Volentine GD *et al.* Shunt surgery vs endoscopic sclerotherapy for long term treatment of variceal bleeding. Early results of a randomized trial. Ann Surg. 1987;206:261–71.
44. Teres J, Bordas JM, Bravo D *et al.* Sclerotherapy vs distal splenorenal shunt in the elective treatment of variceal hemorrhage: a randomized controlled trial. Hepatology. 1987;7:430–6.
45. Warren WD, Henderson JM, Millikan WJ *et al.* Distal splenorenal versus endoscopic sclerotherapy for long term management of variceal bleeding. Preliminary report of a prospective, randomized trial. Ann Surg. 1986;203:454–62.
46. Paquet KJ, Mercado MA, Gad HA. Surgical procedures for bleeding oesophageal varices when sclerotherapy fails: a prospective study. Am J Surg. 1990;160·:43–7.
47. Reichle FA, Fahmy WF, Golsorkhi M. Prospective comparative clinical trial with distal splenorenal and mesocaval shunts. Am J Surg. 1979;137:13–21.

48. Fischer JE, Bower RH, Atamian S, Welling R. Comparison of distal and proximal splenorenal shunts. A randomized prospective trial. Hepatology. 1981;1:151–60.
49. Langer B, Taylor BR, MacKensie DR *et al.* Further report of a prospective randomized trial comparing distal splenorenal shunt with end to side portacaval shunt. An analysis of encephalopathy, survival and quality of life. Gastroenterology. 1985;88:424–9.
50. Millikan W Jr, Warren WD, Henderson JM *et al.* The Emory prospective randomized trial. Selective versus nonselective shunt to control variceal bleeding. Ten year follow up. Ann Surg. 1985;201:712–22.
51. Grace ND, Conn HO, Resnick RH *et al.* Distal splenorenal vs portal-systemic shunts after hemorrhage from varices: a randomized controlled trial. Hepatology. 1988;8:1475–81.
52. Harley HAJ, Morgan T, Edeker AG *et al.* Results of a randomized trial of end to side portacaval shunt and distal splenorenal shunt in alcoholic liver disease and variceal bleeding. Gatroenterology. 1986;91:802–9.
53. Sarfeh IJ, Rypins EB, Fardi M *et al.* Clinical implications of portacaval hemodynamics after small diameter portacaval H graft. Surgery. 1984;96:223–9.
54. Adam R, Diamond T, Bismuth H. Partial portacaval shunt: renaissance of an old concept. Surgery 1992;11:610–16.
55. Starzl TE, Porter KA, Francavilla A. The Eck fistula in animals and humans. Current progress in surgery, 1983; vol. 20. Chicago: Year Book Medical Publishers.
56. Comm Ho, Resnick RH, Grace ND *et al.* Distal splenorenal shunt vs portal systemic shunt: current status of a controlled trial. Hepatology. 1981;1:151–60.
57. Launois B. Unpublished data.
58. Iwastsuki S, Stayl TE, Todd S *et al.* Liver transplantation in the treatment of bleeding esophageal varices. Surgery. 1988;104:697–705.
59. Launois B. Unpublished data.
60. Tunotte JG, Lambert ML. Variceal haemorrhage, hepatic cirrhosis and portacaval shunts. Surgery. 1973;73:810–7.
61. Chandler JG, Vanmeter CH, Kaiser DL, Mills SE. Factors affecting immediate and long-term survival after emergent and elective splanchnic–systemic shunts. Ann Surg. 1985;201:476–87.
62. Bismuth H, Adam R, Mathew S, Sherlock D. Options for elective treatment of portal hypertension in cirrhotic patients in the transplantation era. Am J Surg. 1990;160:105–110.

5

Hyperdynamic circulation in chronic liver disease: significance and pathogenesis

J. REICHEN

INTRODUCTION: FORWARD VERSUS BACKWARD FLOW THEORY

When one observes a cirrhotic liver macroscopically or microscopically, the most striking feature is the increased consistency and the increase in connective tissue. Therefore, it is not surprising that early investigators in the field of portal hypertension were most impressed with the increased resistance. In a seminal paper, Whipple laid the foundation for the 'backward flow theory'[1]: he noted the similarity between patients with portal vein thrombosis and with liver cirrhosis, namely the presence of splenomegaly, elevated portal pressure and oesophageal varices. He stated that obstruction leading to an increase in resistance was the main feature of portal hypertension and proposed correction by the circumvention of the obstruction, i.e. the construction of portosystemic shunts[1].

In the early 1950s it was recognized, however, that hyperdynamic circulation was not an infrequent occurrence in patients with portal hypertension[2,3]; to the best of our knowledge, Kowalski and Abelmann were the first to describe increased cardiac output and decreased peripheral resistance (Fig. 1). It is not universally present in all patients with liver cirrhosis. Thus, Kowalski and Abelmann[2] found it only in about 30% of their patients (Fig. 1); potential factors in this heterogeneity are discussed below. This observation, later confirmed in many studies in patients[3–7] and experimental animals[8,9], is the foundation for the 'forward flow theory' of portal hypertension[8]. This theory states that the increased splanchnic inflow into the portal vein is a main factor in the maintenance of portal hypertension. This theory is important

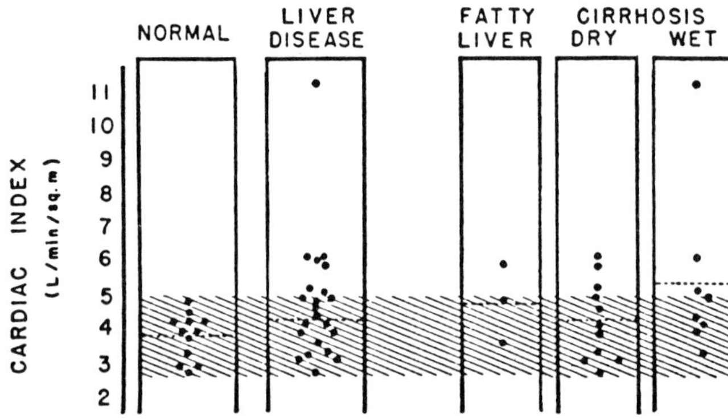

Fig. 1 Cardiac index in patients with different forms of chronic liver disease. An increased cardiac output is noted in 7/22 patients. From ref. 2 (by copyright permission of the American Society for Clinical Investigation)

in the design of novel pharmacological approaches to the treatment of portal hypertension[10].

The two models, backward and forward flow, are not mutually exclusive, both increased resistance and increased portal inflow contributing to the maintenance of portal hypertension. As a matter of fact both factors are needed for the development of splanchnic hyperaemia; this is reflected in the proposed term of 'active congestion'[11]. In the portal vein stenosis rat model, the forward and backward component have been estimated to account for 40% and 60% of the increase in portal pressure, respectively[12].

CLINICAL RELEVANCE

Clinically, the hyperkinetic circulation syndrome manifests itself[3] by evidence of increased peripheral flow (warm, flushed extremities; bounding pulses, capillary pulsations) and of increased cardiac output (tachycardia, active precordial impulse, frequent presence of systolic ejection murmurs). Although high cardiac output failure in patients with cirrhosis has been described[3], this is a rare occurrence[13]. Recently, Bernardi and colleagues have postulated that the hyperdynamic circulation syndrome represents a compensatory mechanism to maintain steady blood pressure levels since in preascitic patients it was observed only in the supine but not the prone position[14].

The hyperdynamic circulation is associated with abnormal oxygen consumption in spite of increased oxygen transport; this is related to the degree of liver failure[15]. Decreased oxygen consumption cannot be corrected by oxygen administration, implying impaired arterial baroreflex control[16]. Hyperdynamic circulation, together with altered oxygen utilization, could be involved in multiple organ failure in end-stage liver disease. These effects will be considered separately in this chapter; the reader is referred to a recent editorial on this topic[17].

In addition to the hyperdynamic circulation there is a major dysregulation of many cardiovascular responses to different stimuli[5]; in particular, reduced reflex tachycardia and muscle baroreflex responses to hypotension or tilting are markedly impaired in experimental animals[18] and patients[19]. These findings are of clinical importance since they could affect the defensive response to shock, and have to be taken into account when using drugs affecting the autonomous nervous system.

The hyperdynamic circulation is important for the pathophysiology of ascites formation; the initial vasodilation is at the heart of modern theories of ascites formation[20,21]; this aspect of the hyperdynamic circulation will not be considered any further here. Renal aspects of hyperdynamic circulation are reviewed in ref. 20.

The cardiac sequelae of portal hypertension have been reviewed in detail by Lee[13]. In spite of the hyperdynamic circulation, high-output cardiac failure is rare in cirrhotic patients[13]. Nevertheless, the heart participates prominently in some aspects of the hyperdynamic state. A limited cardiac preload reserve has been demonstrated in cirrhotic rats[22]; this could limit adaptation of cardiac performance in response to alterations in volume load. The heart also exhibits a decreased chronotropic response to norepinephrine which has been clearly associated with desensitization of myocardial β-receptors[23].

PATHOGENETIC FACTORS IN HYPERDYNAMIC CIRCULATION

A variety of factors have been implicated as being responsible for the hyperkinetic circulation in patients with chronic liver disease (Table 1).

Hepatocellular dysfunction

Increased cardiac output and peripheral evidence of hyperkinetic circulation was initially described in patients with parenchymatous liver disease[2,3,24]. The observation that the syndrome occurs also in patients[25,26] and animals[27,8] with intact liver function raises doubts as to whether hepatic dysfunction plays a major role in the development of the hyperkinetic circulation syndrome. On the other hand, liver dysfunction may contribute to its progression as evidenced by the progression of the hyperkinetic circulation with progression of cirrhosis[4,6,7] and the existence of the syndrome in fulminant hepatic failure[28]. The extent of hyperkinetic circulation has been found to be associated with the degree of dysfunction as measured by Child's classification[6] (see Fig. 2) or by indocyanine green elimination[7].

Table 1 Potential pathogenetic factors in the evolution and maintenance of hyperdynamic circulation in chronic liver disease

1. Hepatocellular dysfunction
2. Portal hypertension
3. Portosystemic shunting
4. Increased plasma volume
5. Increased release of vasodilators
6. Blunted response to vasoconstrictors/deficiency of vasoconstrictors

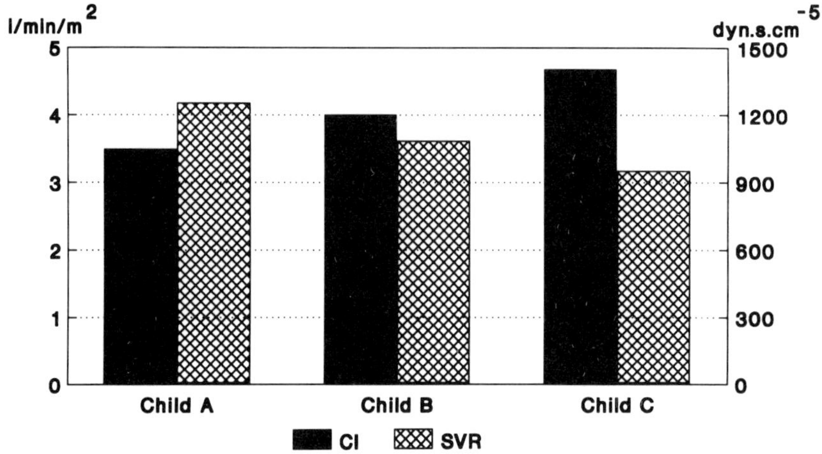

Fig. 2 Hyperdynamic circulation as a function of severity of liver disease assessed by Child's classification. With increasing functional impairment cardiac output (CI) increases and total systemic vascular resistance (SVR) decreases. Redrawn from ref. 6 (with permission from the authors and *British Medical Journal*)

Portal hypertension

Hyperkinetic circulation appears to be primarily related to portal hypertension rather than to cirrhosis since it is found in prehepatic portal hypertension with normal liver function[25] as well as in acute[28], chronic non-cirrhotic[2] and chronic cirrhotic[2,3] parenchymal liver disease. However, portal hypertension is not a necessary condition for the hyperdynamic circulation syndrome, since it is also observed in normal animals after fashioning of a portacaval shunt[27]; it is aggravated in cirrhotic patients after portosystemic shunt surgery. Finally, it persists after orthotopic liver transplantation in the absence of portal hypertension[26]. A similar phenomenon is observed when portal vein obstruction is relieved in the rat[29]. These phenomena suggest that the hyperkinetic circulation syndrome may become fixed at some point in time, whatever the initiating cause.

Portosystemic shunts

In prehepatic portal hypertension – exemplified by the portal vein stenosis model – portosystemic shunts invariably develop[8] in a predictable fashion, related to the degree of portal pressure[30]. The finding that hyperdynamic circulation evolved in both portal vein ligated rats and rats with a portosystemic shunt, led Braillon and colleagues to postulate that portosystemic shunting rather than portal hypertension was the prerequisite for hyperdynamic circulation[31]. Support for this hypothesis comes from the finding that creation of a portosystemic shunt in animals with normal liver histology induced a hyperkinetic circulation syndrome[27,31] and that the hyperkinetic circulation is aggravated in patients after a distal splenorenal shunt[32].

This is not true, however, in cirrhosis, where there is no relationship between portal pressure or hyperdynamic circulation and portosystemic shunts, mostly owing to the high variability of the degree of shunting[9,30]. Also against a significant role of portosystemic shunting is the finding that hyperdynamic circulation occurs before development of significant shunting in rat models of liver cirrhosis[33]. Early pharmacological treatment partially prevents the formation of portosystemic shunts in portal vein ligation but does not prevent the development of hyperdynamic circulation[34].

Portosystemic shunts certainly contribute to maintenance of hyperkinetic circulation. This contention is also supported by the finding that flow in the azygos vein, draining most of the supradiaphragmatic collaterals, is increased more than predicted from the increase in cardiac output alone[6]. Whether the effect of portosystemic shunting is purely haemodynamic – as arteriovenous shunts increase cardiac output – or whether the shunting of vasoactive agents around the liver is the mechanism whereby shunting induces and/or aggravates the hyperkinetic circulation remains unclear at present.

Increased plasma volume

Total blood and plasma volume are increased in cirrhotic patients[3,35,36]. Increased plasma volume most likely contributes to hyperkinetic circulation, although not as a primary pathogenetic event since it increases late in the evolution of portal hypertension induced by portal vein stenosis in the rat[37] (Fig. 3).

The evolution of events as depicted in Fig. 3 also seems to suggest that vasodilation is the earliest event after induction of portal hypertension[37] (see below). This sequence of events suggests that there is early depletion of the 'effective' blood volume as initially suggested by Peters for oedematous states[38]. The apparent inconsistency – decreased effective blood volume in a patient with increased total blood volume – has recently been resolved. Thus, Henriksen demonstrated by an indicator dilution technique that 'central' blood volume – consisting of the heart cavities, lungs and central arterial tree – is reduced in patients with liver cirrhosis[39]. This reduction in 'effective' blood volume sets into motion a whole battery of events such as non-osmotic AVP release[40], activation of the sympathetic nervous system[41] and of the renin–angiotensin–aldosterone system[42].

The increased blood volume is compartmentalized not only within the arterial bed; thus increased total vascular capacity with marked venous dilation has been found in cirrhotic rats[43]; investigations on cardiac performance in cirrhotic patients came to a similar conclusion[44].

Increased release of vasodilators

Modern hypotheses of ascites formation assign a major role to vasodilation[20,21]; this will be discussed in detail elsewhere in this volume. Indeed, humoral factors have been shown to play a major role in the vasodilation in different

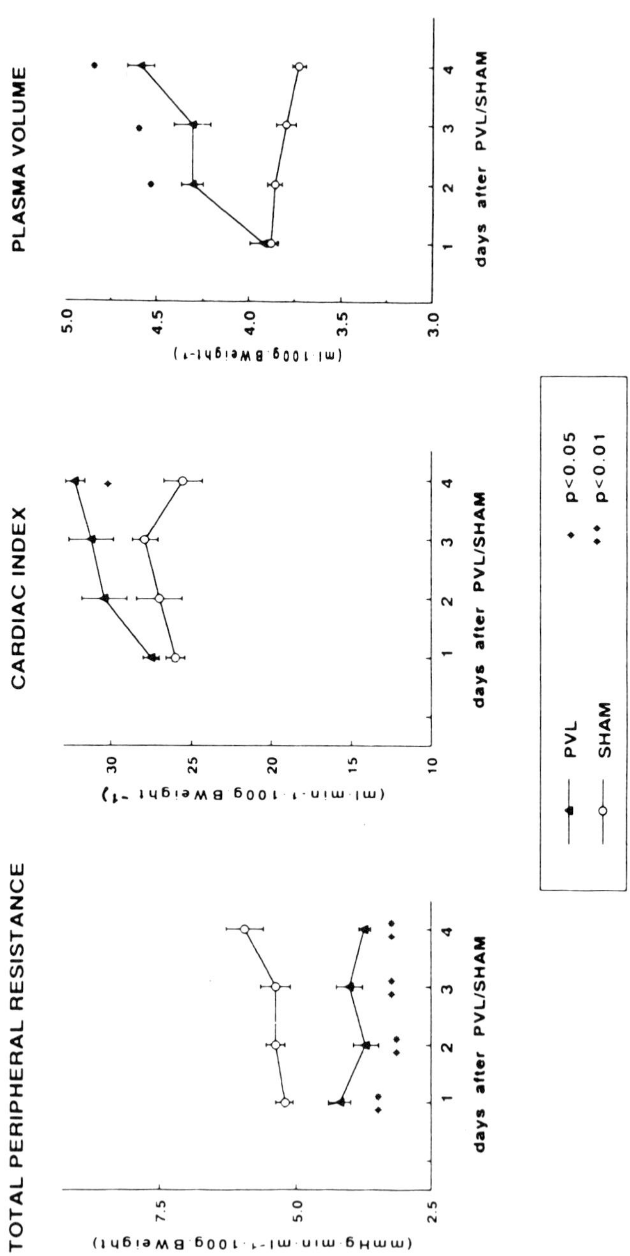

Fig. 3 Temporal evolution of vasodilation, cardiac output and plasma volume in rats with portal vein stenosis. The sequence of events suggests the peripheral vasodilation in the initial event in the hyperkinetic circulation syndrome. Redrawn from ref. 37 (with permission from the authors and from the publisher)

vascular beds including the splanchnic area[45] and the extremities[46]. Different factors have been incriminated in this phenomenon (Table 2).

Nitric oxide

Nitric oxide has recently been identified as the endothelium-derived relaxing factor[47]; it is liberated from L-arginine by nitric oxide synthetase. The enzyme exists in a constitutive and regulated form in many organs including the liver; it can be inhibited by different analogues of L-arginine.

Such inhibitors have been found to decrease cardiac output and normalize peripheral vascular resistance in rats with portal vein stenosis[48]. Nitric oxide could also be involved in the blunted response to different vasodilators[49], although preliminary results from another group seemed to come to different conclusions[50].

Nitric oxide seems an attractive candidate as an early factor in inducing vasodilation and hyperkinetic circulation, since its release is mediated by shear stress[47]. Thus, one could envision that portal hypertension *per se* induces nitric oxide release as the first event, later leading to vasodilation and the hyperkinetic circulation syndrome.

Glucagon

Glucagon is a potent vasodilator in the splanchnic area, and for a while was thought to be the main mediator of the vasodilation in cirrhotic patients. Indeed, glucagon plasma levels are markedly increased in patients with cirrhosis; however, the haemodynamic response to exogenously added glucagon is blunted[51]. This phenomenon may depend on the stage of liver disease, since Lee and collaborators found a response to glucagon only in Child's class A patients, while in more progressed liver disease this response was abolished altogether[52]. In rats with portal vein stenosis glucagon accounts for only 25–30% of the increase in splanchnic blood flow[53]. Thus, glucagon probably contributes to the hyperdynamic circulation, perhaps with a major role early in the development of portal hypertension[52].

Table 2 Vasodilators with potential involvement in the pathophysiology of hyperkinetic circulation in chronic liver disease

1. Nitric oxide
2. Glucagon
3. Calcitonin gene-related peptide
4. Eicosanoids
5. Adenosine
6. Cholephiles (bile salts)
7. Platelet-activating factor
8. Gamma-aminobutyric acid

Adenosine

Whether adenosine, a potent vasodilator mainly in the hepatic arterial bed, is involved in the hyperdynamic circulation remains controversial. In patients with alcoholic liver disease a haemodynamic role for adenosine has been convincingly demonstrated using purine-receptor antagonists[54]. In cirrhotic rats the response to exogenous adenosine was blunted as compared to controls, although the compound clearly aggravated hyperdynamic circulation[55]. However, 8-phenyltheophylline, a powerful adenosine antagonist, had no significant systemic or splanchnic haemodynamic effects[55]. In contrast, Lee and collaborators found that the same antagonist, albeit at a higher dose, increased portal tributary resistance by 60% without exhibiting any systemic haemodynamic effects[56].

Other vasodilator agents

Another potential candidate could be calcitonin gene-related peptide, a potent vasodilator which has been found to be increased in different vascular beds of cirrhotic patients[57]. This increase was found to be due to overproduction rather than to decreased clearance.

Eicosanoids could also contribute to hyperkinetic circulation. Thus, inhibition of prostaglandin synthesis with indomethacin diminishes cardiac output in patients with cirrhosis and increases peripheral vascular resistance[58,59]. Prostacylin-like activity was markedly increased in portal veins early after portal vein ligation[60]. Further studies using more refined analytical techniques and more specific inhibitors of eicosanoid biosynthesis are needed to clarify the role of eicosanoids in the pathogenesis of the circulatory abnormalities in portal hypertension.

Different cholephiles, in particular bile acids, could contribute to some of the vascular abnormalities: Bomzon and colleagues demonstrated that bile acids impaired the contractile response of smooth muscle to adrenergic agents[61]. The role of bile acids in the hyperdynamic state remains controversial, however. Thus, Thomas and colleagues demonstrated that drainage of bile acids in portal vein stenosed rats reduced portal venous inflow[62], while another group ascribed the elevated bile acid levels to portosystemic shunting and could not reduce the hyperdynamic circulation by bile acid drainage[63]. We have described that biliary retention induced portal hypertension in the absence of any major histological changes or functional impairment[64]; these data suggest that a compound(s) normally excreted into bile has vasoactive properties.

An involvement of gamma-aminobutyric acid has been postulated since it is vasoactive and its levels are elevated in cirrhotic patients[65]. Endotoxin levels are frequently elevated in plasma of cirrhotic patients; therefore the role of endotoxin, platelet-activating factor and endorphins has been investigated by several groups. At least in the portal vein stenosis model, endotoxin does not seem to play a major role in the hyperdynamic circulation syndrome[66]. At least in coexisting sepsis, endotoxin via activation of the platelet-activating factor may aggravate hyperkinetic circulation[67]. Indeed, platelet-activating factor is increased in portal blood of cirrhotic rats[68] and part of the hyperdynamic circulation can be abolished by specific antagonists[67,68]. Since endorphins play a role in septic shock, a link between hyperdynamic circulation and endorphin was sought but not found[69].

Blunted response to vasoconstrictors

An activation of the sympathetic nervous system is well established in cirrhotic patients[70,71]; it is involved in maintenance of portal hypertension[72]. Recently, increased sympathetic outflow in cirrhotic patients has been demonstrated directly by intraneural recordings[73]. The main determinant appears to be decreased central blood volume, since catecholamines can be normalized through central blood volume expansion by water immersion[71].

A variety of vasoconstrictor agents has been found to be increased in patients with cirrhosis (Table 3); this is thought to be a response to renal hypoperfusion and central volume depletion. Vasodilation is maintained by a blunted response to the vasoconstrictor agents listed in Table 3. The mechanism(s) for this phenomenon remain unclear (see below). Although the response to many constricting neurotransmitters is blunted, this is by no means universal. Thus, vasoconstriction induced by serotonin is actually increased in portal hypertension[74].

Endothelin

The endothelins are a family of small peptides with marked vasoconstrictor activity (for review see ref. 75). Decreased concentrations of endothelin 1 have been described in cirrhotic subjects[76], suggesting that a lack of endothelin could contribute to hyperdynamic circulation. However, since endothelins act at their site of synthesis in a paracrine fashion, it is unclear to which extent peripheral endothelin levels reflect activity at its site of action. Furthermore, recent preliminary reports indicated that endothelin levels were actually increased, more so in patients with ascites[77] or marked functional impairment[78].

Table 3 Vasoconstrictor substances in chronic liver disease

A. Increased production/blunted response
1. β-adrenergic agents
2. Angiotensin II
3. Vasopressin
4. Endothelin?
B. Increased sensitivity
1. Serotonin
2. Endothelin?

In support of a relative lack of endothelin is the finding that pharmacological doses of endothelin increased arterial pressure more in cirrhotic rats than in controls. It also reversed some of the renal abnormalities in sodium handling[79]. These latter studies could also be explained by a blunted response to endothelin; the contrary has been described, however; namely an increased sensitivity to exogenous endothelin in portal vein strips from cirrhotic rats[80]. Thus, the exact role of endothelin in maintenance of portal hypertension and in the counterregulation to initial vasodilation remains largely to be determined.

β-Adrenergic agents

The response to *β*-adrenergic agents is blunted in patients[5,81] and animal models[61,72,82–85]. Where the evolution of this phenomenon has been investigated, the blunted response was found to be a late event[68,84]. In rats with compensated cirrhosis vascular reactivity to norepinephrine was normal[86]. This is in line with clinical data demonstrating a correlation between impaired response to adrenergic agents and severity of the liver disease[81].

Most studies found a decreased receptor affinity as measured by ED_{50} or similar parameters[61,82,83,87] although a decrease in maximal response has also been described under some circumstances[61,84]. The mechanism of this blunted response remains debated. A down-regulation of *β*-receptors on lymphocytes of cirrhotic patients has been taken as evidence of general receptor down-regulation[88]; this finding has not been confirmed, however[89]. Using different adrenergic agents as well as other vasoconstrictors, MacGilchrist *et al.* suggested that a generalized smooth vascular defect was responsible for the blunted response[83].

This could be due to structural alterations of vessels chronically exposed to increased pressure. As in any other vascular bed, increased pressure induces muscular hypertrophy in the portal vein[90]. In spite of this hypertrophy, the maximum contraction, corrected for the increased cross-sectional area, is reduced[90,91]. Whether this is due to alterations in activation or an intrinsic change in the contractile system itself has not yet been established.

Recently, some doubt has been shed on the concept that activation of the sympathetic nervous system was involved to a major extent in hyperdynamic circulation, since it persisted after pithing of portal hypertensive rats[92]; sympathetic activation is well documented, however (see above) and the persistence of hyperdynamic circulation in pithed rats could also be explained by fixed vasodilation[26]. In contrast to pithing, ganglionic blockade abolishes the reduced sensitivity to phenylephrine in portal vein stenosed rats, suggesting an enhanced heart rate baroreflex response[85].

An important concept, namely that vasodilators could contribute to the blunted response to vasoconstrictors, has recently been formulated. Thus, exogenous glucagon can render normal rats hyposensitive to norepinephrine[87]. A similar phenomenon has been described for nitric oxide where a normal response to *α*-adrenergic agents in splanchnic arteries from portal hypertensive rats could be restored after nitric oxide synthetase inhibition[49].

Other agents

The renin–angiotensin–aldosterone system is stimulated in response to central volume depletion[20,21]; the degree of stimulation is related to the severity of portal hypertension[42]. As with β-adrenergics, a decreased pressor response of cirrhotic patients to angiotensin II has been described[83]. Another important regulator of blood volume is vasopressin, which is also increased in patients with cirrhosis and ascites to maintain arterial pressure[93]. A decreased vascular response to vasopressin due to a post-receptor defect has been described[94].

ATTEMPT AT AN INTEGRATED VIEW

The initial factor inducing hyperkinetic circulation remains elusive; what appears clear from the discussions above is that the syndrome has to be multifactorial with a precarious balance between vasoconstrictors and vasodilators. A potential scenario is depicted in Fig. 4. The initial event is portal hypertension inducing portosystemic shunts. Portal hypertension and/or the portosystemic shunting lead to an increase in vasodilating substances; prime candidates are glucagon and nitric oxide but a variety of other agents has been implicated. The resulting vasodilation induces a reduction in 'central' blood volume, activating the sympathetic nervous system, the renin–angiotensin–aldosterone axis and inducing the release of vasopressin. These mediators are responsible for the increased cardiac output and total blood volume. Increased cardiac output, vasodilation and increased plasma volume are obviously the hallmarks of hyperdynamic circulation. Not yet incorporated into this regulated system in Fig. 4 is endothelin, since it remains

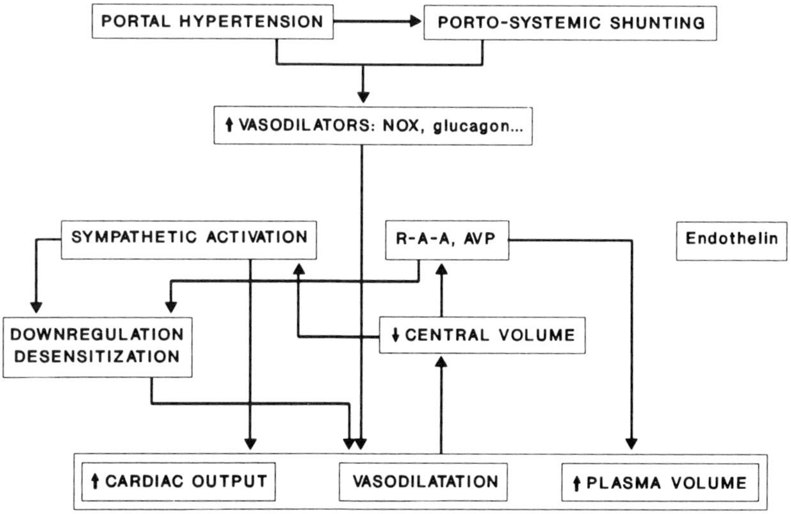

Fig. 4 Schematic proposal for the development and maintenance of the hyperkinetic circulation syndrome. For further details see text

to be determined whether it is actually decreased, as suggested by the early studies, or whether it increases in concentration leading to down-regulation of its receptors and a blunted response. As any simple scheme, the proposed sequence of events is probably wrong, and the list of mediators discussed in this review is certainly incomplete. What appears obvious to this reviewer, however, is that an integrated view on the different events is necessary to further our understanding of the pathophysiology of this fascinating condition, and that a simplistic therapeutic or research approach focusing on only one factor will be misleading and may be harmful to patients.

ACKNOWLEDGEMENTS

This work was supported by a grant from the Swiss National Foundation for Scientific Research (32.30168.90). The artwork by Ms M. Kappeler is gratefully acknowledged.

References

1. Whipple AO. The problem of portal hypertension in relation to the hepatosplenopathies. Ann Surg. 1945;122:449–75.
2. Kowalski HJ, Abelmann WH. The cardiac output at rest in Laennec's cirrhosis. J Clin Invest. 1953;32:1025–33.
3. Murray JF, Sherlock S. Circulatory changes in chronic liver disease. Am J Med. 1958;24:356–67.
4. Siegel JH, Goldwyn RM, Farrell J. Hyperdynamic states and the physiologic determinants of survival. Arch Surg. 1974;108:282–92.
5. Lunzer MR, Manghani KK, Newman SP, Sherlock SP. Bernard AG, Ginsburg J. Impaired cardiovascular responsiveness in liver disease. Lancet. 1975;2:382–5.
6. Braillon A, Cales P, Valla D, Gaudy D, Geoffroy P, Lebrec D. Influence of the degree of liver failure on systemic and splanchnic haemodynamics and on response to propranolol in patients with cirrhosis. Gut. 1986;27:1204–9.
7. Ito K, Ramirez-Schon G, Shah PM, Del Guercio RRM. Functioning hepatic cell mass and the hyperdynamic state in cirrhosis. Surg Gynecol Obstet. 1988;167:180–6.
8. Vorobioff J, Bredfeldt JE, Groszmann RJ. Hyperdynamic circulation in portal-hypertensive rat model: a primary factor for maintenance of chronic portal hypertension. Am J Physiol. 1983;244:G52–7.
9. Vorobioff J, Bredfeldt JE, Groszmann RJ. Increased blood flow through the portal system in cirrhotic rats. Gastroenterology. 1984;87:1120–6.
10. Reichen J. Pharmacological considerations on pathogenesis and treatment of portal hypertension. Hepatology. 1990;11:1066–78.
11. Witte CL, Witte MH, Bair G, Mobley WP, Morton D. Experimental study of hyperdynamic vs. stagnant mesenteric blood flow in portal hypertension. Ann Surg. 1974;179:304–10.
12. Benoit JN, Wocmack WA, Hernandez L, Granger DN. 'Forward' and 'backward' flow mechanisms of portal hypertension. Gastroenterology. 1985;89:1096–9.
13. Lee SS. Cardiac abnormalities in liver cirrhosis. West J Med. 1989;151:530–5.
14. Bernardi M, Di Marco C, Trevisani F, De Collibus C, Fornale L, Baraldini M, Andreone P, Cursaro C, Zaca F, Ligabue A, Gasbarrini G. The hemodynamic status of preascitic cirrhosis: an evaluation under steady state conditions and after postural change. Hepatology. 1992;16:341–6.
15. Moreau R, Lee SS, Soupison T, Roche-Sicot J, Sicot C. Abnormal tissue oxygenation in patients with cirrhosis and liver failure. J Hepatol. 1988;7:98–105.
16. Koshy A, Moreau R, Cerini R, Roulot D, Bacq Y, Hadengue A, Lebrec D. Effects of oxygen inhalation on tissue oxygenation in patients with cirrhosis. J Hepatol. 1989;9:240–5.

17. Sherlock S. Vasodilation associated with hepatocellular disease: relation to functional organ failure. Gut. 1990;31:365–7.
18. Battarbee HD, Farrar GE, Spears RP. Responses to hypotension in conscious rats with chronic portal venous hypertension. Am J Physiol. 1990;259:G48–55.
19. Bernardi M, Trevisani F, Santini C, Liabue A, Capelli M, Gasbarrini G. Impairment of blood pressure control in patients with liver cirrhosis during tilting. Study on adrenergic and renin–angiotensin system. Digestion. 1982;25:124–30.
20. Arroyo V, Bernardi M, Epstein M, Henriksen JH, Schrier RW, Rodes J. Pathophysiology of ascites and functional renal failure in cirrhosis. J Hepatol. 1988;6:239–57.
21. Schrier RW. Pathogenesis of sodium and water retention in high-output and low-output cardiac failure, nephrotic syndrome, cirrhosis and pregnancy. N Engl J Med. 1988;319:1065–72.
22. Ingles AC, Hernandez I, Garcia-Estan J, Quesada T, Carbonell LF. Limited cardiac preload reserve in conscious cirrhotic rats. Am J Physiol. 1991;260:H1912–17.
23. Lee SS, Marty J, Mantz J, Samain E, Braillon A, Lebrec D. Desensitization of myocardial beta-adrenergic receptors in cirrhotic rats. Hepatology. 1990;12:481–5.
24. Martini GA, Hagemann JE. Ueber Fingernagelveraenderungen bei Lebercirrhose als Folge veraenderter peripherer Durchblutung. Klin Wochenschr. 1956;34:23–32.
25. Lebrec D, Bataille C, Bercoff E, Valla D. Hemodynamic changes in patients with portal venous obstruction. Hepatology. 1983;3:550–3.
26. Henderson JM, Mackay GJ, Hooks M, Chezmar JL, Galloway JR, Dodson TF, Kutner MH. High cardiac output of advanced liver disease persists after orthotopic liver transplantation. Hepatology. 1992;15:258–62.
27. Gurll NJ, Reynolds DG, Coon D. Acute and chronic splanchnic blood flow responses to portacaval shunt in the normal dog. Gastroenterology. 1980;78:1432–6.
28. Hecker R, Sherlock S. Electrolyte and circulatory changes in terminal liver failure. Lancet. 1956;2:1121–5.
29. Sikuler E, Groszmann RJ. Interaction of flow and resistance in maintenance of portal hypertension in a rat model. Am J Physiol. 1986;250:G205–12.
30. Geraghty JG, Angerson WJ, Carter DC. Portal venous pressure and portasystemic shunting in experimental portal hypertension. Am J Physiol. 1989;257:G52–7.
31. Braillon A, Lee SSG, Peignoux-Martinot M, Valla D, Lebrec D. Role of portasystemic shunts in the hyperkinetic circulation of the portal hypertensive rat. J Lab Clin Med. 1986;108:543–8.
32. Levi JU, Zeppa R, Hutson DG. Early hemodynamic effects of the distal splenorenal shunt. Surg Forum. 1976;27:370–1.
33. Fernandez-Munoz D, Caramelo C, Santos JC, Blanchart A, Hernando L, Lopez-Novoa JM. Systemic and splanchnic hemodynamic disturbances in conscious rats with experimental liver cirrhosis without ascites. Am J Physiol. 1985;249:G316–20.
34. Lin H-C, Soubrane O, Lebrec D. Prevention of portal hypertension and portosystemic shunts by early chronic administration of clonidine in conscious portal vein-stenosed rats. Hepatology. 1991;14:325–30.
35. Rector WG, Ibarra F. Intravascular volume in cirrhosis. Reassessment using improved methodology. Dig Dis Sci. 1988;33:460–6.
36. Hadengue A, Moreau R, Gaudin C, Bacq Y, Champigneulle B, Lebrec D. Total effective vascular compliance in patients with cirrhosis: a study of the response to acute blood volume expansion. Hepatology. 1992;15:809–15.
37. Colombato LA, Albillos A, Groszmann RJ. Temporal relationships of peripheral vasodilatation, plasma volume expansion and the hyperdynamic circulatory state in portal-hypertensive rats. Hepatology. 1991;15:323–8.
38. Peters JP. The role of sodium in production of edema. N Engl J Med. 1948;239:353–62.
39. Henriksen JH, Bendtsen F, Sorensen TIA, Stadeager C, Ring-Larsen H. Reduced central blood volume in cirrhosis. Gastroenterology. 1989;97:1506–13.
40. Bichet D, Szatalowicz V, Chaimovitz V, Schrier RW. Role of vasopressin in abnormal water excretion in cirrhotic patients. Ann Intern Med. 1982;96:413–17.
41. Bichet DG, VanPutten VJ, Schrier RW. Potential role of increased sympathetic activity in impaired sodium and water excretion in cirrhosis. N Engl J Med. 1982;307:1552–7.
42. Bosch J, Arroyo V, Betriu A, Mas A, Carrilho F, Rivera F, Navarro-Lopez F, Rodes J. Hepatic hemodynamics and the renin–angiotensin–aldosterone system in cirrhosis.

Gastroenterology. 1980;78:92–9.
43. Ingles AC, Hernandez I, Garcia-Estan J, Quesada T, Carbonell LF. Increased total vascular capacity in conscious cirrhotic rats. Gastroenterology. 1992;103:275–81.
44. Lewis FW, Adair O, Rector JWG. Arterial vasodilation is not the cause of increased cardiac output in cirrhosis. Gastroenterology. 1992;102:1024–9.
45. Benoit JN, Barrowman JA, Harper SL, Kvietys PR, Granger DN. Role of humoral factors in the intestinal hyperemia associated with portal hypertension. Am J Physiol. 1984;247:G486–93.
46. Korthuis RJ, Benoit JN, Kvietys PR, Townsley MI, Taylor AE, Granger N. Humoral factors may mediate increased rat hindquarter blood flow in portal hypertension. Am J Physiol. 1985;249:H827–33.
47. Palmer RMJ, Ferrige AG, Moncada S. Nitric oxide release accounts for the biological activity of endothelium derived relaxing factor. Nature. 1987;327:524–6.
48. Pizcueta MP, Pique JM, Bosch J, Whittle BJR, Moncada S. Effects of inhibiting nitric oxide biosynthesis on the systemic and splanchnic circulation of rats with portal hypertension. Br J Pharmacol. 1992;105:184–90.
49. Sieber C, Groszmann RJ. *In vitro* hyporeactivity to methoxamine in portal hypertensive rats: Reversal by nitric oxide blockade. Am J Physiol. 1992;262:G996–1001.
50. Karatapanis S, McCormick PA, Jacobs M, Jeremy J, Stansby J, Collins P, McIntyre N, Burroughs AK. Role of nitric oxide in the altered systemic vascular reactivity in portal vein constricted rats. J Hepatol. 1992;16:S34.
51. Silva G, Navasa M, Bosch J, Chesta J, Pizcueta MP, Casamitjana R, Rivera F, Rodes J. Hemodynamic effects of glucagon in portal hypertension. Hepatology. 1990;11:668–73.
52. Lee SS, Moreau R, Hadengue A, Cerini R, Koshy A, Lebrec D. Glucagon selectively increases splanchnic blood flow in patients with well-compensated cirrhosis. Hepatology. 1988;8:1501–5.
53. Benoit JN, Zimmermann B, Premen AJ, Go VLW, Granger DN. Role of glucagon in splanchnic hyperemia of chronic portal hypertension. Am J Physiol. 1986;251:G674–7.
54. Orrego H, Carmichael FJ, Saldivia V, Giles HG, Sandrin S, Israel Y. Ethanol-induced increase in portal flow: role of adenosine. Am J Physiol. 1988;254:G495–501.
55. Champigneulle B, Braillon A, Kleber G, Gaudin C, Cailmail S, Lebrec D. Adenosine and hemodynamic alterations in cirrhotic rats. Am J Physiol. 1991;260:G543–7.
56. Lee SS, Chilton L, Pak JM. Adenosine receptor blockade reduces splanchnic hyperemia in cirrhotic rats. Hepatology. 1992;15:1107–11.
57. Bendtsen F, Schifter S, Henriksen J. Increased circulating calcitonin gene-related peptide in cirrhosis. J Hepatol. 1990;12:118–23.
58. Bruix J, Bosch J, Kravetz D, Mastai R, Rodes J. Effects of prostaglandin inhibition on systemic and hepatic hemodynamics in patients with cirrhosis of the liver. Gastroenterology. 1985;88:430–5.
59. Sitzmann JV, Li S-S, Adkinson NF. Evidence for role of prostacyclin as a systemic hormone in portal hypertension. Surgery. 1991;109:149–53.
60. Hamilton G, Phing RCF, Hutton RA, Dandona P, Hobbs KEF. The relationship between prostacyclin activity and pressure in the portal vein. Hepatology. 1982;2:236–42.
61. Bomzon A, Finberg JPM, Tovbin D, Naidu SG, Better OS. Bile salts, hypotension and obstructive jaundice. Clin Sci. 1984;67:177–83.
62. Thomas SH, Joh T, Benoit JN. Role of bile acids in splanchnic hemodynamic response to chronic portal hypertension. Dig Dis Sci. 1991;36:1243–8.
63. Genecin P, Polio J, Colombato LA, Ferraioli G, Reuben A, Groszmann RJ. Bile acids do not mediate the hyperdynamic circulation in portal hypertensive rats. Am J Physiol. 1990;259:G21–5.
64. Zimmermann H, Reichen J, Saegesser H, Thenisch B, Zimmermann A. Biliary retention in a chronic choledocho-venous fistula in the rat: Induction of portal hypertension but not of biliary cirrhosis. J Hepatol. 1992: in press.
65. Minuk GY, MacCannell KL. Is the hypotension of cirrhosis a GABA-mediated process? Hepatology. 1988;73–7.
66. Mehta R, Gottstein J, Zeller WP, Lichtenberg R, Blei AT. Endotoxin and the hyperdynamic circulation of portal vein-ligated rats. Hepatology. 1990;12:1152–6.

67. Kleber G, Braillon A, Gaudin C, Champigneulle B, Cailmail S, Lebrec D. Hemodynamic effects of endotoxin and platelet activating factor in cirrhotic rats. Gastroenterology. 1992;103:282–8.
68. Villamediana LM, Sanz E, Fernandez-Gallardo S, Caramelo C, Sanchez M, Braquet P, Lopez-Novoa JM. Effects of the platelet-activating factor antagonist BN 52021 on the hemodynamics of rats with experimental cirrhosis of the liver. Life Sci. 1986;39:201–5.
69. Lee SS, Hadengue A, Moreau R, Girod C, Jiron MI, Lebrec D. Naloxone does not alter haemodynamics in cirrhosis. Studies in humans and rats. J Hepatol. 1987;5:149–53.
70. Henriksen JH, Ring-Larsen H, Kanstrup IL, Christensen NJ. Splanchnic and renal elimination and release of catecholamines in cirrhosis. Evidence of enhanced sympathetic nervous activity in patients with decompensated cirrhosis. Gut. 1984;25:1034–43.
71. Nicholls KM, Shapiro MD, Van Putten VJ, Kluge R, Chung HM, Bichet DG, Schrier RW. Elevated plasma norepinephrine concentrations in decompensated cirrhosis. Association with increased secretion rates, normal clearance rates, and suppressibility by central volume expansion. Circ Res. 1985;56:457–61.
72. Willett IR, Esler M, Jennings G, Dudley FJ. Sympathetic tone modulates portal venous pressure in alcoholic cirrhosis. Lancet. 1986;2:939–43.
73. Floras JS, Legault L, Morali GA, Hara K, Blendis LM. Increased sympathetic outflow in cirrhosis and ascites: direct evidence from intraneural recordings. Ann Intern Med. 1991;114:373–80.
74. Cummings SA, Groszmann RJ, Kaumann AJ. Hypersensitivity of mesenteric veins to 5-hydroxytryptamine- and ketanserin-induced reduction of portal pressure in portal hypertensive rats. Br J Pharmacol. 1986;89:501–13.
75. Randall MD. Vascular activities of the endothelins. Pharmacol Ther. 1991;50:73–9.
76. Veglio F, Pinna G, Melchio R, Rabbia F, Panarelli M, Gagliardi B, Chiandussi L. Plasma endothelin levels in cirrhotic subjects. J Hepatol. 1992;15:85–7.
77. Asbert M, Gines A, Gines P, Jimenez W, Claria J, Salo J, Arroyo V, Rivera F, Rodes J. Increased circulating endothelin levels in cirrhosis. J Hepatol. 1992;16:S31.
78. Zotz RB, Fritschka R, Lange R, Erhard J, Beste M, Skworz K, Bruer N, Goebell H. Increased endothelin plasma concentration in patients with reduced liver function. J Hepatol. 1992;16:S31.
79. Claria J, Jimenez W, Arroyo V, Castro A, Asbert M, Ros J, Rivera F, Rodes J. Doses of endothelin have natriuretic effects in conscious rats with cirrhosis and ascites. Kidney Int. 1991;40:182–7.
80. Hanish E, Lorey T, Weber T, Schulz M, Hermann G. Increased *in vitro* sensitivity of portal veins from cirrhotic vs healthy rats to endothelin-1 and -3 in the presence of equal plasma levels. J Hepatol. 1992;16:S34.
81. Ramond MJ, Comoy E, Lebrec D. Alterations in isoprenaline sensitivity in patients with cirrhosis: evidence of abnormality of the sympathetic nervous activity. Br J Clin Pharmacol. 1986;21:191–6.
82. Kiel JW, Pitts V, Benoit JN, Granger ND, Shepherd AP. Reduced vascular sensitivity to norepinephrine in portal hypertensive rats. Am J Physiol. 1985;248:G192–5.
83. MacGilchrist AJ, Sumner D, Reid JL. Impaired pressor reactivity in cirrhosis: evidence for a peripheral vascular defect. Hepatology. 1991;13:689–94.
84. Bomzon A, Blendis LM. Vascular reactivity in experimental portal hypertension. Am J Physiol. 1987;252:G158–62.
85. Battarbee HD, Farrar GE, Spears RP. Pressor responses in conscious rats with chronic portal venous hypertension. Am J Physiol. 1989;257:G773–81.
86. Villamediana LM, Dieguez G, Santos JC, Garcia-Villlalon AL, Caramelo C, Lopez-Novoa JM. Vascular reactivity to norepinephrine in rats with cirrhosis of the liver. Can J Physiol Pharmacol. 1988;66:567–72.
87. Pizcueta MP, Casamitjana R, Bosch J, Rodes J. Decreased systemic vascular sensitivity to norepinephrine in portal hypertensive rats: role of hyperglucagonism. Am J Physiol. 1990;258:G191–5.
88. Gerbes AL, Remien J, Juengst D, Sauerbruch T, Paumgartner G. Evidence for down-regulation of beta-2-adrenoceptors in cirrhotic patients with severe ascites. Lancet. 1986;1:1409–11.

89. Garcia-Pagan JC, Navasa M, Rivera F, Bosch J, Rodes J. Lymphocyte beta-1-adrenoceptors and plasma catecholamines in patients with cirrhosis. Gastroenterology. 1992;102:2015–23.
90. Johansson B. Structural and functional changes in rat portal veins after experimental portal hypertension. Acta Physiol Scand. 1976;98:381–3.
91. Arner A, Malmqvist U, Uvelius B. Effects of Ca^{2+} on force–velocity characteristics of normal and hypertrophic smooth muscle of the rat portal vein. Acta Physiol Scand. 1985;124:525–33.
92. Abergel A, Braillon A, Gaudin C, Kleber G, Lebrec D. Persistence of hyperdynamic circulation in cirrhotic rats following removal of the sympathetic nervous system. Gastroenterology. 1992;102:656–60.
93. Claria J, Jimenez W, Arroyo V, LaVilla G, Lopez C, Asbert M, Castro A, Gaya J, Rivera F, Rodes J. Effect of V1-vasopressin receptor blockade on arterial pressure in conscious rats with cirrhosis and ascites. Gastroenterology. 1991;100:494–501.
94. Murray BM, Paller MS. Pressor resistance to vasopressin in sodium depletion, potassium depletion, and cirrhosis. Am J Physiol. 1986;251:R525–30.

6

Portal venous hypertension and pathogenesis of ascites

M. NIEDERBERGER, A. WEIGERT and R. W. SCHRIER

INTRODUCTION

Oedema and ascites are typical clinical features appearing during the evolution of liver cirrhosis and are secondary to extracellular fluid and plasma volume expansion induced by an increased renal sodium retention as reflected by a low urinary sodium concentration described in cirrhotic patients in 1950 by Eisenmenger *et al.*[1] Despite this volume expansion, arterial blood pressure is low and cardiac output is high, indicating a decrease in peripheral arterial resistance[2–5] occurring despite stimulation of neurohumoral vasoconstrictor systems.

The difficulty of determining if the renal sodium and water retention is a primary event unrelated to hypovolaemia or is secondary to arterial underfilling has generated different hypotheses to conciliate these apparent contradictory features[6–8]. Since more than 60% of cirrhotic patients develop oedema and ascites during the evolution of their disease, the water and sodium disturbances in liver disease are major problems in therapeutic management and a clarification of their pathogenesis will imply different treatment strategies depending on the mechanisms leading to water and sodium retention. Indeed, if renal sodium and water retention is primary, then rational treatment would consist of diuretic therapy and reversal of a putative initiating event, e.g. an increase in hepatic sinusoidal pressure. If, on the other hand, a primary decrease in peripheral arterial resistance elicits the renal functional abnormalities, then treatment would logically consist of attempts to antagonize the effects of a putative vasodilator factor(s).

THEORIES FOR INITIATION OF SODIUM AND WATER RETENTION IN CIRRHOSIS

As discussed below, three successive hypotheses have been proposed to explain the pathogenesis of the disorders of water and sodium balance occurring in cirrhosis, and they differ mainly in the degree of expansion of the vascular compartment, especially of the arterial tree and in the pathogenetic importance of the portal venous hypertension.

The classical 'underfill' theory

The oldest hypothesis, named the 'underfill' theory, proposed that ascites was formed by fluid transudation from a congested splanchnic vascular bed induced by portal hypertension and led to circulatory hypovolaemia which, by activation of the neurohumoral systems, increased secondary renal sodium and water retention[9]. However, renal sodium retention in experimental models of cirrhosis and reduced capacity for sodium excretion in cirrhotic patients have been demonstrated to occur prior to ascites formation[10–12], thus suggesting that ascites was not the initiating factor of the sodium retention.

The 'overflow' hypothesis

Lieberman *et al.* demonstrated that sodium retention in cirrhosis was not associated with hypovolaemia, but surprisingly with an expansion of the non-splanchnic blood volume[6,13,14] and therefore proposed that the ascites formation occurred secondary to a 'primary' renal sodium and water retention, i.e. not induced by hypovolaemia[14]. This leads to plasma volume expansion and then 'overflow' ascites formation occurs in the presence of portal hypertension. This theory therefore has been called the 'overflow' hypothesis[6]. In dogs with dimethylnitrosamine-induced cirrhosis, Levy *et al.* demonstrated that urinary sodium retention and an increase in non-splanchnic plasma volume preceded ascites formation[15], and no detectable alteration in cardiac output, peripheral vascular resistance or positive sodium could be detected until 2 weeks after ascites was present[11]. López-Novoa *et al.* confirmed that sodium retention preceded ascites formation in rats with carbon tetrachloride-induced cirrhosis[12]; however cirrhotic rats had a hyperdynamic circulatory status prior to ascites formation[16].

In order to assess the role of the portal venous hypertension in the initiation of sodium renal retention, Levy *et al.* prevented the development of portal venous hypertension by an end-to-side portacaval shunt prior to the induction of cirrhosis and demonstrated that renal sodium retention still occurred and preceded ascites formation[17]. Continuous removal of ascites through a LeVeen peritoneovenous shunt induced a marked diuresis and natriuresis associated with a complete mobilization of ascites. However, in spite of the enhanced sodium and water excretion, dogs with a LeVeen shunt given a high sodium load still retained sodium and developed oedema[18]. Unikowsky *et al.* studied dogs with bile duct ligation and an associated side-to-side portacaval anastomosis[19]. Animals with a partial occlusion of this portacaval anastomosis retained sodium and developed ascites with desoxycorticosterone acetate (DOCA) administration and a high salt intake. In contrast, animals with a patent side-to-side portacaval anastomosis showed no sodium retention and escaped from the effects of DOCA. Compared to end-to-side portacaval anastomosis, side-to-side anastomosis was assumed to normalize the intrahepatic pressure. In this same model, Levy and Wexler showed that hepatic denervation could prevent renal sodium retention despite the intrahepatic hypertension[20]. A neuroanatomical basis was provided by Kostreva *et al.* who found baroreceptors in canine liver which responded to an augmented intrahepatic pressure by increasing renal sympathetic activity[21]. Other evidence for the existence of a hepatorenal reflex was provided by Anderson *et al.*, who found that renal vasoconstriction, sodium and water retention and increased renin secretion was induced by acute constriction of the portal vein in dogs without any change in systemic haemodynamics. These effects were abolished by kidney denervation[22]. In contrast to bile duct ligation, however, this model is not associated with an increased intrahepatic venous pressure.

The 'peripheral arterial vasodilation' hypothesis

Although the above studies support a predominant role of portal venous hypertension in sodium and water retention through a hepatorenal reflex, the 'overflow' hypothesis does not explain the progressive stimulation of the neurohumoral vasopressor systems as the cirrhosis progresses. Specifically, the stimulation of the renin–angiotensin–aldosterone system, the non-osmotic release of arginine vasopressin and the sympathetic nervous system which is consistently found in decompensated cirrhosis are not in accordance with the 'overflow' hnypothesis, since plasma volume expansion should suppress these markers of hypovolaemia[23–29]. To reconcile the haemodynamic and the neurohumoral profiles found in liver cirrhosis, a new hypothesis has been proposed by Schrier *et al.* which attributes the renal sodium and water retention to a primary arterial vasodilation[7,8]. This peripheral arterial vasodilation induces, on the one hand, the hyperdynamic circulation with elevated cardiac output and heart rate and, on the other hand, the stimulation of the vasoconstrictor systems which leads to renal vasoconstriction, renal sodium and water retention and body fluid volume expansion in order to maintain an adequate arterial circulatory state (Fig. 1). Due to the associated portal hypertension and hypoalbuminaemia, a transudate collects in the abdominal cavity. As cirrhosis progresses, peripheral arterial resistance continues to fall, thus further stimulating the systemic vasoconstrictor systems which cause progressive renal vasoconstriction. Therefore, it is not surprising that the worst prognosis in cirrhotic patients is associated with the highest plasma hormone concentrations of norepinephrine, renin, aldosterone, and vasopressin and the presence of pretreatment hyponatraemia[27,30].

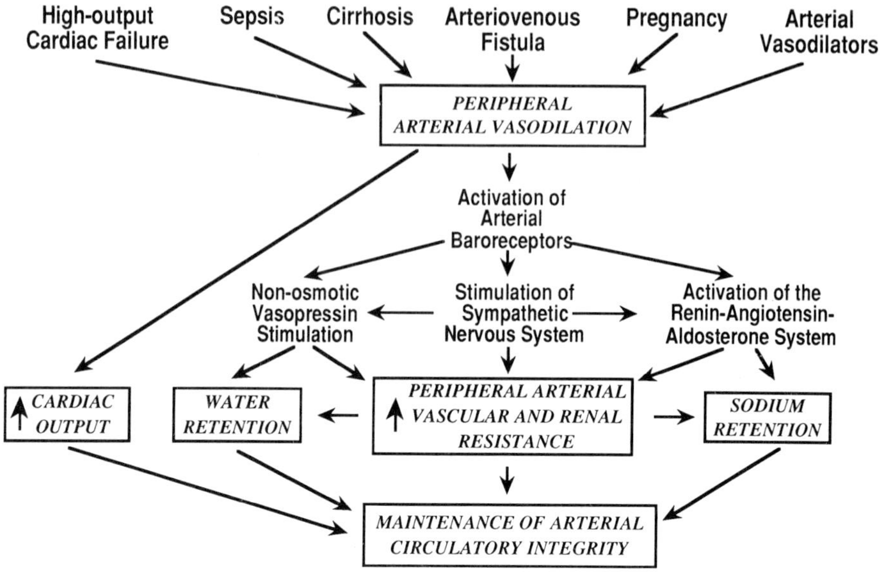

Fig. 1 Sequence of events in which peripheral arterial vasodilation initiates renal sodium and water retention. (Modified from ref. 122 with permission)

There are, however, arguments against the 'peripheral arterial vasodilation' hypothesis, particularly in the initial stages of cirrhosis. As noted earlier, Levy and Allotey could not detect alterations in cardiac output or peripheral vascular resistance until 2 weeks after the appearance of ascites[11]. However, other investigators have shown a fall in peripheral arterial resistance before ascites formation in experimental models[16]. An initial fall in peripheral arterial resistance may also be obscured by secondary constrictor responses which, additionally, may initiate sodium and water retention. In some supine cirrhotic patients, head-out water immersion (HWI) also induced a natriuresis similar to or greater than that observed in control subjects, a finding which might be considered to support the 'overflow' hypothesis[31]. Associated with this natriuresis, the rise in plasma atrial natriuretic peptide (ANP) concentration was shown to be significantly greater in cirrhotic patients that in normal controls[32]. This finding could suggest that the central blood volume is greater in cirrhotic patients. However, due to their increased splanchnic blood volume, it can also be argued that HWI is able to produce a greater central blood volume redistribution in supine cirrhotic patients than in supine normal subjects. This is supported by the fact that cirrhotic patients kept recumbent for 24 h exhibited greater sodium excretion than controls. This increased natriuresis was associated with lower plasma renin activity and increased plasma ANP levels[33].

Another difficulty with the 'peripheral arterial vasodilation' hypothesis is that the arterial blood volume cannot be directly measured. Indeed, detecting an underfilled arterial compartment is technically complex since total plasma volume tends to increase in cirrhotic patients. A recent technique has been used to measure central blood volume, defined as the blood volume in the heart cavities, lungs and central arterial tree[34]. Using this technique, central blood volume was found to be significantly reduced, despite an increased total plasma volume, in patients with cirrhosis as compared to controls.

NEUROHUMORAL RESPONSES INDUCED BY THE PERIPHERAL ARTERIAL VASODILATION

In decompensated cirrhotic humans and animals pharmacological blockade of angiotensin II, arginine vasopressin, and sympathetic nervous system, respectively by angiotensin II receptor antagonists or converting enzyme inhibitors, V_1-vasopressin antagonists and α-adrenergic antagonists, have been shown to decrease blood pressure[35–39].

The role of increased angiotensin II in sodium retention was investigated by pharmacological inhibition with saralasin, but the systemic hypotension induced in cirrhotic patients precludes any interpretation of changes in renal blood flow[35]. Moreover, when angiotensin II is infused to cirrhotic patients with ascites in doses sufficient to raise the renal perfusion pressure, urinary sodium excretion is greatly enhanced[40].

Although plasma aldosterone concentrations are frequently elevated in patients with decompensated cirrhosis, important differences have been reported in studies comparing normals to compensated and decompensated cirrhotic subjects[41–43]. Notable differences in sodium intake, plasma potassium concentrations, posture, diuretic treatment, and diurnal variation may explain the discordance in results between the studies. However, increased plasma aldosterone concentrations are mostly found in cirrhotic patients with ascites.

A correlation between plasma aldosterone and the severity of sodium retention is difficult to establish. Some investigators have assumed that, even if normal plasma aldosterone levels are measured, these levels are relatively high for the degree of plasma volume expansion observed in decompensated cirrhotic patients. Rosoff *et al.* administered aminoglutethimide (a potent inhibitor of adrenal steroid synthesis) to three patients with cirrhosis and ascites, and observed a persistence of avid sodium retention despite a profound decrease in plasma aldosterone[41]. Antagonism of the tubular action of aldosterone with a high dose of spironolactone, however, was associated with reversal of ascites over 3–4 weeks in 80–90% of patients[44]. Using HWI, Epstein *et al.* demonstrated that the suppression of plasma aldosterone was not associated with a natriuresis in half of the patients[31]. The natriuretic response to HWI, however, was greatly enhanced by spironolactone administration, thus suggesting that aldosterone contributes to the sodium retention in cirrhosis[45]. In contract to normal subjects, some cirrhotic patients fail to escape from the sodium-retaining effects of synthetic mineralocorticoid hormones. A recent study by La Villa *et al.* found that patients who failed to demonstrate mineralocorticoid escape had lower peripheral arterial resistance than patients who escaped[46]. As shown in Fig. 2, cirrhosis-induced peripheral arterial vasodilation activates many factors that decrease distal tubular sodium delivery[47]. In this regard, angiotensin II has been shown,

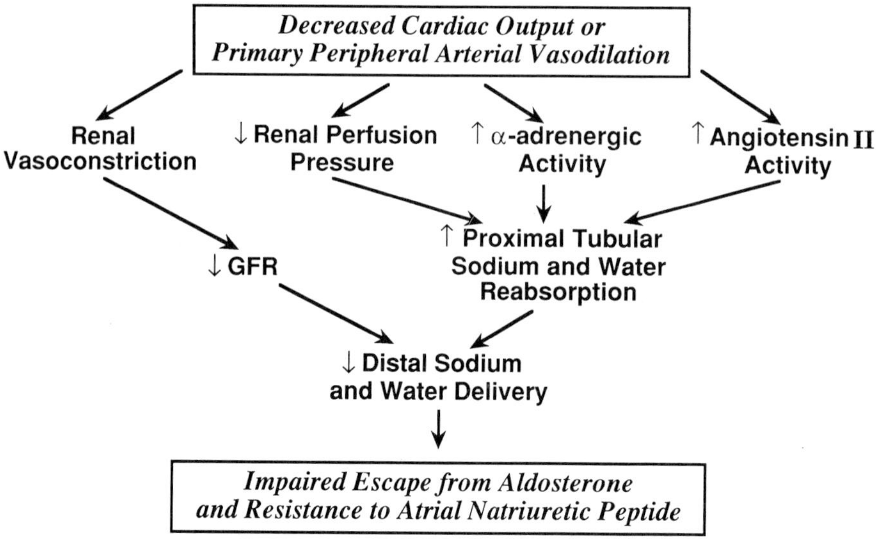

Fig. 2 Mechanisms whereby peripheral arterial vasodilation impairs aldosterone escape and causes resistance to atrial natriuretic factor by decreasing distal sodium delivery. (Modified from ref. 47 with permission)

along with adrenergic stimulation, to have a direct effect to increase sodium reabsorption in the renal proximal tubules[48]. It can therefore be proposed that the decrease in distal tubular sodium delivery induced by the diminished filtered load of sodium and the increased proximal tubular reabsorption in cirrhosis impairs the escape from the sodium-retaining effect of aldosterone. This mechanism has also been advocated to explain the renal unresponsiveness to ANP in cirrhotic patients. Indeed, plasma ANP levels are elevated in cirrhotic patients with ascites on a low-sodium diet as compared to normal subjects on the same diet[49–51]. However, decompensated cirrhotic patients have been constantly shown to be unresponsive to ANP infusions. Recent studies have demonstrated a restoration of the blunted response to ANP by renal denervation in cirrhotic rats[52]. Moreover, inverse relationships between baseline sympathetic nerve activity and the natriuretic response to ANP and between sympathetic nerve activity and lithium clearance have been shown, thus suggesting a decreased distal delivery of sodium in cirrhotic patients[53]. Since ANP, like aldosterone, acts in the collecting duct, distal sodium delivery can modulate its effect. Aldosterone therefore appears to have a pivotal role in the sodium retention of cirrhosis, and its effect is modulated by the rate of distal sodium delivery as influenced by the degree of peripheral vasodilation.

Renal water retention is a feature of cirrhotic patients with ascites; this inability to excrete water is best detected with an acute water load[23,54]. Decompensated cirrhotic patients are most likely to show an abnormal response to an oral water challenge. While Klinger *et al.* could not separate compensated from decompensated cirrhotic patients by assessing the renal water handling[54], Bichet *et al.* observed a much higher incidence of ascites in those cirrhotic patients with impaired water excretion[23,24]. Non-excretor patients were defined by their inability to excrete more than 80% of the load over 5 h. These non-excretors were shown to have higher plasma levels of arginine vasopressin, renin, aldosterone and norepinephrine. When HWI was performed in these patients, water and sodium excretion was consistently improved and arginine vasopressin, renin, aldosterone and norepinephrine were suppressed[25]. A complete normalization of sodium and water excretion occurred with HWI and the infusion of norepinephrine[27]. Since suppression of arginine vasopressin was similar with this combined manoeuvre as compared to HWI alone, the normalization of water excretion caused by HWI and norepinephrine infusion was probably caused by an increase in distal fluid delivery.

The impairment in renal water excretion in cirrhosis finds its clinical expression in hyponatraemia and hypo-osmolality in decompensated cirrhotic patients who have consistently elevated plasma arginine vasopressin levels[23,24]. These findings therefore suggest that non-osmotic release of arginine vasopressin, as mediated by an increased sympathetic stimulation through central adrenergic pathways, is a major factor in the water retention associated with cirrhosis. Plasma arginine vasopressin levels correlate in cirrhosis with plasma norepinephrine concentrations and with free water excretion[55]. When expansion of intravascular volume was achieved with HWI, Epstein *et al.*, however, found that, despite the improvement in water excretion, arginine vasopressin was not suppressed in all patients[56]. Due to low basal vasopressin levels reported in this study, however, the failure to demonstrate detectable suppression with HWI may be explicable by methodological difficulties. Bichet *et al.* showed that arginine vasopressin suppression could be obtained when non-excretor cirrhotic patients were examined, thus suggesting that the non-osmotic stimulation of arginine vasopressin was involved in the abnormal water excretion[25]. Because these patients often have a reduced glomerular filtration rate, water retention was considered to be induced both by arginine vasopressin and a diminished delivery of water to the distal tubule. Recent studies performed in cirrhotic rats using a V_2-vasopressin receptor antagonist demonstrated, however, that the renal water excretion could be normalized[57], thus suggesting a primary role for vasopressin. The use of effective V_2-vasopressin antagonists in human cirrhosis has to be attempted.

In patients with cirrhosis and ascites, increased renal norepinephrine release was demonstrated by measuring renal arterial and venous concentrations of this catecholamine[58,59]. Bichet *et al.* also found a negative correlation between plasma norepinephrine and urinary sodium excretion[24]. HWI has been shown to suppress plasma norepinephrine in cirrhotic patients in association with increased sodium excretion[26]. Lumbar sympathetic blockade has also been shown to increase sodium excretion in cirrhotic patients[60]. In cirrhotic models, renal denervation increases the sodium excretion[61]. The difference between normal and cirrhotic animals is best found in studies conducted in animals on a low dietary sodium intake[62]. Recently Simon *et al.* also found a greater increase in plasma norepinephrine concentration in cirrhotic than in normal humans during sodium restriction[63]. These findings are therefore most compatible with activation of the above compensatory mechanisms in response to arterial underfilling, even though total plasma volume is expanded.

SODIUM AND WATER RETENTION: RELATION TO THE PORTAL HYPERTENSION

Many investigators have attempted to find a relationship between hepatic haemodynamics and renal sodium retention. Obstruction to hepatic venous outflow with portal hypertension and a positive sodium balance are recognized as the principal factors in the pathogenesis of ascites formation. The role of portal hypertension is supported by the disappearance of ascites which can occur following portacaval anastomosis even when abnormal renal sodium retention persists[17]. Other studies, as reported above, support the primary role of a neural hepatorenal reflex in early sodium and water retention in cirrhosis. However, in human studies the degree of sodium retention is weakly correlated with portal pressure[64] and no relationship to the degree of portosystemic shunting was found by Rector *et al.*[65]. In addition to the severity of hepatic damage, specific causes of the liver disease can influence sodium balance regulation. For example, in contrast to patients with alcohol-induced cirrhosis, patients with primary biliary cirrhosis manifest less renal avidity for sodium despite comparably severe portal hypertension. Chaimovitz *et al.* have demonstrated that the diuretic and natriuretic responses to a sodium chloride load in patients with primary biliary cirrhosis exceeded those observed in both healthy volunteers and patients with a compensated alcohol-induced cirrhosis, perhaps secondary to the renal effect of greater bile salt accumulation[66].

POTENTIAL CAUSES OF PERIPHERAL ARTERIAL VASODILATION AND ARTERIAL UNDERFILLING

Many factors have been suggested as being involved in the pathogenesis of the peripheral arterial vasodilation in cirrhosis. Since peripheral arteriovenous fistulae are known to induce peripheral arterial vasodilation and renal sodium retention[67], it has been suggested that cirrhosis-induced vasodilation is a result of the portosystemic shunts and arteriovenous fistulae which appear in splanchnic, pulmonary, muscular and cutaneous vascular beds during the evolution of the cirrhotic process[68]. Although venovenous and arteriovenous shunts in cirrhosis are in part responsible for the increased vascular capacity, they generally complicate the later stages of cirrhosis and thus are unlikely factors in the initiation of the sodium and water retention.

It has been suggested that the early vasodilation observed in experimental models of cirrhosis reflects the release of a vasodilatory substance in response to a stimulus induced by the liver cirrhosis, and that progression of the hepatic disease is associated with a further increase in the release of the vasodilator(s). Vasoactive intestinal peptide[69,70], false neurotransmitters[71,72], calcitonin gene-related peptide[73], glucagon[74,75], platelet-activating factor[76], prostaglandins[77–80] and bradykinin[81] have been considered as potential factors in cirrhosis-induced vasodilation but no definitive conclusions have been reached. HWI in cirrhotic patients was shown to produce an increase in ANP secretion which could explain the further increase in peripheral arterial vasodilation observed during this manoeuvre[82]. However, the importance of ANP in the systemic vasodilation observed in cirrhotic patients has yet to be demonstrated, particularly since some investigators suggest a vascular unresponsiveness to ANP in cirrhosis[53]. ANP by its ability to shift fluid from the intravascular to the interstitial space may also be involved in oedema formation in cirrhosis[83].

Nitric oxide (NO)

A recent hypothesis suggests that increased NO synthesis in response to chronic endotoxaemia could explain the peripheral arterial vasodilation in cirrhosis[84]. Indeed, NO is a potent vasodilator produced by the action of a family of enzymes, the nitric oxide synthases[85] (NOS), on the amino acid L-arginine. Endothelial cells express a constitutive isoform of this enzyme[86–89] and may also express an inducible one[90–92]. The inducible isoform is ubiquitous and may be expressed in different cell types, like macrophages and vascular smooth muscle cells. It can be induced by a large number of substances, particularly by endotoxin[93–95] and cytokines[96–98]. The effect of NOP is mediated by a stimulation of the soluble guanylate cyclase leading to the formation of cyclic guanosine monophosphate (cGMP)[99]. Urinary cGMP was shown to be increased in cirrhotic patients and was not always associated with increased plasma ANP levels[100]. This is an important observation relative to the role of NO, since cGMP is the secondary messenger of both NO and of ANP[101]. Controversial results have, however, been obtained when endotoxin was measured in the portal and systemic circulation of healthy and cirrhotic subjects; these inconsistencies are probably explained by methodological differences[102]. Additionally, the levels of cytokines, like tumour necrosis factor-α, are increased in the plasma of cirrhotic patients[103,104], further suggesting that induction of the NOS is likely. NO was shown to play a role in the control of the splanchnic circulation of chronic portal hypertensive rats, but no effect on the hyperdynamic circulation was observed by Iwata *et al.*[105]. Pizcueta *et al.*, however, described an attenuation of the hyperdynamic circulatory state using NO inhibitors[106]. The absence of effect on systemic circulation observed by Iwata *et al.*[105] could be explained by the fact that the portal vein ligation does not induce endotoxaemia, at least during the early stages[107]. Recent studies using NO inhibitors in cirrhotic rats tend to support a role for NO in the arterial hypotension[108]. Further studies are, however, necessary to confirm the role of NO in the cirrhosis-induced vasodilation.

Endothelin

This recently described peptide[109,110] is the most powerful vasoconstrictor known, and was found to be released by endothelial cells when stimulated by endotoxin[111]. The levels of endothelin are increased in patients with cirrhosis, and very high levels are reached when these patients develop the hepatorenal syndrome[112]. The action of this peptide could account for the differential vasoconstriction seen in certain vascular beds (e.g. renal, portal) despite generalized vasodilation. The reason for these vascular systems reacting differently is unclear, but could include different regional levels of the peptide, increased sensitivity to endothelin, synergism of concomitant vasoconstrictors (e.g. thromboxane) or relative deficiency of antagonistic vasodilators (e.g. prostacyclin or nitric oxide).

Angiotensin II

Studies with angiotensin II infusions have consistently shown a decreased pressor response in cirrhotic humans and animals, and this angiotensin resistance may be involved in the peripheral arterial vasodilation of cirrhosis[40,80]. Pretreatment of cirrhotic rats with an angiotensin-converting enzyme inhibitor (captopril) to reduce circulating angiotensin II failed to normalize the response to angiotensin II. Studies of angiotensin II binding by mesenteric artery smooth muscle showed that in cirrhotic animals receptor affinity for angiotensin II was significantly lower than in controls; receptor number, however, was significantly increased[80]. The total binding of angiotensin II by vascular receptors from cirrhotics was not different from that in controls, since the decrease in affinity was counterbalanced by the increase in receptor number. Prereceptor alterations[4], increased receptor occupancy[113], receptor down-regulation[114] and postreceptor abnormalities[80] are several possible explanations for these decreased pressor effects of angiotensin. A decreased pressor response to norepinephrine has also been obtained in cirrhosis but results are not uniform[40,80,115].

Local factors associated with peripheral arterial vasodilation also may explain why arterial underfilling is resistant to correction with volume expansion, even when colloids are used. Increased capillary leakage of water, electrolytes and albumin is related to an increase in capillary surface area and to an increase in capillary hydrostatic pressure associated with diminished resistance in precapillary arterioles[116]. Thus, the peripheral arterial vasodilation favours interstitial oedema formation, which in turn aggravates the arterial underfilling.

Accumulation of bile salts in cirrhosis has been shown to exert a negative inotropic effect on the heart[117]. Alcoholic cardiomyopathy also has a deleterious effect on cardiac function[118]. In both situations the expected increase in cardiac output in response to the peripheral vasodilation is attenuated, thus further diminishing arterial filling. In cirrhosis, when low systemic resistance was elevated to normal levels by intravenous administration of angiotensin II, pulmonary wedge pressures rose significantly; this observation indicated left ventricular dysfunction[119]. Moreover, after angiotensin II administration cardiac output in cirrhotic rats decreased by $\approx 10\%$, whereas in control animals it increased by $\approx 11\%$[120]. Renal blood flow was particularly impaired by angiotensin II in cirrhotic animals, whereas flow to muscles was maintained. In late stages of cirrhosis a decreased venous return caused by inferior vena caval compression by tense ascites may also decrease the cardiac preload and thus attenuate a compensatory increase in cardiac output[121].

SUMMARY

The 'peripheral arterial vasodilation' hypothesis most completely explains the clinical spectrum of cirrhosis ranging from compensated to decompensated to the hepatorenal syndrome (Fig. 3). As the systemic peripheral vasodilation increases, the neurohumoral responses to arterial underfilling are stimulated with resultant renal vasoconstriction, sodium and water retention. Hypoalbuminaemia and portal hypertension, as well as local effects of vasodilation at the capillary level, also contribute to ascites formation and peripheral oedema. The suppressed plasma renin activity and aldosterone concentrations and exaggerated natriuresis observed in some patients with early cirrhosis during HWI, and the supine position, probably indicate greater central translocation of fluid in these volume-expanded cirrhotic patients as compared to normal subjects. This interpretation is supported by the greater increases in ANP during HWI in these patients as compared to controls. The neurohumoral responses to arterial vasodilation in cirrhosis combine to decrease distal sodium and water delivery, an event which impairs escape from the sodium-retaining effects of aldosterone and causes resistance to the

	COMPENSATED CIRRHOSIS (NO ASCITES)	DECOMPENSATED CIRRHOSIS (ASCITES)	HEPATORENAL SYNDROME
Peripheral Arterial Vasodilation	↑	↑↑	↑↑↑
Plasma Hormones (AVP, Renin, Aldosterone, NE)	Normal	↑	↑↑
Plasma Volume	↑	↑↑	↑↑↑

Fig. 3 Stages of progression of cirrhosis. AVP, arginine vasopressin; NE, norepinephrine. *These normal plasma hormone concentrations are relatively elevated given the degree of plasma volume expansion. **The progressive renal sodium and water retention increases extracellular fluid, interstitial fluid, and plasma volume. However, the concomitant occurrence of hypoalbuminaemia in decompensated cirrhosis and hepatorenal syndrome may attenuate the degree of plasma volume expansion. (From Schrier RW. The edematous patient. In: Schrier RW, editor. Manual of nephrology. 3rd edn. Boston: Little, Brown; 1990:1–19)

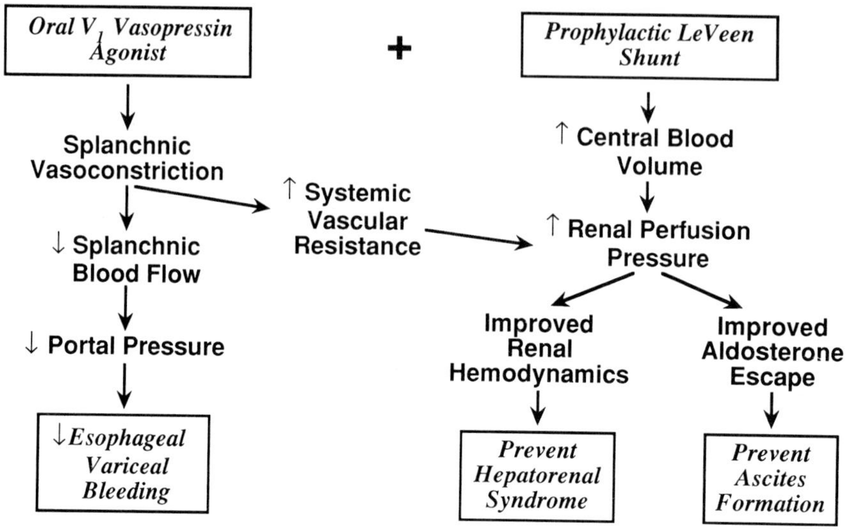

Fig. 4 Proposed future treatment strategy for decompensated cirrhosis. (From ref. 123 with permission)

distal tubular effect of ANP (Fig. 2). As discussed, the peripheral arterial vasodilation of cirrhosis is no doubt multifactorial in nature, and the resultant arterial underfilling may be worsened by events which impair the cardiac response to afterload reduction, including bile salt accumulation, alcoholic cardiomyopathy and tense ascites decreasing cardiac preload. This pathogenetic schema of cirrhosis is compatible with the unifying body fluid volume hypothesis (Fig. 1) which we have recently proposed[122,123]. In Fig. 4 is a proposed therapeutic strategy for the treatment of patients with cirrhosis, which is based on this pathogenetic schema. Such a therapeutic approach has the potential to decrease morbidity and mortality in cirrhosis[123].

ACKNOWLEDGEMENTS

The authors are grateful to Ms Norma Worland for manuscript preparation. Michel Niederberger is supported by a grant from the Swiss National Science Foundation.

References

1. Eisenmenger WJ, Blondheim SH, Bongiovanni AM, Kunkel HG. Electrolyte studies on patients with cirrhosis of the liver. J Clin Invest. 1950;29:1491–9.
2. Murray JF, Dawson AM, Sherlock S. Circulatory changes in chronic liver disease. Am J Med. 1958;24:358–67.
3. Mashford ML, Mahon WA, Chalmers TC. Studies of the cardiovascular system in the hypotension of liver failure. N Engl J Med. 1962;267:1071–4.

4. Lunzer MR, Newman SP, Bernard AG, Manghani KK, Sherlock SP, Ginsburg J. Impaired cardiovascular responsiveness in liver disease. Lancet. 1975;2:382–5.
5. Fernandez-Seara J, Prieto J, Quiuroga J, Zozaya JM, Cobos MA, Rodriguez-Eire JL, Garcia-Plaza A, Leal J. Systemic and regional hemodynamics in patients with liver cirrhosis and ascites with and without functional renal failure. Gastroenterology. 1989;97:1304–12.
6. Lieberman FL, Denison EK, Reynolds TB. The relationship of plasma volume, portal hypertension, ascites, and renal sodium retention in cirrhosis: the overflow theory of ascites formation. Ann NY Acad Sci. 1970;170:202–12.
7. Schrier RW, Arroyo V, Bernardi M, Epstein M, Henricksen JH, Rodes J. Peripheral arterial vasodilation hypothesis: a proposal for the initiation of renal sodium and water retention. Hepatology. 1988;8:1151–7.
8. Schrier RW. Pathogenesis of sodium and water retention in high-output and low-output cardiac failure, nephrotic syndrome, cirrhosis, and pregnancy. N Engl J Med. 1988;319:1065–72, 1127–34.
9. Papper S. The role of the kidney in Laennec's cirrhosis of the liver. Medicine. 1958;37:299–316.
10. Papper S, Rosenbaum JD. Abnormalities in the excretion of water and sodium in 'compensated' cirrhosis of the liver. J Lab Clin Med. 1950;40:523–30.
11. Levy M, Allotey JBK. Temporal relationships between urinary salt retention and altered systemic hemodynamics in dogs with experimental cirrhosis. J Lab Clin Med. 1978;92:560–9.
12. López-Novoa JM, Rengel MA, Hernando L. Dynamics of ascites formation in rats with experimental cirrhosis. Am J Physiol. 1980;238:F353–7.
13. Lieberman FL, Reynolds TB. Plasma volume in cirrhosis of the liver: its relation to portal hypertension, ascites, and renal failure. J Clin Invest. 1967;46:1297–308.
14. Lieberman FL, Ito S, Reynolds TB. Effective plasma volume in cirrhosis with ascites. Evidence that a decreased value does not account for renal sodium retention, a spontaneous reduction in glomerular filtration rate (GFR), and a fall in GFR during drug-induced diuresis. J Clin Invest. 1969;48:975–81.
15. Levy M. Sodium retention and ascites formation in dogs with experimental portal cirrhosis. Am J Physiol. 1977;233:F572–85.
16. Fernandez-Munoz D, Caramelo C, Santos JC, Blanchart A, Hernando L, López-Novoa JM. Systemic and splanchnic hemodynamic disturbances in conscious rats with experimental liver cirrhosis without ascites. Am J Physiol. 1985;249:G316–20.
17. Levy M, Wexler MJ. Renal sodium retention and ascites formation in dogs with experimental cirrhosis but without portal hypertension or increased splanchnic vascular capacity. J Lab Clin Med. 1978;91:520–36.
18. Levy M, Wexler MJ, McCaffrey C. Sodium retention in dogs with experimental cirrhosis following removal of ascites by continuous peritoneovenous shunting. J Lab Clin Med. 1979;94:933–46.
19. Unikowsky B, Wexler MJ, Levy M. Dogs with experimental cirrhosis of the liver but without intrahepatic hypertension do not retain sodium or form ascites. J Clin Invest. 1983;72:1594–604.
20. Levy M, Wexler MJ. Hepatic denervation alters first-phase urinary sodium excretion in dogs with cirrhosis. Am J Physiol. 1987;253:F664–71.
21. Kostreva DR, Castaner A, Kampine JP. Reflex effects of hepatic baroreceptors on renal and cardiac sympathetic nerve activity. Am J Physiol. 1980;238:R390–4.
22. Anderson RJ, Cronin RE, McDonald KM, Schrier RW. Mechanisms of portal hypertension-induced alterations in renal hemodynamics, renal water excretion, and renin secretion. J Clin Invest. 1976;58:964–70.
23. Bichet D, Szatalowicz V, Chaimovitz C, Schrier RW. Role of vasopressin in abnormal water excretion in cirrhotic patients. Ann Intern Med. 1982;96:413–17.
24. Bichet DG, Van Putten VJ, Schrier RW. Potential role of increased sympathetic activity in impaired sodium and water excretion in cirrhosis. N Engl J Med. 1982;307:1552–7.
25. Bichet DG, Groves BM, Schrier RW. Mechanisms of improvement of water and sodium excretion by immersion in decompensated cirrhotic patients. Kidney Int. 1983;24:788–94.
26. Nicholls KM, Shapiro MD, Van Putten VJ, Kluge R, Chung HM, Bichet DG, Schrier RW. Elevated plasma norepinephrine concentrations in decompensated cirrhosis. Association with increased secretion rates, normal clearance rates and suppressibility by central blood volume expansion. Circ Res. 1985;56:457–61.

27. Shapiro MD, Nicholls KM, Groves BM, Kluge R, Chung HM, Bichet DG, Schrier RW. Interrelationship between cardiac output and vascular resistance as determinants of effective arterial blood volume in cirrhotic patients. Kidney Int. 1985;28:206–11.
28. Nicholls KM, Shapiro MD, Kluge R, Chung HM, Bichet DG, Schrier RW. Sodium excretion in advanced cirrhosis: effect of expansion of central blood volume and suppression of plasma aldosterone. Hepatology. 1986;6:235–8.
29. Perez-Ayuso RM, Arroyo V, Camps J, Rimola A, Costa J, Gaya J, Rivera F, Rodes J. Renal kallikrein excretion in cirrhotics with ascites: relationship to renal hemodynamics. Hepatology. 1984;4:247–52.
30. Nicholls KM, Shapiro MD, Groves BS, Schrier RW. Factors determining renal response to water immersion in non-excreter cirrhotic patients. Kidney Int. 1986;30:417–21.
31. Epstein M, Levinson R, Sancho J, Haber E, Re R. Characterization of the renin-aldosterone system in decompensated cirrhosis. Circ Res. 1977;41:818–29.
32. Campbell PJ, Leung WM, Logan AG, Debowski TE, Blendis LM, Skorecki KL. Hyperresponsiveness to water immersion in sodium retaining cirrhotics: the role of atrial natriuretic factor. Clin Invest Med. 1988;11:392–5.
33. Trevisani F, Bernardi M, Gasbarrini A, Tame MR, Giancane S, Andreone P, Baraldini M, Cursaro C, Ligabue A, Gasbarrini G. Bed rest-induced hypernatriuresis in cirrhotic patients without ascites: does it contribute to maintain 'compensation'? J Hepatol. 1992;16:190–6.
34. Henricksen JH, Bendtsen F, Sorensen TIA, Stadeager C, Ring-Larsen H. Reduced central blood volume in cirrhosis. Gastroenterology. 1989;97:1506–13.
35. Schroeder ET, Anderson GH, Goldman SH, Streeten DHP. Effect of blockade of angiotensin II on blood pressure, renin and aldosterone in cirrhosis. Kidney Int. 1976;9:511–19.
36. Arroyo V, Bosch J, Mauri M, Ribera F, Navarro-López F, Rodes J. Effect of angiotensin-II blockade on systemic and hepatic haemodynamics and on the renin–angiotensin–aldosterone system in cirrhosis with ascites. Eur J Clin Invest. 1981;11:221–9.
37. Pariente EA, Bataille C, Bercoff E, Lebrec D. Acute effects of captopril on systemic and renal hemodynamcis and on renal function in cirrhotic patients with ascites. Gastroenterology. 1985;88:1255–9.
38. Claria J, Jimenez W, Arroyo V, La Villa G, López C, Asbert M, Castro A, Gaya J, Rivera F, Rodes J. Effect of V_1-vasopressin receptor blockade on arterial pressure in conscious rats with cirrhosis and ascites. Gastroenterology. 1991;100:494–501.
39. Epstein M, Berk DP, Hollenberg NK, Adams DF, Chalmers TC, Abrams HL, Merrill JP. Renal failure in the patient with cirrhosis. The role of active vasoconstriction. Am J Med. 1970;49:175–85.
40. Laragh JH, Cannon PJ, Bentzel CJ, Sicinski AM, Meltzer JI. Angiotensin II, norepinephrine, and renal transport of electrolytes and water in normal man and in cirrhosis with ascites. J Clin Invest. 1963;42:1179–92.
41. Rosoff L Jr, Zia P, Reynolds T, Horton R. Studies of renin and aldosterone in cirrhotic patients with ascites. Gastroenterology. 1975;69:698–705.
42. Wernze H, Spech HJ, Muller G. Studies on the activity of the renin-angiotensin-aldosterone system (RAAS) in patients with cirrhosis of the liver. Klin Wochenschr. 1978;56:389–97.
43. Bernardi M, De Palma R, Trevisani F, Santini C, Capani F, Baraldini M, Gasbarrini G. Chronobiological study of factors affecting plasma aldosterone concentration in cirrhosis. Gastroenterology. 1986;91:683–91.
44. Gregory PB, Broeckelschen PH, Hill MD, Lipton AB, Knauer CM, Egger M, Miller R. Complications of diuresis in the alcoholic patient with ascites: a controlled trial. Gastroenterology. 1977;73:534–8.
45. Epstein M, Pins DS, Schneider N, Levinson R. Determinants of deranged sodium and water homeostasis in decompensated cirrhosis. J Lab Clin Med. 1976;87:822–39.
46. La Villa G, Salmeron JM, Arroyo V, Bosch J, Gines P, Garcia-Pagan JC, Gines A, Asbert M, Jimenez W, Rivera F, Rodes J. Mineralocorticoid escape in patients with compensated cirrhosis and portal hypertension. Gastroenterology. 1992;102:2114–19.
47. Schrier RW, Better OS. Pathogenesis of ascites formation: mechanism of impaired aldosterone escape in cirrhosis. Eur J Gastro Hepatol. 1991;3:721–9.
48. Schuster VL, Kokko JP, Jacobson HR. Angiotensin II directly stimulates sodium transport in rabbit proximal convoluted tubules. J Clin Invest. 1984;73:507–15.

49. Campbell PJ, Skorecki KL, Logan AG, Wong PY, Leung WM, Greig P, Blendis LM. Acute effects of peritoneovenous shunting on plasma atrial natriuretic peptide in cirrhotic patients with massive refractory ascites. Am J Med. 1988;84:112–19.
50. Laffi G, Pinzani M, Meacci E, La Villa G, Renzi D, Baldi E, Cominelli F, Marra F, Gentilini P. Renal hemodynamic and natriuretic effects of human atrial natriuretic factor infusion in cirrhosis with ascites. Gastroenterology. 1989;96:167–77.
51. Gines P, Jimenez W, Arroyo V, Navasa M, López C, Tito L, Serra A, Bosch J, Sanz G, Rivera F, Rodes J. Atrial natriuretic factor in cirrhosis with ascites: plasma levels, cardiac release and splanchnic extraction. Hepatology. 1988;8:636–42.
52. Koepke JP, Jones S, DiBona GF. Renal nerves mediate blunted natriuresis to atrial natriuretic peptide in cirrhotic rats. Am J Physiol. 1987;252:R1019–23.
53. Morali GA, Floras JS, Legault L, Tobe S, Skorecki KL, Blendis LM. Muscle sympathetic nerve activity and renal responsiveness to atrial natriuretic factor during the development of hepatic ascites. Am J Med. 1991;91:383–92.
54. Klinger EL Jr, Vaamonde CA, Vaamonde LS, Lancestremere RG, Morosi HJ, Frisch E, Papper S. Renal function changes in cirrhosis of the liver. A prospective study. Arch Intern Med. 1970;125:1010–15.
55. Grossman SH, Davis D, Gunnells JC, Shand DG. Plasma norepinephrine in the evaluation of baroreceptor function in humans. Hypertension. 1982;4:566–71.
56. Epstein M, Weitzmann RE, Preston S, DeNunzio G. The relationship between plasma arginine vasopressin and renal water handling in decompensated cirrhosis. Miner Electrolyte Metab. 1984;10:155–65.
57. Claria J, Jimenez W, Arroyo V, Guarner F, López C, La Villa G, Asbert M, Rivera F, Rodes J. Blockade of the hydroosomotic effect of vasopressin normalizes water excretion in cirrhotic rats. Gastroenterology. 1989;97:1294–9.
58. Henricksen J, Ring-Larsen H, Kanstrup IL, Christensen NJ. Splanchnic and renal elimination and release of catecholamines in cirrhosis. Evidence of enhanced sympathetic nervous activity in patients with decompensated cirrhosis. Gut. 1984;25:1034–43.
59. Ring-Larsen H, Hesse B, Henricksen JH, Christensen NJ. Sympathetic nervous activity and renal and systemic hemodynamics in cirrhosis: plasma norepinephrine concentration, hepatic extraction, and renal release. Hepatology. 1982;2:304–10.
60. Solis-Herruzo JA, Duran A, Favela V, Castellano G, Madrid JL, Munoz-Yogue MT, Morillas JD, Estenoz J. Effects of lumbar sympathetic block on kidney function in cirrhotic patients with hepatorenal syndrome. J Hepatol. 1987;5:167–73.
61. Chaimovitz C, Massry SG, Friedler RM, Coburn JW. Effect of renal denervation and α-adrenergic blockade on sodium excretion in dogs with chronic ligation of the common bile duct. Proc Soc Exp Biol Med. 1974;146:764–70.
62. DiBona GF, Sawin LL. Role of renal nerves in sodium retention of cirrhosis and congestive heart failure. Am J Physiol. 1991;260:R298–305.
63. Simon MA, Diez J, Prieto J. Abnormal sympathetic and renal response to sodium restriction in compensated cirrhosis. Gastroenterology. 1991;101:1354–60.
64. Wood LJ, Massie D, McLean AJ, Dudley FJ. Renal sodium retention in cirrhosis: tubular site and relation to hepatic dysfunction. Hepatology. 1988;8:831–6.
65. Rector WG Jr, Lewis F, Robertson AD, Everson GT. Renal sodium retention complicating alcoholic liver disease: relation to portosystemic shunting and liver function. Hepatology. 1990;12:455–9.
66. Chaimovitz C, Rochman J, Eidelman S, Better OS. Exaggerated natriuretic response to volume expansion in patients with primary biliary cirrhosis. Am J Med Sci. 1977;274:173–8.
67. Epstein FH, Post RS, McDowell M. The effect of an arteriovenous fistula on renal hemodynamics and electrolyte excretion. J Clin Invest. 1953;32:233–41.
68. Dal Palu C, Donaggio G, Dal Zotto I, Pessina AC. Arteriovenous shunts in cirrhotic patients studied with human serum albumin macroaggregates tagged with I^{131} (MMA ^{131}I). Scand J Gastroenterol. 1968;3:425–31.
69. Henricksen JH, Staun-Olsen P, Borg Mogensen N, Fahrenkrug J. Circulating endogenous vasoactive intestinal polypeptide (VIP) in patients with uraemia and liver cirrhosis. Eur J Clin Invest. 1986;16:211–16.
70. Calam J, Unwin RJ, Dorudi S, Taylor C, Springer CJ, Peart WS. Effects of vasoactive intestinal polypeptide infusions on renal function in patients with liver disease. Clin Exp

Pharmacol Physiol. 1988;15:491–5.
71. Fischer JE, Baldessarini RJ. False neurotransmitters and hepatic failure. Lancet. 1971;2:75–80.
72. Thornton JR, Dean H, Losowsky MS. Is ascites caused by impaired hepatic inactivation of blood borne endogenous opioid peptides? Gut. 1988;29:1167–72.
73. Bendtsen F, Schiffer S, Henricksen JH. Increased circulating calcitonin gene-related peptide (CGRP) in cirrhosis. J Hepatol. 1991;12:118–23.
74. Marco J, Diego J, Villanueva ML, Diaz-Fierros M, Valverde I, Segovia JM. Elevated plasma glucagon levels in cirrhosis of the liver. N Engl J Med. 1973;289:1107–11.
75. Romeo JM, López Farré A, Martin-Paredero V, López-Novos JM. A role for glucagon in the splanchnic and systemic hemodynamic changes induced by portal-systemic blood shunting. Clin Physiol Biochem. 1990;8:144–52.
76. Caramelo C, Fernandez-Gallardo S, Santos JC, Inarrea P, Sanchez-Crespo M, López-Novoa JM, Hernando L. Increased levels of platelet-activating factor in blood from patients with cirrhosis of the liver. Eur J Clin Invest. 1987;17:7–11.
77. Hamilton G, Phing RCF, Hutton RA, Dandona P, Hobbs KEF. The relationship between prostacyclin activity and pressure in the portal vein. Hepatology. 1982;2:236–42.
78. Hashizume M, Inokuchi K, Tanaka K. The role of prostacyclin in patients with portal hypertension. Liver. 1985;5:89–93.
79. Zipser RD, Hoefs JC, Speckart PF, Zia PK, Horton R. Prostaglandins: modulators of renal function and pressor resistance in chronic liver disease. J Clin Endocrinol Metab. 1979;48:895–900.
80. Murray BM, Paller MS. Decreased pressor reactivity to angiotensin II in cirrhotic rats. Evidence for a post-receptor defect in angiotensin action. Circ Res. 1985;57:424–31.
81. Wong PY, Talamo RC, Williams GH. Kallikrein-kinin and renin–angiotensin systems in functional renal failure of cirrhosis of the liver. Gastroenterology. 1977;73:1114–18.
82. Epstein M, Loutzenhiser R, Norsk P, Atlas S. Relationship between plasma ANF responsiveness and renal sodium handling in cirrhotic humans. Am J Nephrol. 1989;9:133–43.
83. Epstein M. Atrial natriuretic factor in patients with liver disease. Am J Nephrol. 1989;9:89–100.
84. Vallance P, Moncada S. Hyperdynamic circulation in cirrhosis: a role for nitric oxide? Lancet. 1991;337:776–8.
85. Lowenstein CJ, Snyder SH. Nitric oxide, a novel biologic messenger. Cell. 1992;70:705–7.
86. Marsden PA, Schappert KT, Chen HS, Flowers M, Sundell CL. Wilcox JN, Lamas S, Michel T. Molecular cloning and characterization of human endothelial nitric oxide synthase. FEBS Lett. 1992;307:287–93.
87. Lamas S, Marsden PA, Li GK, Tempest P, Michel T. Endothelial nitric oxide synthase, molecular cloning and characterization of a distinctive constitutive enzyme isoform. Proc Natl Acad Sci USA. 1992;89:6348–52.
88. Janssens SP, Shimouchi A, Quertermous T, Bloch DB, Bloch KD. Cloning and expression of a cDNA encoding human endothelium-derived relaxing factor/nitric oxide synthase. J Biol Chem. 1992;267:14519–22.
89. Sessa WC, Harrison JK, Barber CM, Zeng D, Durieux ME, D'Angelo DD, Lynch KR, Peach MJ. Molecular cloning and expression of a cDNA encoding cell endothelial nitric oxide synthase. J Biol Chem. 1992;267:15274–6.
90. Radlomski NW, Palmer RMJ, Moncada S. Glucocorticoids inhibit the expression of an inducible, but not the constitutive, nitric oxide synthase in vascular endothelial cells. Proc Natl Acad Sci USA. 1990;87:10043–7.
91. Lamas S, Michel T, Brenner BM, Marsden PA. Nitric oxide synthesis in endothelial cells: evidence for pathway induced by TNF-alpha. Am J Physiol. 1991;261:C634–41.
92. Mulsch A, Bassenge E, Busse R. Nitric oxide synthesis in endothelial cytosol: evidence for a calcium-dependent and a calcium-independent mechanism. Naunyn-Schmiedeberg's Arch Pharmacol. 1989;340:767–70.
93. Julou Schaeffer G, Gray GA, Fleming I, Schott C, Parrat JR, Stoclet JC. Loss of vascular responsiveness induced by endotoxin involves L-arginine pathway. Am J Physiol. 1990;259:H1038–43.
94. Beasley D, Cohen RA, Lewinsky NG. Endotoxin inhibits contraction of vascular smooth muscle *in vitro*. Am J Physiol. 1990;258:H1187–92.
95. Weigert AL, Schini VB, Vanhoutte PM. Lipopolysaccharide causes relaxation of the rat aorta by inducing the L-arginine–nitric oxide pathway in smooth muscle. FASEB J. 1991;5:86.

96. Busse R, Mulsch A. Induction of nitric oxide synthase by cytokines in vascular smooth muscle cells. FEBS Lett. 1990;275:87–90.
97. Schini VB, Junquero DC, Scott-Burden T, Vanhoutte PM. Interleukin I-beta induces the production of an L-arginine-derived relaxing factor from cultured smooth muscle cells from rat aorta. Biochem Biophys Res Commun. 1991;176:114–21.
98. Beasley D, Schwartz JF, Brenner BM. Interleukin 1 induces prolonged L-arginine dependent cyclic guanosine monophosphate and nitrite production in rat vascular smooth muscle. J Clin Invest. 1991;87:602–8.
99. Gruetter CA, Bary BK, Gruetter DY, Kadowitz PJ, Ignarro LJ. Relaxation of bovine coronary artery and activation of arterial guanylate cyclase by nitric oxide, nitroprussate and carcinogenic nitrosamine. J Cyclic Nucleotide Res. 1979;5:211–24.
100. Miyase S, Fujiyama S, Chikazawa H, Sato T. Atrial natriuretic peptide in liver cirrhosis with mild ascites. Gastroenterol Jpn. 1990;25:356–62.
101. Leitman DC, Agnost VL, Tuan JJ, Andresen JW, Murad F. Atrial natriuretic factor and sodium nitroprusside increase cyclic GMP in cultured rat lung fibroblasts by activating different forms of guanylate cyclase. Biochem J. 1987;244:69–74.
102. Bourgoignie JJ, Valle GA. Endotoxin and renal dysfunction in liver disease. In: Epstein M, editor. The kidney in liver disease. 3rd edn. Baltimore: Williams & Wilkins; 1998:486–507.
103. Yoshioka K, Kakumu S, Arao S, Tsutsumi Y, Inoue M. Tumor necrosis factor-alpha production by peripheral blood mononuclear cells of patients with chronic liver disease. Hepatology. 1989;10:769–73.
104. Deviere J, Content J, Denys C, Vandenbussche P, Schandene L, Wybran J, Dupont E. Excessive *in vitro* bacterial lipopolysaccharide-induced production of monokines in cirrhosis. Hepatology. 190;11:628–34.
105. Iwata F, Joh T, Kawai T, Itoh M. Role of EDRF in splanchnic blood flow of normal and chronic portal hypertensive rats. Am J Physiol. 1992;263:G149–54.
106. Pizcueta MP, Pique JM, Bosch J, Whittle BJR, Moncada S. Effects of inhibiting nitric oxide biosynthesis on the systemic and splanchnic circulation of rats with portal hypertension. Br J Pharmacol. 1992;105:184–90.
107. Mehta R, Gottstein J, Zeller WP, Lichtenberg R, Blei AT. Endotoxin and the hyperdynamic circulation of portal vein-ligated rats. Hepatology. 1990;12:1152–6.
108. Claria J, Jimenez W, Ros J, Asbert M, Castro A, Arroyo V, Rivera F, Rodes J. Pathogenesis of arterial hypotension in cirrhotic rats with ascites: role of endogenous nitric oxide. Hepatology. 1992;15:343–9.
109. Yoshizawa T, Shinmi O, Giaid A, Yanagisawa M, Gibson SJ, Kimura S, Uchiyama Y, Polak JM, Masaki T, Kanazawa I. Endothelin: a novel peptide in the posterior pituitary system. Science. 1990;247:462–4.
110. Inoue A, Yanagisawa M, Kimura S, Kasuya Y, Miyauchi T, Goto K, Masaki T. The human endothelin family: three structurally and pharmacologically distinct isopeptides predicted by three separate genes. Proc Natl Acad Sci USA. 1989;86:2863–7.
111. Sugiura M, Inagami T, Kon V. Endotoxin stimulates endothelin release *in vivo* and *in vitro* as determined by radioimmunoassay. Biochem Biophys Res Commun. 1989;161:1220–7.
112. Moore KP, Wendon J, Frazer M, Gimson AES, Karani J, Williams R, Badr KF. Plasma endothelin levels in acute and chronic renal failure, chronic renal disease and hepatorenal syndrome. J Am Soc Nephrol. 1991;2:652.
113. Thurston H, Laragh JH. Prior receptor occupancy as a determinant of the pressor activity of infused angiotensin II in the rat. Circ Res. 1975;36:113–17.
114. Gerbes AL, Jungst D, Remieu J, Sauerbruch T, Paumgartner G. Evidence for down-regulation of β-2-adrenoreceptors in cirrhotic patients with severe ascites. Lancet. 1986;1:1409–11.
115. Kiel JW, Pitts V, Benoit JN, Granger DN, Shepherd AP. Reduced vascular sensitivity to norepinephrine in portal-hypertensive rats. Am J Physiol. 1985;248:G192–5.
116. Caramelo C, Fernandez-Munoz D, Santos JC, Blanchart A, Rodriguez-Puyol D, López-Novoa JM, Hernando L. Effect of volume expansion on hemodynamics, capillary permeability and renal function in conscious, cirrhotic rats. Hepatology. 1986;6:129–34.
117. Binah O, Rubinstein I, Bomzon A, Better OS. Effects of bile acids on ventricular muscle contraction and electrophysiological properties: studies in rat papillary muscle and isolated ventricular myocytes. Naunyn Schmiedebergs Arch Pharmacol. 1987;335:160–5.

118. Rubin E. Alcoholic myopathy in heart and skeletal muscle. N Engl J Med. 1979;301:28–33.
119. Limas CJ, Guiha NH, Lekagul O, Cohn JN. Impaired left ventricular function in alcoholic cirrhosis with ascites. Ineffectiveness of ouabain. Circulation. 1974;49:755–60.
120. Fernandez-Munoz MD, Villamediana LM, Blanchart A, Caramelo C, Hernando L, López-Novoa JM. Haemodynamic effects of angiotensin II in conscious, non-ascitic cirrhotic rats. Clin Physiol Biochem. 1988;6:36–43.
121. Guazzi M, Polese A, Magrini F, Fiorentini C, Olivari MT. Negative influence of ascites on the cardiac function of cirrhotic patients. Am J Med. 1975;59:165–70.
122. Schrier RW. Body fluid volume regulation in health and disease: a unifying hypothesis. Ann Intern Med. 1990;113:155–9.
123. Schrier RW. An odyssey into the milieu intérieur: pondering the enigmas. J Am Soc Nephrol. 1992;2:1549–59.

7

Treatment of ascites

J. RODES, V. ARROYO and P. GINES

The most important factors in the mechanism involved in the pathogenesis of ascites are portal hypertension and renal sodium and water retention[1]. The development of ascites carries a bad prognosis among cirrhotic patients and it constitutes one of the most indicative signs for hepatic transplantation in these patients. In the past few years several studies have investigated the survival and prognostic factors in cirrhotics with ascites indicating that systemic and renal haemodynamic alterations and renal function are even better predictors than liver function tests. In fact, mean arterial pressure lower than 82 mmHg, marked renal sodium retention (urinary sodium excretion < 10 mEq/day), low glomerular filtration rate (< 50 ml/min) and very high plasma levels of renin and norepinephrine are the most important factors in predicting survival (Table 1)[2].

Treatment of ascites is directed to eliminating the intra-abdominal fluid by increasing urinary excretion of water and sodium and/or through

Table 1 Prognostic factors in hepatic cirrhosis with ascites

Clinical parameters		
Liver function	*Renal function*	*Haemodynamic and hormonal parameters*
Previous ascites	Glomerular filtration rate	Mean arterial pressure
Previous encephalopathy	Serum creatinine	Plasma renin activity
Hepatomegaly	BUN	Plasma norepinephrine concentration
Nutritional status	Plasma sodium concentration	
Serum bilirubin	Urinary sodium excretion	
Serum albumin	Urinary potassium excretion	
Serum gamma globulin	Urinary osmolality	
Protein concentration in ascitic fluid		

paracentesis. This chapter comprises an overview of diuretic treatment, paracentesis and peritoneovenous shunt.

LOW-SODIUM DIET AND BED REST

The standard position in cirrhotics with ascites is associated with an intense activation of the renin–angiotensin–aldosterone and sympathetic nervous systems, a reduction of glomerular filtration rate and urinary sodium excretion, and a decrease in response to loop diuretics. Therefore, it seems rational to believe that bed rest could be beneficial in the management of patients with ascites[3].

The main goal of medical treatment of ascites is the mobilization of intra-abdominal fluid by producing a negative sodium balance. This can be achieved simply by reducing sodium intake in the diet (40–60 mEq/day). Approximately 20% of the cirrhotic patients with ascites are able to spontaneously excrete relatively high amounts of sodium in the urine (more than 40 mEq/day). In these patients ascites may be eliminated with only bed rest and low-sodium diet. The remaining 80% of the patients require diuretic therapy to increase urinary sodium excretion to over their sodium ingestion, thereby achieving a net negative sodium balance. Patients receiving diuretics with a positive response without decreasing ascitic volume are probably not following the correct diet[3].

DIURETICS

Cirrhotic patients with ascites are mainly treated with distal diuretics, principally spironolactone and loop diuretics, especially furosemide. Pharmacological studies have clearly demonstrated that loop diuretics are the most powerful, impairing sodium reabsorption in the ascending limb of the loop of Henle and a high dose may increase urinary sodium excretion to up to 30% of filtered sodium. This response is principally related to the inhibitory effect on the specific cotransport system (Na^+–2Cl–K^+ transport) localized in the luminal membrane of the epithelial cells in the ascending limb of the loop of Henle[4]. Spironolactone and other distal diuretics (triamterene, amyloride) are less powerful than loop diuretics. Spironolactone inhibits sodium reabsorption in the collecting tubule by antagonizing the action of aldosterone; therefore, it is particularly effective in those patients with hyperaldosteronism[5]. The administration of spironolactone is more useful than loop diuretics. In fact, loop diuretics alone in cirrhotic patients with ascites show a satisfactory response in only 50% of patients without renal failure[6]. In contrast, spironolactone increases urinary sodium excretion in most of these patients.

Loop diuretics have a rapid effect. The maximum diuretic response is obtained within the first 1–2 h and decreases at 3–4 h after administration.

On the contrary, the natriuretic effect of spironolactone is much slower, since following its administration there is a latent period of 3–4 days. The simultaneous administration of furosemide and spironolactone may increase the diuretic effect of both drugs. In addition, this association may reduce the incidence of hypokalaemia or hyperkalaemia when these agents are administered alone[7]. The therapeutic schedule recommended may be to start with 100 mg/day of spironolactone. In patients lacking good response the dose should be increased to 200 mg/day in association with 40 mg/day of furosemide. In patients not responding to these doses after 4–5 days, the dose should progressively increase up to 160 mg/day of furosemide and 400 mg/day of spironolactone. Patients not responding to this therapeutic schedule should be considered as having ascites refractory to diuretic therapy. Most patients with this lack of response present functional renal failure. After the disappearance of ascites the doses of diuretics should be individually adjusted to maintain the patients free of fluid retention[3].

About 11–70% of cirrhotic patients treated with diuretics develop complications[8]; about 20% of the patients present with renal failure due to a depletion of intravascular volume. This diuretic-induced renal failure is moderate and is always reversible after suppression of the drug. Peripheral oedema is more easily reabsorbed than ascitic fluid. This explains why diuretic-induced renal failure is less frequent in patients with ascites and oedema than in those with ascites alone. In this latter group of patients a loss of more than 500 g body weight per day is not advisable, otherwise the excess loss of body weight may lead to hypovolaemia and consequently renal failure. Hyperkalaemia and/or metabolic acidosis may be seen in those patients receiving high doses of spironolactone, particularly in those with functional renal failure. Hyponatraemia, occasionally important, is another usual complication of the diuretic regime[9]. Finally, diuretics may induce the development of hepatic encephalopathy by mechanisms still poorly understood (Table 2)[10].

Table 2 Diuretics most commonly used in the treatment of ascites

	Dosage (mg/day)	*Secondary effects*	*Comments*
Spironolactone	100–400	Gynaecomastia Hyperkalaemia Metablic acidosis	May induce hyperkalaemia in patients with functional renal failure
Furosemide	20–160	Hypokalaemia Encephalopathy Muscular cramps Metabolic acidosis	Combine with spironolactone Treatment with quinidine
Amyloride	5–10	Hyperkalaemia Metabolic acidosis	Alternative to spironolactone when there is painful gynaecomastia
Triamterene	100–300	Hyperkalaemia	May be useful only in patients with moderate sodium retention

PERITONEOVENOUS SHUNT

This technique was introduced in 1974. This prosthesis consists of a multiple perforated intra-abdominal tube connected to a one-way pressure-sensitive valve which, in turn, connects to a silicone tube traversing the subcutaneous tissue up to the neck. It is introduced into the superior vena cava, through the internal jugular vein near the right atrium. The valve is maintained open when intra-abdominal pressure is greater than 3–5 cm H_2O of the right atrium pressure. In these circumstances the ascitic fluid flows towards the intravascular compartment, achieving a continuous expansion of plasma volume[11]. This technique produces a marked increase of plasma volume and cardiac output, and inhibitis renin, aldosterone, norepinephrine and antidiuretic hormone concentrations, therefore leading to an increase in diuresis, natriuresis and free water clearance. It has been shown that the glomerular filtration rate and renal plasma flow of patients with functional renal failure increase. The latter is considered essential to increase the natriuretic effect of diuretics in patients with refractory ascites[12].

Unfortunately, the peritoneovenous shunt is associated with complications, some being very severe[13–18]. The most important are bacterial infections, particularly *Staphylococcus aureus*, although its incidence has significantly diminished upon the routine use of preoperative prophylactic antibiotic therapy. Other severe complications include pulmonary oedema and gastrointestinal bleeding due to rupture of oesophageal varices. These complications are due to the massive passage of ascitic fluid which suddenly increases plasma volume. These two complications may be prevented by the evacuation of ascitic fluid preoperatively, or during surgery before shunt insertion.

Disseminated intravascular coagulation is observed in practically every cirrhotic patient treated with this procedure. However, it is important to point out that this complication is fortunately a laboratory finding. Patients with clinical manifestations of disseminated intravascular coagulation are very uncommon. These laboratory changes include a decrease in plasma fibronogen and platelet concentrations, prolongation of prothrombin, partial thromboplastin and thrombin times, and a rise in the plasma levels of fibrin and fibrinogen degradation products. It is considered that the mechanism of disseminated intravascular coagulation is due to the passage of tissue thromboplastin and clotting factors plasminogen activators, endotoxin, fibrin split products, and collagen to the general circulation from the ascitic fluid. This could also be prevented by elimination of ascitic fluid prior to surgery.

The most frequent complication of peritoneovenous shunt is obstruction of the prosthesis[12,13]. This is observed among 30–40% of patients during the first year. The obstruction may be due to thrombosis of the superior vena cava, thrombosis of the venous limb of the prosthesis or deposition of fibrin in the valve or around the intravenous catheter. Although thrombosis of the superior vena cava is usually incomplete, total obstruction may occur producing a superior vena cava syndrome. Furthermore, this vascular thrombosis may also produce pulmonary embolism. Shunt occlusion is followed, although not necessarily, by reaccumulation of ascitic fluid. The diagnosis of this complication may be made by Doppler ultrasonography or by $^{99}Tc^{m}$ scintigraphy after intraperitoneal radioisotope injection. If the obstruction is confirmed, a shuntogram should be performed after the injection of contrast medium into the proximal subcutaneous limb of the shunt to identify the site of occlusion. It has been suggested that the insertion of a titanium tip into the venous end of the shunt may prevent thrombotic obstruction[12]; however, this requires further controlled clinical trials. Finally, another unsolved complication is the development of peritoneal fibrosis induced by the intra-abdominal segment of the prosthesis leading to intestinal obstruction. The aetiology of this complication is unknown. Although the peritoneovenous shunt was initially thought to be an excellent therapy for cirrhotic patients with ascites, the evidence of development of the above-mentioned complications has recently led to the consideration that this procedure may be useful only in very selected patients, particularly in those with preserved hepatic function and refractory ascites. Moreover, it is well established that the peritoneovenous shunt does not improve the survival of patients with cirrhosis and ascites[14].

PARACENTESIS

Paracentesis is the oldest treatment of ascites and an easy way to compensate these patients. This technique was abandoned at the end of the 1950s upon the introduction of diuretics, mainly spironolactone. At that time it was considered that paracentesis had a high rate of complications, such as systemic haemodynamic and renal function alterations, electrolyte disturbances and hepatic encephalopathy. However, this assumption was never substantiated by carefully controlled prospective investigations.

Several prospective studies have recently been published re-evaluating the usefulness of therapeutic paracentesis in the management of patients with cirrhosis and ascites. The first study consisted of a controlled trial comparing repeated large-volume paracentesis (4–6 l/day) until disappearance of ascites plus intravenous albumin infusion (40 g after each tap) with standard diuretic therapy in 117 patients with tense ascites and avid sodium retention admitted to several hospitals in the Barcelona area[19,20]. Patients with severe liver impairment (hepatic encephalopathy, serum bilirubin of over 10 mg/dl, and prothrombin activity less than 40%) or overt renal failure (serum creatinine greater than 3 mg/dl) were excluded. The results of this study demonstrated that:

1. Paracentesis was more effective than diuretics in eliminating ascites.
2. Paracentesis plus intravenous albumin infusion did not induce significant changes in hepatic and renal function, serum electrolytes, and cardiac output, plasma volume, plasma renin activity and plasma concentration of noradrenaline and antidiuretic hormone in the whole group of 58 patients treated with this technique, or in the subgroup of patients with moderate functional renal failure or without peripheral oedema.

3. The incidence of hyponatraemia, renal impairment, and hepatic encephalopathy was significantly lower in patients treated with paracentesis than in those treated with diuretics.
4. The duration of hospital stay was lower in the paracentesis group.
5. There were no significant differences in the probability of readmission of patients to hospital during follow-up, causes of readmission, probability of survival, and causes of death between the two groups of patients.

These results were later confirmed in a similar trial performed in Milan[20].

The next randomized controlled trial, also from the Barcelona group, aimed at establishing whether intravenous albumin infusion is necessary in cirrhotic patients treated with large-volume paracentesis, also confirmed the efficacy and safety of this technique[21]. In this study the incidence of hyponatraemia, renal impairment and hepatic encephalopathy in the group of 52 patients treated with repeated large-volume paracentesis plus intravenous albumin infusion was lower than in that reported in patients treated with diuretics. In this group of patients the mobilization of ascites by paracentesis associated with intravenous albumin infusion was also not associated with significant changes in renal and hepatic function and hormonal levels. In contrast, the incidence of these complications (hyponatraemia and renal impairment) in the group of 53 patients treated with repeated large-volume paracentesis without intravenous albumin infusion was significantly higher. In all these patients the mobilization of ascites was associated with a marked increase in the plasma levels of renin, indicating impairment in systemic haemodynamics. A subsequent investigation by Simon *et al.*[22] confirmed that complete mobilization of ascites by large-volume paracentesis without intravenous albumin infusion increases the activity of the renin–angiotensin system and impairs renal and systemic haemodynamics. Recent studies have demonstrated that the administration of Dextran-70 and Haemaccel 5%, less expensive plasma volume expanders, may substitute albumin infusion[23]. These studies have shown that large-volume paracentesis associated with intravenous infusion of Dextran or Haemaccel is not associated with significant changes in renal and hepatic function. The incidence of hyponatraemia, renal impairment and hepatic encephalopathy in patients receiving Dextran or Haemaccel was comparable to patients receiving albumin. Recently, Cabrera *et al.*[24] have shown that large-volume paracentesis associated with intravenous isotonic saline solution may be an alternative therapy for tense ascites. In this study it was demonstrated that plasma renin activity and plasma aldosterone concentration do not increase after this procedure, indicating that intravenous isotonic saline solution prevents the development of effective hypovolaemia. If this is confirmed by further studies, the procedure may be a less expensive alternative treatment of tense ascites in cirrhotic patients. It is important to point out that patients treated with paracentesis should be discharged from hospital with diuretics to avoid the reaccumulation of ascitic fluid. Tító *et al.*[25] investigated whether ascites could be safely mobilized in 38 patients by total paracentesis (complete removal of ascites in a single paracentesis session) plus intravenous albumin infusion (6–8 g per litre of ascitic fluid removed). The aim of the study was to assess if cirrhotic patients with tense ascites could be treated in a 1-day hospitalization regime. A mean of 10.7 l was removed in approximately 1 h, with no significant changes being observed in renal and hepatic function or in the plasma levels of noradrenaline, renin, and aldosterone over a period of 6 days during which patients were hospitalized without diuretics. In this series of patients the incidence of hyponatraemia, renal impairment and hepatic encephalopathy (3.0% and 1.0% respectively) as well as the clinical course of the disease, estimated by the probability of survival, and causes of deaths, were comparable to those reported by the same group in patients treated with large-volume paracentesis.

A multicentre randomized study carried out in Spain has recently been reported, in which repeated large-volume paracentesis associated with intravenous albumin infusion was compared with LeVeen shunt[26]. The study included 89 patients with refractory ascites (no response to 400 mg/day of spironolactone and 160 mg/day of furosemide) or recidivant ascites (more than three episodes of ascites within 9 months despite adequate diuretic therapy). Thirty-three patients had renal failure. Forty-one patients received treatment with paracentesis while 48 received the LeVeen shunt and were subsequently discharged from hospital with diuretics to avoid reaccumulation of ascites. The mobilization of ascites was effective with both types of treatments. Hospital stay was significantly shorter in the paracentesis group than in the LeVeen shunt group, whereas there were no significant differences with regards to the proportion of patients who developed complications during hospitalization or the number of deaths between the two groups. During follow-up 37 patients in each group were rehospitalized. In the paracentesis group the number of rehospitalizations for any reason or for ascites was significantly higher, and the median time to a first readmission for any reason, or for ascites, was significantly shorter than in the peritoneovenous shunt group. The total numbers of times in hospital during follow-up, however, were similar in the two groups. Three patients had shunt obstruction during their first hospitalization and 15 patients had a total of 20 obstructions during follow-up. The probability of shunt obstruction 1 year after the insertion of the prosthesis was 40%. This aspect is very important, since shunt obstruction may require reoperation. The conclusion of this trial was that the LeVeen shunt and paracentesis are equally effective in relieving refractory ascites, although the former may provide better long-term control of ascites but shunt occlusion is common and survival is not improved.

Paracentesis is a simple procedure, although several precautions should be considered to avoid complications. The procedure should be performed under strict sterile conditions. The skin of the abdomen should be disinfected and draped in a sterile manner. Sterile gown, gloves, cap, and mask should be used by the physician during the entire procedure. The use of a modified Kuss needle is advised. This needle consists of a sharp-pointed blind-metal needle within a 7 cm long 17 gauge metal blunt-edged cannula with side-holes. The needle is inserted in the left lower abdominal quadrant under local anaesthesia. Afterwards the inner part of the needle is removed and the cannula is connected to a large-volume capacity suction pump. The duration of the procedures ranges from 20 to 90 min, depending on the amount of ascitic fluid removed. In patients submitted to total paracentesis the total procedure is finished when the flow from the cannula becomes intermittent despite gentle mobilization of the cannula within the abdominal cavity and turning the patient to the left side. After paracentesis patients should recline for 2 h on the side opposite to the paracentesis site to prevent leakage of ascitic fluid. The intravenous administration of albumin or other plasma volume expanders should be initiated immediately after the procedure. Following the mobilization of ascites peripheral oedema rapidly reabsorbs in most patients, and usually disappears within the first 2 days after treatment. Most of the peripheral oedema goes to the intraperitoneal cavity, therefore it is not uncommon for patients with peripheral oedema to require a second paracentesis to remove the fluid shifted from the interstitial space to the intraperitoneal compartment.[27]

THERAPEUTIC SCHEDULE OF ASCITES

In summary the following schedule for ascites may be considered[28].

1. Patients with tense ascites: bed rest, low-sodium diet (40 mEq/day). If there is no response, total paracentesis associated with intravenous albumin infusion (6–8 g of albumin per litre of ascitic fluid removed) is indicated. After paracentesis, spironolactone may be initiated (100–400 mg/day) plus furosemide (20–160 mg/day). In patients with a positive response the doses of diuretics should be adjusted with individual response. Patients not responding to the high dose of diuretics should be considered as patients with refractory ascites.
2. Patients with slight or moderate ascites: bed rest, low-sodium diet (40 mEq/day). If there is no response, spironolactone (100–200 mg/day). In patients with positive response the doses of diuretics should be individually adjusted. In patients not responding to spironolactone alone, furosemide (40–160 mg/day) should be added. In patients responding to this diuretic regime the doses should be individually adjusted. Patients with negative response should be considered as patients with refractory ascites.
3. Patients with refractory ascites: patients should receive bed rest and low-sodium diet. The first choice of treatment should be total paracentesis associated with albumin infusion (6–8 g of albumin per litre of ascitic fluid removed); after paracentesis patients should be treated with spironolactone (300–400 mg/day) plus furosemide (120–160 mg/day). If there is re-accumulation of ascitic fluid repeated paracentesis is required. Perito-neovenous shunting should be considered with patients with frequent episodes of tense ascites.

References

1. Schrier RW, Arroyo V, Bernardi M *et al.* Peripheral arterial vasodilation hypothesis: a proposal for the initiation of renal sodium and water retention in cirrhosis. Hepatology. 1988;8:1151–7.
2. Llach J, Ginés P, Arroyo V *et al.* Prognostic value of arterial pressure, edogenous vasoactive

systems and renal function in cirrhosis with ascites. Gastroenterology. 1988;94:482–7.
3. Arroyo V, Rodés J. A rational approach to the treatment of ascites. Postgrad Med J. 1975;51:558–62.
4. Reeves WB, Molony DA. The physiology of loop diuretics. Sem Nephrol. 1988;8:225–33.
5. Horisberger JD, Giebisch G. Potassium-sparing diuretics. Renal Physiol. 1987;10:198–220.
6. Pérez-Ayuso RM, Arroyo V, Planas R *et al.* Randomized comparative study of efficacy of furosemide versus spironolactone in nonazotemic cirrhosis with ascites: relationship between the diuretic response and the activity of the renin-angiotensin-aldosterone system. Gastroenterology. 1983;84:961–8.
7. Roose LS, Underwook RH, Newmark SR, Kisch ES, Williams GH. Pathophysiology of spironolactone-induced gynecomastia. Ann Intern Med. 1977;87:398–403.
8. Strauss E, De Sa MF, Lacet CM, Cartapattida da Silva E, Regina do Santos W. Standardization of a therapeutic approach for ascites due to chronic liver disease: a prospective study of 100 cases. GED 1985;4:79–86.
9. Rodés J, Bosch J, Arroyo V. Clinical types and drug therapy of renal impairment in cirrhosis. Postgrad Med J. 1985;55:492–7.
10. Arroyo V, Bosch J, Casamitjana R *et al.* Use of piretanide, a new loop diuretic, in cirrhosis with ascites. Gut. 1980;21:855–9.
11. LeVeen HH, Christoudias B, Ip M *et al.* Peritoneovenous shunting for ascites. Ann Surg. 1974;180:580–5.
12. Smajda C, Franco D. The LeVeen shunt in the elective treatment of intractable ascites in cirrhosis. A prospective study on 140 patients. Ann Surg. 1985;201:488–93.
13. Bories P, Garcia Compean D, Michel H *et al.* The treatment of refractory ascites by the LeVeen shunt: a multi-centre controlled trial (57 patients). J Hepatol. 1986;3:212–18.
14. Stanley MM, Ochi S, Lee KK *et al.* Peritoneovenous shunting as compared with medical treatment in patients with alcoholic cirrhosis and massive ascites. N Engl J Med. 1989;321:1632–8.
15. Scholz DG, Nagomey DM, Londor KD. Poor outcome from peritoneovenous shunts for refractory ascites. Am J Gastroenterol. 1989;84:540–3.
16. Bemhoft RA, Pellegrini CA, Way LW. Peritoneovenous shunt for refractory ascites: operative complications and long-term results. Arch Surg. 1982;117:631–5.
17. Prokesch RC, Rimiand D. Infectious complications of the peritoneovenous shunt. Am J Gastroenterol. 1983;78:235–40.
18. Womser GP, Hubbard RC. Peritonitis in cirrhotic patients with LeVeen shunts. Am J Med. 1981;71:358–62.
19. Quintero E, Ginés P, Arroyo V *et al.* Paracentesis versus diuretics in the treatment of cirrhotics with tense ascites. Lancet. 1985;1:611–13.
20. Salerno F, Badalamenti S, Incerti P *et al.* Repeated paracentesis and IV albumin infusion to treat 'tense' ascites in cirrhotic patients: a safe alternative therapy. J Hepatol. 1987;5:102–8.
21. Ginés P, Tító LL, Arroyo V *et al.* Randomized comparative study of therapeutic paracentesis with and without intravenous albumin in cirrhosis. Gastroenterology. 1988;94:1493–502.
22. Simon DM, McCain JR, Bonkovky HL *et al.* Effects of therapeutic paracentesis on systemic and heaptic hemodynamics and on renal and hormonal function. Hepatology. 1987;7:423–9.
23. Planas R, Ginés P, Arroyo V *et al.* Dextran-70 versus albumin as plasma expanders in cirrhotic patients with tense ascites treated with total paracentesis: results of a randomized study. Gastroenterology. 1990;99:1–9.
24. Cabrera J, Inglada L, Quintero E *et al.* Large volume paracentesis and intravenous saline: effects on the renin–angiotensin system. Hepatology. 1991;14:1025–8.
25. Tító LL, Ginés P, Arroyo V *et al.* Total paracentesis associated with intravenous albumin in the management of patients with cirrhosis and ascites. Gastroenterology. 1990;98:146–52.
26. Ginés P, Arroyo V, Vargas V *et al.* Paracentesis with intravenous infusion of albumin as compared with peritoneovenous shunting in cirrhosis with refractory ascites. N Engl J Med. 1991;325:829–35.
27. Arroyo V, Ginés P, Jiménez W, Rodés J. Ascites, renal failure, and electrolyte disorders in cirrhosis: pathogenesis, diagnosis, and treatment. In: McIntyre N *et al.*, editors. Oxford textbook of clinical hepatology. Oxford: Oxford Medical Press; 1991:429–70.
28. Ginés P, Arroyo V, Rodés J. Pharmacotherapy of ascites associated with cirrhosis. Drugs. 1992;43:316–32.

Section II

Liver and nervous system

8

Encephalopathy in acute liver failure

P. FERENCI

The occurrence of brain dysfunction in patients with severe acute liver disease is the hallmark of fulminant hepatic failure. It is unknown whether the pathogenesis of brain dysfunction in acute liver disease differs from that in chronic liver diseases or not. In terms of clinical management, however, there are major differences.

Brain dysfunction in acute liver disease includes a potentially reversible metabolic encephalopathy (commonly referred to as 'hepatic encephalopathy', HE) which is complicated by the development of brain oedema in later stages (see Fig. 1). These two conditions are direct consequences of liver failure. However, fulminant liver failure is a disease which also affects other organs such as the cardiocirculatory system, the lungs and the kidneys, leading to

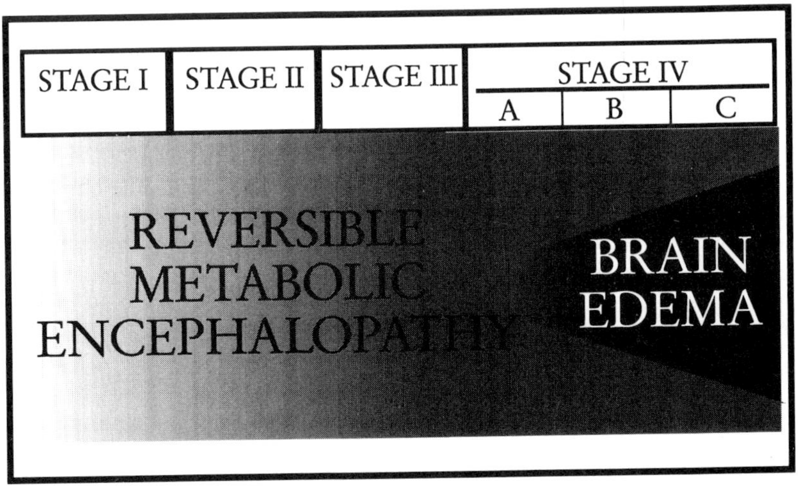

Fig. 1. Brain dysfunction in acute liver failure

conditions which by themselves may impair brain function (hypotension, hypoxaemia, uraemia). The outcome of the patients does not depend on the treatment of HE alone. However, in this chapter only HE and brain oedema will be discussed.

CLINICAL FEATURES AND DIAGNOSIS

Hepatic encephalopathy is a clinical diagnosis. No single laboratory test or electrophysiological examination can substitute for the careful clinical–neurological examination of the patient. The clinical features of HE include a wide range of neuropsychiatric symptoms ranging from minor not readily discernible signs of altered brain function, overt psychiatric and/or neurological symptoms to deep coma. It should be stressed, however, that none of these symptoms is specific for HE, and that the simultaneous presence of both neuropsychiatric symptoms and liver disease is not sufficient for the diagnosis of HE.

The simplest assessment of HE is to grade the mental state based on clinical findings. Several grading scales have been proposed. The most commonly used grading system is that of Parsons-Smith[1] with the modifications by Conn[2], which grades HE in stages I to IV and is based on changes in consciousness and intellectual function. In stages III and IV the Glasgow Coma scale is an additional useful clinical parameter.

Electroencephalography (EEG)

The evolving EEG changes associated with increasingly severe HE consist initially of a bilaterally synchronous decrease in wave frequency and an increase in wave amplitude, associated with the disappearance of readily discernible normal alpha-rhythm (8–13 c.p.s.). Preterminally, there is a loss of wave amplitude. Triphasic waves are characteristic paroxysmal waves in the EEG trace that often appear in stage III HE. Their presence is suggestive of the diagnosis of HE but triphasic waves have been described in several other encephalopathies and are not always present in HE. Thus, EEG assessment may not be sufficient for diagnosis of HE, but it may be particularly helpful when repeated EEG recordings are performed. A more refined assessment can be done using computer-assisted techniques of analysing the EEG that allow variables in the EEG to be quantitated, such as the mean dominant EEG frequency and the power of a particular EEG rhythm[3].

Evoked potentials

Evoked potentials are externally recorded potentials which reflect synchronous volleys of discharges through neuronal networks in response to various

Table 1 Multimodality evoked potentials for diagnosis of hepatic encephalopathy

	Discrimination between			
Method	*Controls and subclinical HE*	*Controls and clinical HE*	*Various stages of HE*	*Comments*
Flash-evoked VEPs	N3 latency	N3 latency waveform	Waveform	Reversible
Pattern-reversal VEPs	P100 latency	P100 latency	P100 latency in stages II to IV	Reversible, cannot be used
Somatosensory evoked potentials (late components)	?	N1–N3 interpeak latency	N1–N3 interpeak latency Loss of N3 in brain oedema	Reversible
Acoustic evoked potentials	—	—	—	
Event-related acoustic evoked potentials	P300	—	—	Cannot be used in stage II to IV

afferent stimuli. According to the type of the stimulus they are visual (VEPs), somatosensory (SEPs), or acoustic evoked (AEPs) responses. Table 1 lists the various methods used and their value in discriminating between normal subjects, patients with subclinical HE and between the various stages of clinical HE. Usually the latency of the various peaks occurring after the stimulus is measured. The late components of SEPs are useful for staging of clinical HE. The N1–N3 interpeak latency correlates with the clinical stage of HE[4]. In late stages of HE the SEP trace is not only quantitatively but also qualitatively different from a normal SEP trace. In particular P3 and N3 are lost in stage IV HE. The changes in SEPs are reversible and are useful to document effects of treatment in patients with HE[5]. Similarly, flash-evoked VEPs discriminate subclinical and clinical HE by prolongations of the N3 latency and changes in the waveform[6] but have a higher degree of variation than SEPs. Using even more sophisticated techniques such as event-related responses (i.e. the P300 wave) even subtle changes of brain function can be detected and used for diagnosis of subclinical HE[7].

Imaging techniques

A *CT scan* should be performed in every patient with HE to exclude other diseases associated with coma or confusion. For diagnosis of generalized or localized cerebral oedema CT scans are less sensitive than direct intracranial pressure monitoring[8].

NMR tomography seems to be superior to CT scans in diagnosing brain oedema and increased cerebral water content in liver failure. Furthermore, very typical changes have been observed on T1-weighted pictures with a strong signal in the basal ganglia, possibly reflecting severe metabolic changes[9]. By ^{1}*H-NMR spectroscopy* cerebral amino acid concentrations can be estimated *in vivo*.

Positron emission tomography offers the possibility to study *in vivo* certain neurotransmitter systems such as dopamine or benzodiazepine receptors. So far no systematic studies have been reported in HE. Furthermore ^{11}C-deoxyglucose may be helpful to study cerebral glucose oxidation *in vivo*.

Intracranial pressure monitoring

Increased intracranial pressure is a frequent complication of fulminant hepatic failure and is one of the important causes of death in these patients. By subdural pressure transducers intracranial pressure can be monitored continuously and this enables the physician to start specific treatment as early as possible[10]. However, continuous monitoring of intracranial pressure should be only performed in highly specialized centres and is currently not part of clinical routine.

PATHOGENESIS OF HEPATIC ENCEPHALOPATHY IN ACUTE LIVER FAILURE

The various hypotheses of the pathogenesis of HE are not mutually exclusive. Most likely many of the described abnormalities may be present at the same time, and may ultimately be responsible for the development of HE. The synergistic action of multiple toxins is well documented, and ammonia together with other toxins may account for many of the abnormalities occurring in liver failure, such as the changes in the blood to brain transport of neurotransmitter precursors, in the metabolism of amino acid neurotransmitters, and in cerebral glucose oxidation. These changes may lead to an activation of inhibitory (GABA, serotonin) and an impairment of excitatory (glutamate, catecholamines) neurotransmitter systems, resulting in an imbalance of neurotransmission towards increased neural inhibition.

Alterations of the blood–brain barrier

The term 'blood–brain barrier' describes complex physiological processes by which the brain is protected from metabolic changes in the body. The blood–brain barrier in mammals is located at the endothelial cells of the cerebral capillary. Because these cells are joined by tight junctions, substrates must pass through capillary endothelial cells to reach brain extracellular fluid. Transport depends on lipid solubility or on mediation by specific carriers present in the capillary cell membranes. Small molecules such as glucose or amino acids have distinct carrier systems. Large molecules such as proteins are completely excluded from the brain by the blood–brain barrier.

Blood–brain barrier function can be studied by the administration of substances which are normally not taken up by the brain, such as tryptophan-blue, sucrose, γ-aminoisobutyric acid or horseradish peroxidase. In several models of acute liver failure an increased brain uptake of these compounds was demonstrated. The breakdown of the normal blood–brain barrier is commonly observed in acute HE. The reason for this non-specific increase in blood–brain barrier permeability is unknown. An increased permeability of the blood–brain barrier will expose the brain to a variety of neurotoxic substances circulating in the blood, and may result in brain oedema (see later).

NEUROTOXINS

Ammonia (the ammonia hypothesis)

Ammonia is the best-characterized neurotoxin which may precipitate HE. In about 90% of patients with HE concentrations of ammonia are increased in arterial blood[11]. Furthermore, in certain inborn errors of the urea cycle, excessive hyperammonaemia is associated with encephalopathy. The increase in blood ammonia is a direct consequence of impaired liver function.

Ammonia interferes with brain function at several sites. It may induce changes of blood to brain transport of amino acids[12], metabolic changes resulting in decreased cerebral concentration of the excitatory amino acid neurotransmitter glutamate[13] and alterations of brain energy metabolism[13–15]. Furthermore, ammonia directly alters neuronal electric activity by inhibiting the generation both of excitatory and inhibitory postsynaptic potentials[15].

However, there are several shortcomings of the ammonia hypothesis of the pathogenesis of HE. Arterial ammonia levels are normal in about 10% of patients with HE but are increased also in many patients with chronic liver disease levels without signs of overt HE[11]. In animals administration of ammonium salts results in neurological symptoms different from HE. Initially an excitatory state is observed, and coma occurs only after seizure activity. Even these neurotoxic effects of ammonia occur only at ammonia concentrations which are substantially higher than those observed in humans with HE.

Mercaptans (the synergism hypothesis)

Mercaptans such as methanethiol and dimethyldisulphide are neurotoxic compounds derived from the catabolism of sulphur-containing amino acids.

Methanethiol can potentiate ammonia toxicity[17]. Accordingly, a synergism between methanethiol and ammonia may explain several shortcomings of the ammonia hypothesis. A similar synergism may exist between ammonia and other toxins such as short-chain fatty acids (C4 to C8) or phenolic compounds derived from the catabolism of tyrosine and phenylalanine[18]. Evaluation of this hypothesis in humans is hampered by methodological difficulties in the measurements of these toxins. Using a well-established assay blood levels of methanethiol are increased in patients with HE but are apparently of no major pathogenetic importance for the development of HE[19].

Impairment of neurotransmission

In the past two decades studies on the pathogenesis of HE have concentrated on possible changes in neurotransmission. Various methods have been applied including neurochemical and neurobehavioural studies (see Table 2). Each of these methods had been developed to study normal brain function and the action of certain drugs. It is uncertain whether these methods can also be applied to the study of abnormal brain function in certain diseases. There are important limitations for the interpretations of neurochemical data which cannot be discussed sufficiently in this chapter.

Table 2 Altered neurotransmission in hepatic encephalopathy

Neurotransmitter system	*Neurochemistry*	*Neurobehavioural studies*
$GABA_A$-benzodiazepine	Receptors ↑ (??) 'Endogenous' BZDs	Increased sensitivity to BZD agonists Improvement of HE by inverse agonists
Glutamate	Concentration ↓ (??) Receptors ↓ (??)	n.d.
Aspartate	Concentration ↑ Receptors ↓	n.d.
Noradrenaline	Concentration ↓ Metabolites ↑	n.d.
Dopamine	Concentration ⊥ Metabolites ⊥ Octopamine ↑	n.d.
Serotonin	Concentration ↑ Metabolites ↑↑	Improvement of HE by 5-HT antagonists
Acetylcholine	Unchanged	n.d.
Opiates	Concentration ↓	Improvement of HE by naloxone

n.d. = Not done, ↑ = increased, ↓ = decreased, ⊥ = unchanged, ?? = conflicting results

ACTIVATION OF GABA-ERGIC NEUROTRANSMISSION

Experimental observations

Neurobehavioural and neurophysiological observations have suggested an increased tone of the inhibitory $GABA_A$-benzodiazepine neurotransmitter system in liver failure. The postsynaptic $GABA_A$-benzodiazepine receptor is closely linked with two other receptor proteins, one for benzodiazepines and the other for picrotoxin. All of these receptor sites regulate a chloride ionophore. Influx of chloride ions into the postsynaptic neuron is followed by the generation of an inhibitory postsynaptic potential. GABA-mediated chloride fluxes can be augmented by benzodiazepines or barbiturates, thus these drugs increase GABA-mediated neural inhibition. Accordingly the similarities of changes of visual evoked potentials in rabbits and rats with HE and those induced in normal animals by drugs acting through the $GABA_A$-benzodiazepine receptor complex indicate a possible involvement of this neurotransmitter system in the pathogenesis of HE[20]. Rats with acute liver failure are more sensitive to the sedative effects of benzodiazepines than normal rats (see Fig. 2). In contrast, administration of antagonists of this receptor complex to animals with fulminant hepatic failure and HE led to a transient clinical improvement which was associated with a normalization of abnormal visual evoked potentials[21,22]. These observations can be readily explained by the presence of increased GABA-ergic tone in this syndrome.

The mechanisms causing the activation of the $GABA_A$-ergic neurotransmission are unknown. Schafer and Jones[23] suggested that gut-derived GABA accumulates in the blood and crosses an abnormally permeable blood–brain

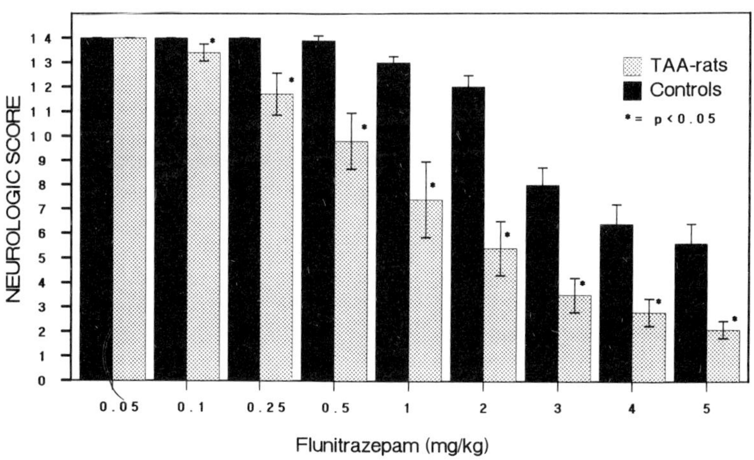

Fig. 2 Effect of the benzodiazepine agonist flunitrazepam on rats with thioacetamide (TAA)-induced liver failure and control rats. The experiments were carried out before development of clinically overt HE, 60 h after the first administration of TAA. Rats received increasing doses of flunitrazepam i.p. and were thereafter evaluated by a standardized clinical neurological examination (for details see ref. 25). A normal rat has a neurological score of 14, which decreases to 0 in surgical coma

barrier and interacts with 'supersensitive' postsynaptic GABA receptors. Subsequent studies yielded conflicting results regarding the status of postsynaptic GABA receptors in HE[24–28], the blood–brain permeability[29], and the increase of plasma and CSF GABA concentrations[30]. Baraldi and Zeneroli[31] attributed the supersensitivity of postsynaptic $GABA_A$-receptors to a degeneration of presynaptic GABA-ergic terminals mediated by some toxins, excess glutamate, or zinc deficiency[32]. So far no other study has reported that neuronal degeneration occurs in HE.

'Endogenous' benzodiazepines

Single-cell recordings from Purkinje neurons revealed an increased sensitivity in HE to the inhibitory effects of benzodiazepine agonists. In contrast, benzodiazepine antagonists augmented neuronal firing action in cerebella of rabbits with HE but not of control rabbits[33]. This effect may be explained by the displacement from the $GABA_A$-benzodiazepine receptor of a benzodiazepine-like ligand not present in normal brains. Such compounds were isolated, characterized and positively identified by gas chromatography–mass spectroscopy as benzodiazepines[34–37] in brains, sera and CSF of humans and experimental animals with liver failure. In humans the concentration of benzodiazepines was higher than in experimental animals with liver failure[36]. At least in animals the presence of benzodiazepines (including diazepam and desmethyl-diazepam) cannot be explained by exogenous benzodiazepine administration. In human studies the use of benzodiazepines prior to HE was carefully excluded[36]. Other sources of benzodiazepines may be plant[38] synthesis by gut bacteria[39].

The role of 'endogenous' benzodiazepines to induce HE may be addressed by neurobehavioural studies using benzodiazepine receptor ligands. They can be classified according to their effects on the chloride ionophore to three different classes. The first class are benzodiazepine agonists such as diazepam. They increase the affinity of GABA to its receptor and/or the coupling of the $GABA_A$ receptor to the chloride ionophore. The second type are inverse agonists such as β-carbolines. They decrease the affinity of GABA receptors and GABA-induced chloride fluxes. The third type of benzodiazepine ligands are antagonists. These drugs stabilize the benzodiazepine receptor in a neutral state and competitively antagonize the binding of other benzodiazepine ligands. Consequently antagonists tend to normalize changes in GABA-ergic tone induced by agonists or inverse agonists. However, most benzodiazepine receptor antagonists have intrinsic effects (partial agonistic (CGS 8216, Ro 15-4513, Ro 15-3505) or partial inverse agonistic (flumazenil). While flumazenil and 'pure' antagonists are ineffective in experimental HE, antagonists with partial inverse agonistic properties unequivocally improve various neurobehavioural features of HE[35,40–43]; see Table 3. This improvement can be blocked by the concomitant administration of 'pure' benzodiazepine antagonists. Thus, for the amelioration of HE the inverse agonistic effects seem to be more important than a displacement of endogenous benzodiazepine ligands

Table 3 Effect of benzodiazepine antagonists on experimental hepatic encephalopathy

Author	*Model*	*Ro 15-1788*	*Ro 15-3505*	*Ro 15-4503*	*CGS 8216*
Baraldi	Gln rat	n.t.	n.t.	n.t.	+++
Gammal	Gln rabbit	+++	+++	+++	n.t.
Steindl	TAA rat	–	+++	+++	n.t.
Bosman	LIS rat	0	+++	+++	n.t.
Zieve	HAL rat	n.t.	n.t.	n.t.	0

Gln: galactosamine; LIS: liver ischaemia; TAA: thioacetamide; +++ = improvement; – = worsening; 0 = no effect; n.t. = not tested

from the receptor. These observations do not support a direct role of 'endogenous' benzodiazepines in the pathogenesis of HE.

The beneficial effects on HE of benzodiazepine antagonist with partial inverse agonistic properties HE do not necessarily imply an overactivity of the $GABA_A$-benzodiazepine neurotransmitter system. Another possible explanation would be an imbalance of excitatory and inhibitory neurotransmission.

Imbalance of inhibitory and excitatory neurotransmission

The most likely affected excitatory neurotransmitter system in HE is the glutamate-ergic system[44]. Similar to other neurotransmitters glutamate is present in various compartments. Only glutamate present in the neuronal compartment is biologically active whereas glutamate in the glial compartment is an important metabolite and is intimately involved in ammonia fixation in the brain. Therefore it has been suggested that hyperammonaemia is associated with a depletion of cerebral glutamate, at least in the metabolic compartments[22]. ^{1}H-NMR spectroscopy in hyperammonaemic rats and in rats with acute liver failure following liver ischaemia confirmed the decrease in concentrations of glutamate and the increase of glutamine concentrations *in vivo*[45]. Although it is unknown whether this decrease also applies to neuronal glutamate these findings point to an imbalance of excitatory and inhibitory neurotransmission in HE. Besides its role as a neurotransmitter glutamate is a potent neurotoxin. Its neurotoxic properties are mediated by a subgroup of glutamate receptors, the kainic acid binding site. By brain dialysis an increased release of glutamate was documented in experimental hyperammonaemia[46]. In the early stages of liver failure this increased release of glutamate may induce seizures, and later neuronal degeneration.

Catecholamines

Noadrenaline and dopamine are important neurotransmitters in the mammalian brain. Noradrenergic neurons are found in most brain areas including the cerebral cortex and the hippocampus. Dopaminergic neurons are concentrated in certain ganglia such as the striatum or the nucleus accumbens. In other brain areas dopamine is present as the direct metabolic precursor of noradrenaline.

The finding of decreased noradrenaline concentrations in the brains of various animals with acute or chronic liver failure is fairly consistent. This decrease may be either due to decreased synthesis or to an increased release of noradrenaline. Recent measurements of concentration of precursors and metabolites of noradrenaline in various brain regions of rats with HE (see Fig. 3) indicate that the decreased brain noradrenaline content is the consequence of an overactivity of noradrenergic neurotransmission, possibly induced by hyperammonaemia[47]. In contrast, measurements of dopamine concentrations in various animal models yielded conflicting results. In most animal models of HE, and in the brains of humans with HE, the concentration of dopamine is within the normal range[47,48]. Thus, there is no firm evidence that impaired dopaminergic neurotransmission contributes to any appreciable extent to the development of HE.

Serotonin

Serotonin is an important neurotransmitter in many brain areas. In the reticular formation it regulates the cortical arousal reaction and thus may be important in the maintenance of consciousness and the regulation of the sleep–wake cycle. Therefore this neurotransmitter system is of particular interest for the study of HE. In all studies a 2–4-fold increased cerebral concentration of the serotonin metabolite 5-hydroxyindoleacetic acid, and in some a minor increase of serotonin itself was observed in HE[47] (for review see ref. 48). These findings indicate that in HE cerebral serotonin turnover is increased. It may be mediated by the increased availability of tryptophan (the precursor of serotonin). However, it is unknown whether increased serotonin turnover is also associated with increased serotoninergic function. The presence of an activated serotoninergic neurotransmission is supported by the observation that the serotonin antagonist methysergid improves the motor activity of rats with thioacetamide-induced liver failure and HE[49].

Altered brain energy metabolism

Undisturbed energy supply and energy metabolism is a prerequisite for normal brain function. Glucose is the most important cerebral energy fuel; to a small extent also ketones can be used by the brain. In terminal stages of liver failure hypoglycaemia may be present as a consequence of impaired hepatic gluconeogenesis, but administration of glucose is not sufficient to normalize brain function in HE. Several studies have addressed cerebral glucose utilization in HE. By quantitative autoradiography of brain slices following ^{14}C-deoxyglucose administration to rats with portacaval shunt Lockwood *et al.*[15] found a 74% increase of the glucose metabolic rate in the reticular formation and 12–18% in the cerebral cortex. A similar increase in glucose metabolism was observed following infusion of ammonia to normal

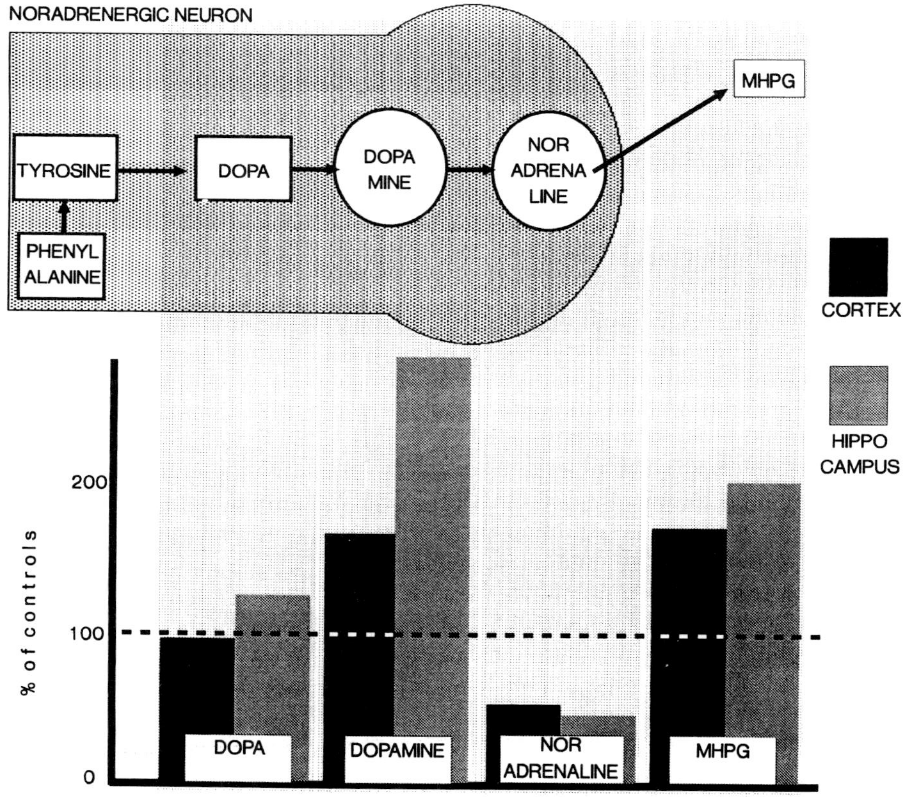

Fig. 3 Changes in the concentration of noradrenaline and of its metabolites in the cerebral cortex and the hippocampus of rats with hepatic encephalopathy. Data taken from Yurdaydin *et al.*[47]. MHPG = 3-methoxy-4-hydroxyphenylglycol

rats. Using an identical experimental design Mans *et al.*[14] reported exactly the opposite results, namely a 5–34% decrease of cerebral glucose utilization in 38 brain areas examined. These conflicting results can be explained by the different mathematical models used to quantitate cerebral glucose metabolism. The depression in cerebral metabolic rate of glucose caused by hyperammonaemia correlated more closely with glutamine, than with ammonia itself. Ammonia is without effect at concentrations of less than 1 mol/ml if it is not converted into glutamine. The deleterious effect of chronic hyperammonaemia seems to begin with the increased synthesis of glutamine[50]. Using ammonia intoxication as model of HE, Hindfelt *et al.*[13] found a major reduction of ATP levels in the reticular formation of comatose rats, indicating a marked impairment of brain energy metabolism. However, these changes were found only in agonal stages and may therefore represent final events unrelated to the evolution of encephalopathy. Clearly, more studies on brain energy metabolism in HE are needed, including new techniques such as positron emission tomography or ^{1}H-NMR spectroscopy.

PATHOGENESIS OF BRAIN OEDEMA IN FULMINANT HEPATIC FAILURE

This complication of hepatic failure is usually seen in patients who were already comatose due to advanced HE. Early recognition and treatment of this condition may considerably improve the outcome of patients. The pathogenesis of brain oedema in liver failure is not fully understood, but similar mechanisms may be responsible as for the occurrence of metabolic encephalopathy. Brain oedema can arise from two broad mechanisms. In vasogenic oedema a breakdown of the blood–brain barrier may lead to leak of plasma contents through an abnormally permeable capillary epithelium; in cellular (or cytotoxic) oedema, net intracellular water accumulation occurs as the result of impaired cellular osmoregulation. Both types may share molecular mechanisms at the endothelial cell level that differ in sequence and strength and thus make the distinction between cytotoxic and vasogenic oedema less precise. By electron microscopic examination of brain biopsy specimens both types of brain oedema were found in patients with fulminant hepatic failure but changes suggesting cytotoxic oedema (such as glial cell swelling) were more pronounced than signs of increased permeability of brain capillaries[51].

In liver failure four mechanisms were suggested to contribute to the development of brain oedema: inhibition of Na^{+}/K^{+} ATPase by toxic compounds with digoxin-like immunoreactivity present in the serum[52]; an increased permeability of the blood–brain barrier[53]; osmotic effects of glutamine and of other non-essential amino acids accumulating in the brain during liver failure[54]; and finally by a primary injury of astrocytes by toxins (ammonia, octanoic acid). Possibly all four conditions are present in liver failure. The osmotic effects by increased intracellular glutamine concentrations are of special relevance in acute liver failure: degree of increase in glutamine concentration in liver failure is similar to that in experimental hyperammonaemia[45] and seems to be direct consequence of cerebral ammonia fixation. Inhibition of glutamine synthetase prevented accumulation of glutamine and the increase in brain water content in dogs infused with ammonia[55].

TREATMENT OF BRAIN DYSFUNCTION IN ACUTE LIVER DISEASE

If patients with acute liver disease develop signs of HE they should be considered as candidates for orthotopic liver transplantation (Fig. 4)[56]. Since the decision has to be made within a short time a transplant centre should be notified immediately, and the patient should be referred to an intensive-care unit specializing in treatment of acute liver failure. Intensive-care management is aimed at stabilizing the patient until a donor liver becomes available, and emergency liver transplantation should be performed if the patient fails to improve.

Treatment of HE is only part of the intensive-care management of patients with fulminant liver failure. Patients should be carefully monitored for changes in cardiocirculatory function, respiration, metabolic parameters (hypoglycaemia, electrolyte imbalances) and any changes must be appropriately corrected. Sepsis must be vigorously watched for by daily cultures of biological fluids. Selective bowel decontamination and prophylactic antibiotic treatment may prevent septic complications. Various extracorporeal liver support systems have been proposed. They should be used only in clinical trials in experienced units. Direct intracranial pressure (ICP) monitoring with an extradural pressure transducer allows early diagnosis of increased ICP and prompt immediate treatment. For sustained increases in ICP above 25 mmHg for more than 5 min mannitol (0.5 g/kg body weight as a bolus over 10 min) should be given. Mannitol administration (up to a maximum

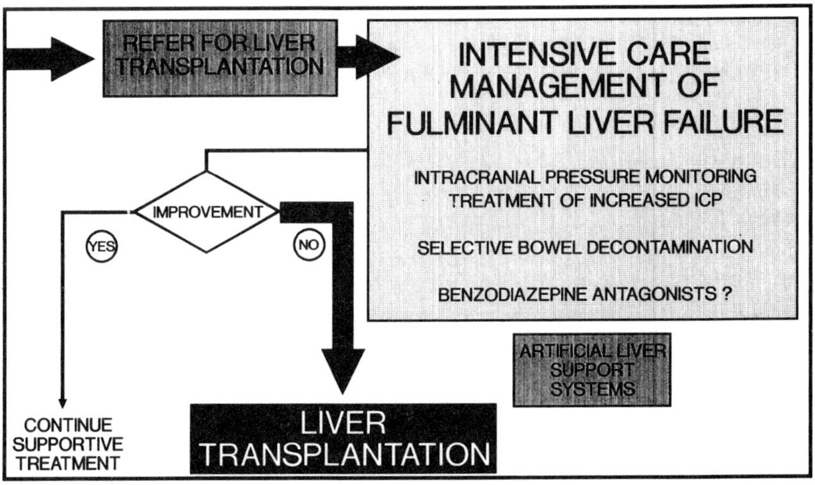

Fig. 4 Treatment of hepatic encephalopathy in acute liver failure

of 100 g) can be repeated in patients with stable renal function. In non-responders thiopental (initial 250–500 mg i.v. every 15 min, followed by a continuous infusion with 20–250 mg/h) can be tried[57].

None of the drugs commonly used for treatment of hepatic encephalopathy has been tested by randomized controlled trials in patients with acute liver failure. In most treatment protocols they were even excluded. The role of ammonia-lowering measures such as lactulose or non-absorbable antibiotics, or of amino acid infusions with high content in branched-chain amino acids is unknown. Benzodiazepine antagonists may be of value for symptomatic treatment of HE in acute liver failure.

In the largest study so far[5], the favourable response to 15 mg flumazenil infused intravenously over 3 h was similar in patients with fulminant hepatic failure or cirrhosis. The favourable clinical response was also documented by marked improvement of SEPs. In five of the eight episodes not reacting to flumazenil patients had marked signs of increased intracranial pressure due to brain oedema. One other potentially useful indication for flumazenil may be differentiation of benzodiazepine-induced coma from HE. Furthermore, prompt improvement by flumazenil may be a favourable prognostic sign[58]. Thus, flumazenil may be a valuable new therapeutic approach in patients with acute HE, but the efficacy of flumazenil treatment remains to be studied by appropriate trials. Furthermore, other benzodiazepines with better pharmacokinetic properties or other pharmacological profiles should be investigated.

References

1. Parsons-Smith BG, Summerskill WHJ, Dawson AM, Sherlock S. The electroencephalograph in liver disease. Lancet. 1957;2:867–71.
2. Conn HO, Lieberthal MM. The hepatic coma syndromes and lactulose. Baltimore: Williams & Wilkins; 1979.
3. Holm E, Krämer W, Reith HJ, Magin T, Mezitis NHE. Electrophysiological and psychometric studies in hepatic encephalopathy. In: Varro V, Balint GA, Creutzferdt W, editors: Current views in gastroenterology. 1977;I:597–613.
4. Yang SS, Chu NS, Liaw YF. Somatosensory evoked potentials in hepatic encephalopathy. Gastroenterology. 1985;89:625–30.
5. Grimm G, Ferenci P, Katzenschlager R *et al.* Improvement of hepatic encephalopathy treated with flumazenil. Lancet. 1988;2:1392–4.
6. Zeneroli ML, Pinelli G, Gollini G *et al.* Visual evoked potentials: a diagnostic tool for the assessment of hepatic encephalopathy. Gut. 1984;25:291–9.
7. Davies MG, Rowan MJ, McMathuina P *et al.* The auditory P300 event-related potential: an objective marker of the encephalopathy of chronic liver disease. Hepatology. 1990;12:688–94.
8. Munoz SJ, Robinson M, Northrup B *et al.* Elevated intracranial pressure and computed tomography of the brain in fulminant hepatic failure. Hepatology. 1991;13:209–12.
9. Zeneroli ML, Cioni G, Vezzalli C *et al.* Brain magnetic resonance imaging in liver cirrhosis patients with encephalopathy. J Hepatol. 1990;10(Suppl. 1):S28.
10. Martin P, Pappas SC. Fulminant hepatic failure. Dig Dis. 1990;8:138–51.
11. Stahl J. Studies of the blood ammonia in liver disease. Its diagnostic, prognostic and therapeutic significance. Ann Intern Med. 1963;58:1–24.
12. Grippon P, Le Poncin-Laffite M, Boschat M *et al.* Evidence for the role of ammonia in the intracerebral transfer and metabolism of tryptophan. Hepatology. 1986;6:682–6.
13. Hindfelt B, Plum F, Duffy TE. Effect of acute ammonia intoxication on cerebral metabolism

in rats with portocaval shunts. J Clin Invest. 1977;59:386–96.
14. Mans AM, Biebuyck JF, Davis DW, Bryan RM, Hawkins RA. Regional cerebral glucose utilization in rats with portocaval anastomosis. J Neurochem. 1983;40:986–91.
15. Lockwood AH, Ginsberg MD, Rhoades HM, Gutierrez MT. Cerebral glucose metabolism after portocaval shunting in the rat. Pattern of metabolism and implications for the pathogenesis of hepatic encephalopathy. J Clin Invest. 1986;78:123–31.
16. Raabe W. Neuronal effects of ammonia. In: Soeters P, Wilson JHP, Meijer AF, Holm E, editors. Advances in ammonia metabolism and hepatic encephalopathy. Amsterdam: Elsevier; 1988:349–55.
17. Zieve L, Doizaki WM, Zieve FJ. Synergism between mercaptanes and ammonia and fatty acids in the production of coma: a possible role for mercaptanes in the pathogenesis of hepatic coma. J Lab Clin Med. 1974;83:16–28.
18. Windus-Podehl G, Lyftogt L, Zieve L. Encephalopathic effect of phenol in rats. J Lab Clin Med. 1983;101:586–92.
19. Blom HJ, Ferenci P, Grimm G *et al.* The role of methanthiol in the pathogenesis of hepatic encephalopathy. Hepatology. 1991;13:376–9.
20. Schafer DF, Pappas SC, Brady LE, Jacobs R, Jones EA. Visual evoked potentials in a rabbit model of hepatic encephalopathy. I: Sequential changes and comparisons with drug induced comas. Gastroenterology. 1984;86:540–5.
21. Baraldi M, Zeneroli ML, Ventura E *et al.* Supersensitivity of benzodiazepine receptors in hepatic encephalopathy due to fulminant hepatic failure in the rat: reversal by a benzodiazepine antagonist. Clin Sci. 1984;67:167–75.
22. Bassett ML, Mullen KD, Skolnik P, Jones EA. Amelioration of hepatic encephalopathy by pharmacologic antagonists of the $GABA_A$-benzodiazepine receptor complex in a rabbit model of fulminant hepatic failure. Gastroenterology. 1987;93:1069–77.
23. Schafer DF, Jones EA. Hepatic encephalopathy and the γ-amino butyric acid neurotransmitter system. Lancet. 1982;2:18–19.
24. Ferenci P, Zieve L, Ebner J *et al.* Postsynaptic gamma-amino butyric acid receptors in hepatic coma following portacaval shunt and hepatic artery ligation in the rat. Metabol Brain Dis. 1987;2:195–200.
25. Zimmermann Ch, Ferenci P, Pifl Ch *et al.* Hepatic encephalopathy in thioacetamide-induced acute liver failure in rats: Characterization of an improved model and study of amino-acid-ergic neurotransmission. Hepatology. 1989;9:594–601.
26. Maddison JE, Dodd PR, Johnston GAR, Farrell GC. Brain GABA receptor binding is normal in rats with thioacetamide-induced hepatic encephalopathy despite elevated plasma GABA-like activity. Gastroenterology. 1987;93:1062–9.
27. Ferenci P, Riederer P, Jellinger K *et al.* Changes in cerebral receptors for gamma-aminobutyric acid in patients with hepatic encephalopathy. Liver. 1988;8:225–30.
28. Butterworth RF, Lavoie J, Giguere JF, Pomier Layrargues M. Affinities and densities of ^{3}H-muscimol ($GABA_A$) binding sites and of central benzodiazepine receptors are unchanged in autopsied brain tissue from cirrhotic patients with hepatic encephalopathy. Hepatology. 1988;8:1084–8.
29. Knudsen GM, Poulsen HE, Paulson OB *et al.* Blood brain barrier permeability in galactosamine induced hepatic encephalopathy: no evidence for increased GABA transport. J Hepatol. 1988;6:187–92.
30. Ferenci P, Ebner J, Zimmermann Ch *et al.* Overestimation of serum concentrations of gamma-aminobutyric acid (GABA) in patients with hepatic encephalopathy by the GABA-radioreceptor assay. Hepatology. 1988;8:69–72.
31. Baraldi M, Zeneroli ML. Experimental hepatic encephalopathy – changes in gamma-amino-butyric acid. Science. 1982;216:427–31.
32. Baraldi M, Caselgrandi E, Borella P, Zeneroli ML. Decrease of brain zinc in experimental hepatic encephalopathy. Brain Res. 1983;258:170–2.
33. Basile AS, Gammal SH, Mullen KD *et al.* Differential responsiveness of cerebellar Purkinje neurons to GABA and benzodiazepine receptor ligands in an animal model of hepatic encephalopathy. J Neurosci. 1988;8:2414–21.
34. Mullen KD, Martin JV, Mendelson WB. Could an endogenous benzodiazepine ligand contribute to hepatic encephalopathy? Lancet. 1988;1:457–9.
35. Basile AS, Pandl L, Jaouni T *et al.* Brain concentrations of benzodiazepines are elevated

in an animal model of hepatic encephalopathy. Proc Natl Acad Sci USA. 1990;87:5263–7.
36. Basile AS, Hughes RD, Harrison IM *et al.* Elevated brain concentrations of 1,4-benzodiazepines in fulminant hepatic failure. N Engl J Med. 1991;325:475–8.
37. Olasmaa M, Rothstein JD, Guidotti A *et al.* Endogenous benzodiazepine receptors ligands in human and animal hepatic encephalopathy. J Neurochem. 1990;55:2015–23.
38. Klotz U. Occurrence of 'natural' benzodiazepines. Life Sci. 1991;48:209–15.
39. Rothstein JD, Garland W, Puia G *et al.* The role of endogenous benzodiazepine receptor ligands in physiology and pathophysiology. In: Barnard EA, Costa E, editors. Transmitter amino acid receptors: structures, transduction and models for drug development. Stuttgart: Thieme Medical Publishers; 1991:325–39.
40. Bosman DK, Van den Buijs CACG, de Haan JG *et al.* Inverse benzodiazepine receptor agonists temporally restore hepatic encephalopathy in the rat. Gastroenterology. 1991;101:772–81.
41. Steindl P, Püspök A, Druml W, Ferenci P. Beneficial effect of pharmacological modulation of the $GABA_A$-benzodiazepine receptor on hepatic encephalopathy in the rat – comparison with uremic encephalopathy. Hepatology. 1991;14:963–8.
42. Gammal SH, Basile AS, Geller D *et al.* Reversal of the behavioural and electrophysiological abnormalities of an animal model of hepatic encephalopathy by benzodiazepine receptor ligands. Hepatology. 1990;11:371–8.
43. Zieve L, Ferenci P, Rzepczynski D, Ebner J, Zimmermann Ch. Benzodiazepine antagonist does not alter course of hepatic encephalopathy nor neural GABA binding. Metabol Brain Dis. 1987;2:201–5.
44. Ferenci P, Pappas SC, Munson PJ, Jones EA. Changes in glutamate receptors on synaptic membranes associated with hepatic encephalopathy or hyperammonemia in the rabbit. Hepatology. 1984;4:25–9.
45. Bosman DK, Deutz NEP, de Graaf AA *et al.* Changes in brain metabolism during hyperammonemia and acute liver failure: Results of a comparative ^{1}H-NMR spectroscopy and biochemical investigation. Hepatology. 1990;12:281–90.
46. Moroni F, Lombardi G, Moneti G, Cortesini C. The release and neosynthesis of glutamic acid are increased in experimental models of hepatic encephalopathy. J Neurochem. 1983;40:850–4.
47. Yurdaydin C, Hörtnagl H, Steindl P *et al.* Increased serotoninergic and noradrenergic activity in hepatic encephalopathy in rats with thioacetamide induced acute liver failure. Hepatology. 1990;12:695–700.
48. Bugge M. Brain monoamine metabolism in experimental hepatic encephalopathy. Thesis. Bulletin No. 65, Lund, Sweden: Department of Surgery, Lund University; 1987.
49. Yurdaydin C, Hörtnagl H, Pifl Ch *et al.* Modulation of hepatic encephalopathy in rats due to thioacetamide induced liver failure by serotonin agonists and antagonists. Gastroenterology. 1989;96:A675.
50. Hawkins RA, Jessy J. Hyperammonaemia does not impair brain function in the absence of net glutamine synthesis. Biochem J. 1991;277:697–703.
51. Kato M, Hughes RD, Keays RT, Williams R. Electron microscopic study of brain capillaries in cerebral edema from fulminant hepatic failure. Hepatology. 1992;15:1060–5.
52. Yang SS, Hughes RD, Williams R. Digoxin-like immunoreactive substances in severe acute liver disease due to viral hepatitis and paracetamol overdose. Hepatology. 1988;8:93–7.
53. Horowitz ME, Schafer DF, Molnar P *et al.* Increased blood brain transfer in a rabbit model of acute liver failure. Gastroenterology. 1983;84:1003–11.
54. Swain M, Butterworth R, Blei A. Brain aminoacids and brain edema in experimental acute liver failure. Hepatology. 1990;12:858.
55. Takahashi H, Koehler RC, Brusilow SW, Traystman RJ. Inhibition of brain glutamine accumulation prevents cerebral edema in hyperammonemic rats. Am J Physiol. 1991;261:H825–9.
56. Peleman RR, Gavaler JS, van Thiel DH *et al.* Orthotopic liver transplantation for acute and subacute hepatic failure in adults. Hepatology. 1987;7:484–9.
57. Forbes A, Alexander GJ, O'Grady JG *et al.* Thiopental infusion in the treatment of intracranial hypertension complicating fulminant hepatic failure. Hepatology. 1989;10:306–10.
58. Bansky G, Meier PE, Riederer E *et al.* Effects of the benzodiazepine receptor antagonist flumazenil in hepatic encephalopathy in humans. Gastroenterology. 1989;97:744–53.

9

Liver disorders and sensory function

W. VOGT and J. SCHÖLMERICH

INTRODUCTION

An impairment of sensory function is a well-known symptom with metabolic disorders such as diabetes mellitus. Patients with this disorder are regularly assessed for polyneuropathy or retinopathy. Most hepatologists consider liver disorders a metabolic disease. However, in contrast to other metabolic disorders most physicians will not look for any impairment of sensory functions in spite of the fact that this can be a problem of socioeconomic relevance, i.e. disturbed dark adaptation which may produce dangers in street traffic for the patient and others.

ZINC DEFICIENCY AND VITAMIN A DEFICIENCY WITH LIVER DISORDERS

The liver is a very important storage organ for vitamins and trace elements. Vitamin A is stored in the liver after intestinal absorption and transport with chylomicrons as retinylpalmitate, and can be distributed on demand as retinol into the circulation. A decreased vitamin A serum concentration has been found in patients with liver diseases independent of the aetiology[1,2]. Lieber and co-workers demonstrated a decreased vitamin A content of the liver in patients with alcoholic liver diseases which was correlated with the severity of organ damage. Besides malnutrition in alcoholics a further cause of this deficiency is malabsorption of the fat-soluble vitamins with cholestatic liver disease. Furthermore vitamin A release from the liver is dependent on the complex formation with retinol-binding protein (RBP), which in turn is zinc-dependent. Vallee *et al.* (1956) were the first to demonstrate zinc deficiency in patients with alcoholic liver cirrhosis which was also dependent on the severity of the disease[3]. This has since also been found for liver diseases of other aetiology[4–7]. A decreased intestinal absorption of zinc and an increased renal loss have been proposed as major causes. This, however, is not undisputed[8–10]. The increased renal clearance is a consequence of decreased hepatic zinc extraction. There is a correlation between urinary zinc loss and the presence of portosystemic shunts (Fig. 1).

Zinc and vitamin A are involved in numerous regulatory mechanisms in the human organism. There is a close relationship between zinc metabolism and vitamin A metabolism, which is evident from zinc-dependent vitamin A release from the liver. A further example is the fact that the enzyme responsible for the production of retinal pigment from retinol, namely retinoldehydrogenase, is a zinc-dependent metalloenzyme. In addition to this impairment of dark adaptation a number of other symptoms, in particular disturbances of taste and hearing, can occur with zinc and/or vitamin A deficiency.

DARK ADAPTATION

As early as 1939 Patek could demonstrate a disturbed dark adaptation in 19 out of 24 patients with liver cirrhosis of different aetiology independently of the presence of cholestasis (Fig. 2). Oral or parenteral application of high

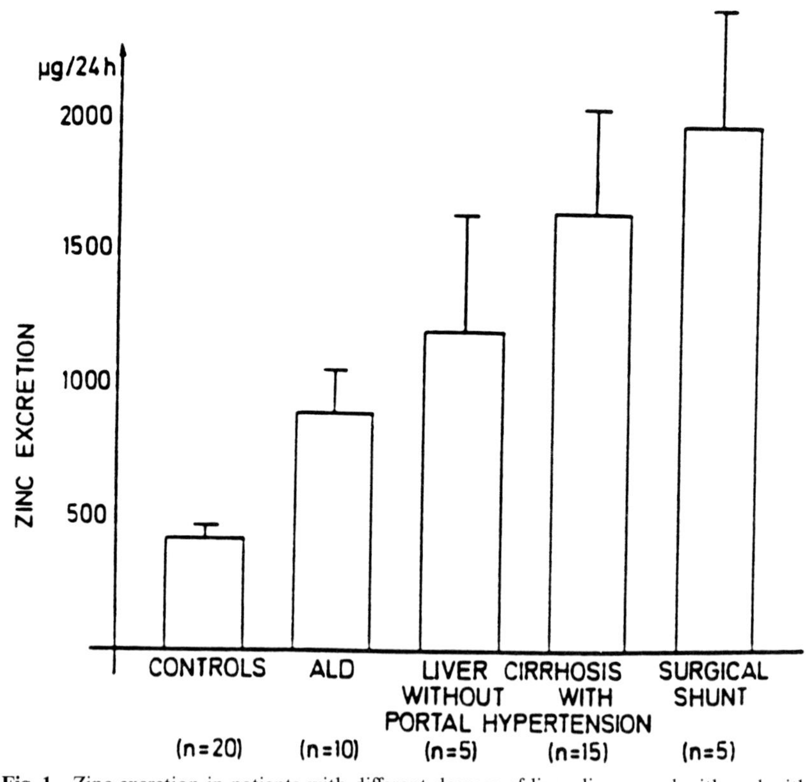

Fig. 1 Zinc excretion in patients with different degrees of liver disease and with and without portosystemic shunt (ALD = alcoholic liver disease without cirrhosis)

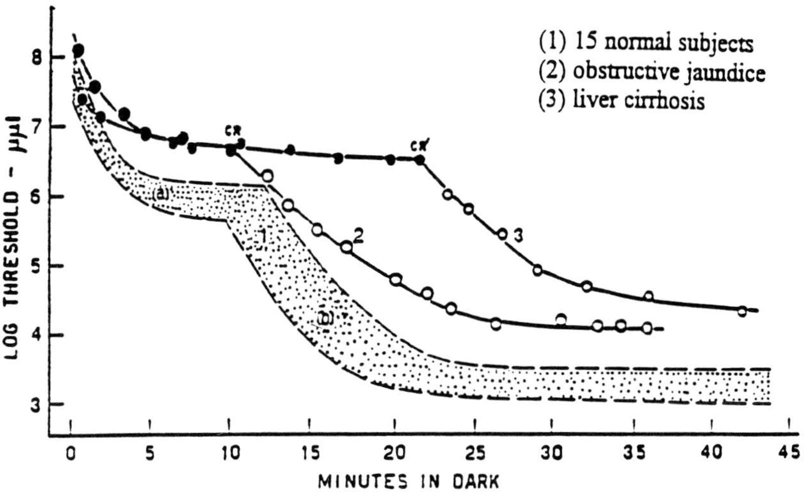

Fig. 2 Dark adaptation curves in normal subjects, patient with obstructive jaundice and patient with liver cirrhosis[11]

doses of vitamin A led to an improvement. This, however, was not true for all patients, which brought the author to the conclusion that a different vitamin A availability could be present. A possible explanation could be the simultaneous presence of zinc deficiency which was not assessed at that time.

Arguments for zinc deficiency-induced disturbance of dark adaptation came from studies of Keeling and co-workers (1982)[38]. In our own study a zinc deficiency defined as serum zinc < 65 μg/dl (normal: > 80 μg/dl) was

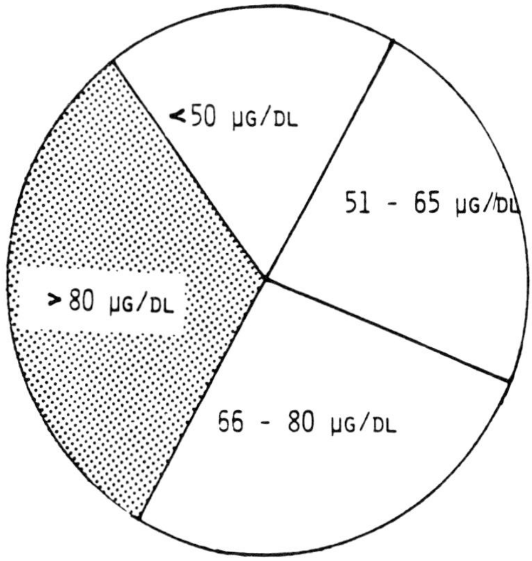

Fig. 3 Incidence of zinc deficiency in 419 patients with liver cirrhosis. Normal serum values > 80 μg/dl, zinc deficiency is suggested by a serum concentration < 65 μg/dl; 31% of these patients had an abnormal dark adaptation

found in 41% of all patients with liver cirrhosis; 31% of these patients had a disturbed dark adaptation (Fig. 3).

Herlong found in nine of 11 patients with primary biliary cirrhosis (PBC) an impaired dark adaptation. Vitamin A treatment resulted in a significant improvement in four of seven patients, the remaining three patients needing zinc substitution in addition[12]. Since vitamin A substitution in patients with liver cirrhosis is potentially dangerous[13], treatment studies have been done mostly with zinc. The positive effect on dark adaptation has been found in studies from Russell *et al.*[14], as well as in our placebo-controlled trial (Fig. 4).

TASTE

In patients with nervous anorexia a disturbed taste function has been found[15]. Patients with chronic liver diseases are frequently cachectic and complain of decreased taste sensibility. This could be objectively shown by assessment of thresholds for different taste qualities[16–18]. Smith and co-workers[16] found a disturbed taste not only in patients with chronic liver diseases but also in those with acute viral hepatitis (Table 1). With improvement of liver function, in the case of viral hepatitis, taste recovered (Fig. 5). Causes for the disturbed taste function are not known; zinc deficiency or vitamin A deficiency has been discussed. However, Sturniolo[17] did not find a correlation between decreased taste sensibility and zinc-plasma concentration. Results of therapeutic studies are contradictory. Sturniolo found no effect of zinc substitution in a placebo-controlled trial. However, in our own study zinc application over 3 months led to a significant improvement of taste thresholds[24].

HEARING

Ruedi (1954) presented evidence for a correlation between inner-ear deafness and vitamin A deficiency[19]. In one-fourth of patients vitamin A substitution improved inner-ear function. These results have been confirmed by several other authors[20–22].

In patients with alcohol-related liver disorders a pathological hearing loss can be demonstrated[23]. In the majority of cases it is a high-frequency deafness, the differences compared to age-matched controls are significant from 2000 Hz upwards. The age-dependent increase of hearing impairment is

Table 1 Objective measurements (mmol/l) of gustatory acuity in patients with liver disease. CLD = chronic liver disease; VH = viral hepatitis[16]

	Detection thresholds		
	NaCl	*Sucrose*	*Urea*
Volunteers ($n = 47$)	13 ± 1	20 ± 3	97 ± 4
CLD ($n = 16$)	80 ± 13	66 ± 17	449 ± 83
VH ($n = 22$)	54 ± 5	43 ± 4	332 ± 50

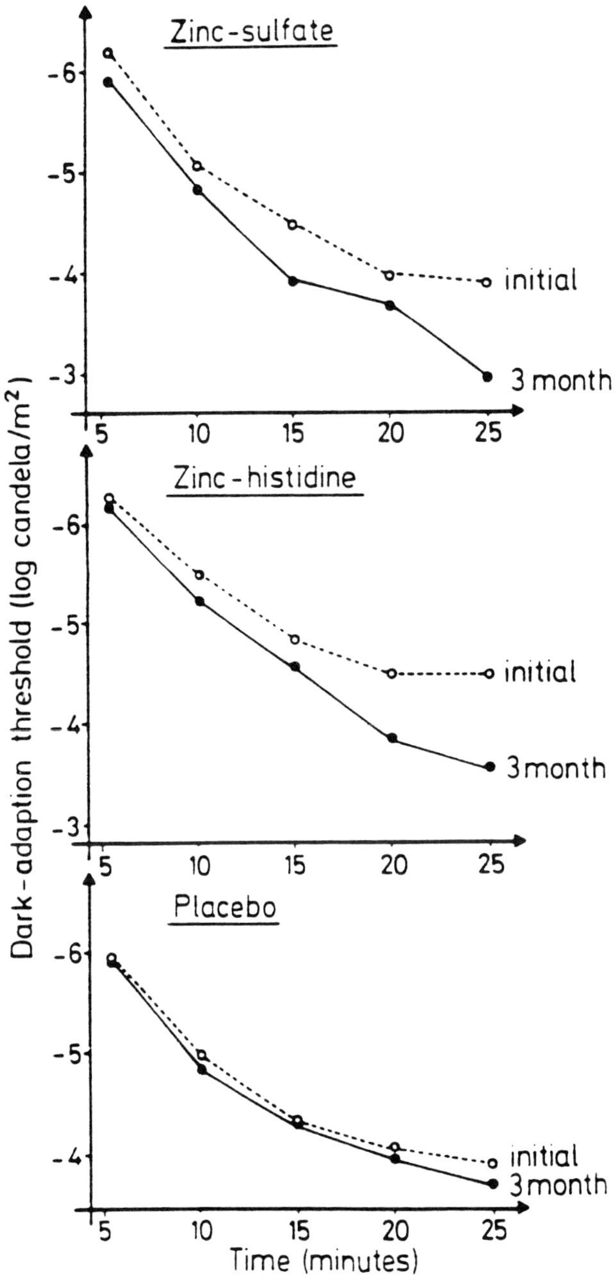

Fig. 4 Placebo-controlled study with zinc substitution for 3 months in 44 patients with liver cirrhosis. Normalization in both zinc groups (group 1: substitution with zinc sulphate; group 2: zinc histidine), but not in placebo group

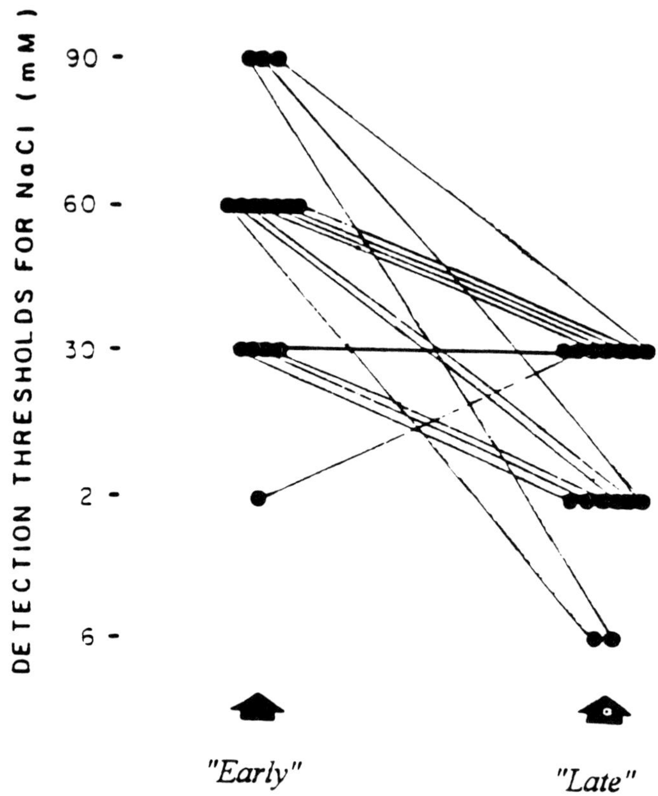

Fig. 5 Changes of gustatory acuity for NaCl with changing liver function in patients with acute viral hepatitis studied a mean of 10 days after the onset of symptoms and again a minimum of 5 weeks later[16]

significantly more pronounced in alcoholics as compared to their age-matched controls (Fig. 6). In these patients significant lower zinc and vitamin A-plasma concentrations have been observed. However, there is no improvement of inner-ear function after 3 months zinc substitution[24].

POLYNEUROPATHY

Eppinger and Arnsteiner (1912) were the first to report the occurrence of polyneuropathy in patients with liver cirrhosis. Later, alcohol was proposed as common aetiological factor. Mühler[26] found in alcoholics, in 40% of all cases, a polyneuropathy, while this was only so in 13% of patients with liver cirrhosis of other aetiology. The pathogenesis of alcoholic polyneuropathy implies several factors. Vitamin B_1 deficiency is predominant and can lead to Wernicke's encephalopathy with the consequence of disturbed sensory function (ataxia and visual abnormalities due to cerebellar and eye muscle defects).

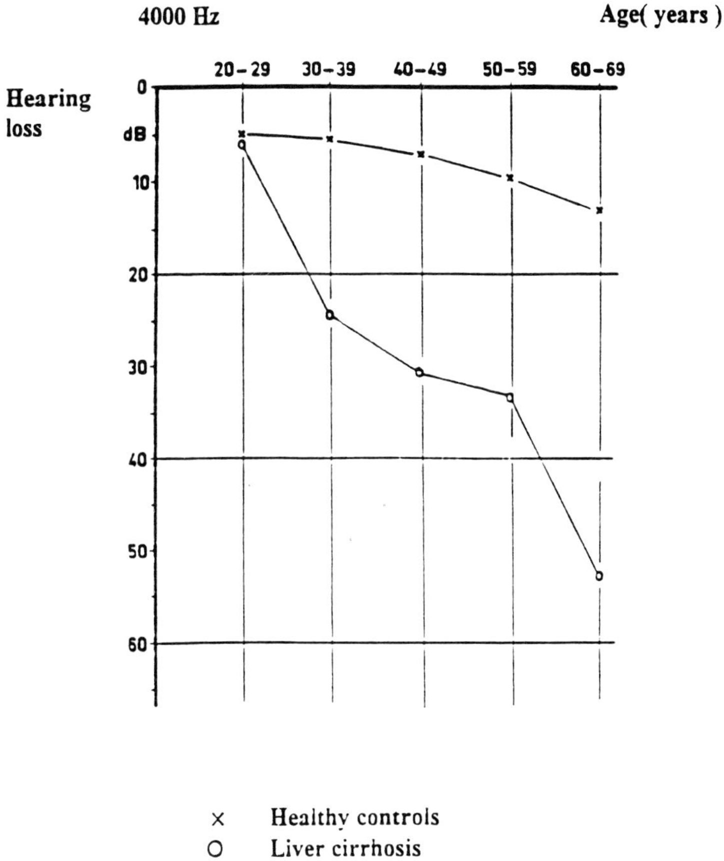

Fig. 6 Age-dependent hearing thresholds (4000 Hz) in patients with liver cirrhosis and healthy controls

The presence of polyneuropathy in chronic liver diseases is not due only to alcohol. Davan and Williams have described a segmental demyelination of nerve fibres; damage to Schwann's cells has been suggested as the cause. Since this damage is also found in diabetes mellitus, disturbed insulin metabolism has been discussed as a pathogenetic factor. If patients with abnormal glucose metabolism are excluded, however, signs of polyneuropathy in liver disease are found which are obviously independent from glucose metabolism[28]; 68% of patients in this study had sensory polyneuropathy, 20% in addition motoric abnormalities with a decrease of nerve conduction velocity. Kardel and Nielsen (1974) found in 91% of patients a disturbed function of peripheral nerves, in particular affecting vibration sense[29]. A correlation with the aetiology of liver disease or with severity could not be found. All patients with surgical portosystemic shunt had polyneuropathy, which led to the suggestion that toxic metabolites may be the cause of this abnormality. Further arguments for this suggestion can be taken from an experimental study in rats by Hindtfeld and Holmin[30]. After surgical shunt

Table 2 Maximal motor nerve conduction velocity (MCV) in controls and PC-shunted animals. Mean ± 1 SD[30]

	MCV (m/s)
Unoperated controls ($n = 6$)	43.3 ± 2.1
Sham operated controls ($n = 9$)	44.0 ± 5.3
PC – 3 weeks ($n = 6$)	35.7 ± 4.3
PC – 8 weeks ($n = 7$)	37.6 ± 3.8
PC – 16 weeks ($n = 8$)	41.8 ± 4.4

in these rats motoric nerve conduction velocity was decreased (Table 2). However, this effect was not present 16 weeks after surgery, which might be due to the improvement of liver function after this time period.

In patients with primary biliary cirrhosis a sensory polyneuropathy has been found with different frequency[31–33]. Patients complain predominantly of paraesthesiae and distally attenuated pain in the legs. Several other genetic mechanisms have been discussed. Thomas and Walker[32] suggested a disturbed nerve architecture as a consequence of histologically proven xanthomatous lipid deposits in the perineural tissue. Charron *et al.*[33] were not able to confirm this suggestion in a single case report. Immune mechanisms in this autoimmune disorder have also been discussed.

New studies have analysed vitamin E metabolism in patients with PBC and other cholestatic liver disorders[34–36]. Jeffrey *et al.*[34] found, in 44% of patients with PBC and in 32% of patients with other cholestatic liver disorders, a vitamin E deficiency. After prolonged presence of vitamin E deficiency neurological abnormalities can be found: areflexia, ataxia, disturbances of sensitivity for vibration and touch, as well as a disturbed eye movement[37]. In the study of Jeffrey *et al.* five of 12 patients with decreased vitamin E levels presented with a mild sensory polyneuropathy. Histologically neither lipid deposits nor inflammatory infiltrates as signs of vasculitis could be found. Therefore the vitamin E deficiency could be a cause of this abnormality. However, vitamin E substitution did not result in improvement of symptoms.

SUMMARY

Disturbances of sensory functions are a frequent symptom of chronic liver disorders independent of the aetiology. A correlation with liver function is only partially present, i.e. in taste abnormalities. From the disturbed sensory function problems with clinical or socioeconomic relevance can occur. The ability to drive in the dark can be severely compromised. A lack of compliance, for example, with sodium chloride restriction in patients with ascites may be understandable due to the decreased taste thresholds. A correlation with vitamin or trace element deficiencies has been suggested (vitamins A and E, and zinc). Results of therapeutic interventions are contradictory; further studies are needed before clear-cut therapeutic recommendations can be given.

References

1. Bell H, Nilsson A, Korum KR, Pedersen LB, Raknerud N, Rasmussen M. Retiniol and retinyl esters in patients with alcoholic liver disease. J Hepatol. 1989;8:26–31.
2. Leo MA, Arai M, Sato M, Lieber CS. Hepatic vitamin A depletion in alcoholic liver injury. N Engl J Med. 1982;307:597–601.
3. Vallee BL, Wacker WE, Bartholomay AF, Robin ED. Zinc metabolism in hepatic dysfunction. Serum zinc concentrations in Laennec's cirrhosis and their validation by sequential analysis. N Engl J Med. 1956;255:403–8.
4. Schölmerich J, Becher MS, Köttgen E *et al.* The influence of portosystemic shunting on zinc and vitamin A metabolism in liver cirrhosis. Hepatogastroenterology. 1983;30:143–7.
5. Kahn AM, Helwig HL, Redeker AG, Reynolds TB. Urine and serum-zinc abnormalities in disease of the liver. Am J Clin Pathol. 1965;44:426–35.
6. Kiilerich S, Dietrischson O, Loud FB *et al.* Zinc depletion in alcoholic liver disease. Scand J Gastroenterol. 1980;15:363–7.
7. Schölmerich J, Löhle E, Köttgen E, Gerok W. Zinc and vitamin A deficiency in liver cirrhosis. Hepatogastroenterology. 1983;30:119–25.
8. Mills PR, Fell GS, Bessent RG, Nelson LM, Russell RI. A study of zinc metabolism in alcoholic cirrhosis. Clin Sci. 1983;64:527–35.
9. Walker BE, Dawson JB, Kelleher J, Losowsky MS. Plasma and urinary zinc in patients with malabsorption syndromes or hepatic cirrhosis. Gut. 1973;14:943–8.
10. Solis-Herruzo JA, De Cuenca B, Munoz-Rivero MC. Intestinal zinc absorption in cirrhotic patients. Z Gastroenterol. 1989;27:335–8.
11. Patek AJ, Haig C. The occurrence of abnormal dark adaption and its relation to vitamin A metabolism in patients with cirrhosis of the liver. J Clin Invest. 1939;18:609–16.
12. Herlong HF, Russell RM, Maddrey WC. Vitamin A and zinc therapy in primary biliary cirrhosis. Hepatology. 1981;1:348–51.
13. Leo MA, Arai M, Sato M, Lieber CS. Hepatotoxicity of vitamin A and ethanol in the rat. Gastroenterology. 1982;82:194–205.
14. Russell RM, Morrison SA, Smith FR, Oaks EV, Carney EA. Vitamin A reversal of abnormal dark adaption in cirrhosis. Ann Intern Med. 1978;88:622–6.
15. Caspar RC, Kirschner B, Sandstead HH, Jacob RA, Davis JM. An evaluation of trace metals, vitamins and the function in anorexia function. Am J Clin Nutr. 1981;33:1801–8.
16. Smith FR, Henkin RI, Dell RB. Disordered gustatory acuity in liver disease. Gastroenterology. 1976;70:568–71.
17. Sturniolo GC, D'Incà RD, Giacomazzi F, Montino MC, D'Odorico A, Soranzo P, Naccarato R. Taste alterations in liver cirrhosis: are they related to zinc deficiency? J Trace Elem Electrolytes Health Dis. 1992;6:15–19.
18. Burck RE, Sachin DA, Jetton MM. Decreased taste and smell acuity in cirrhosis. Ann Intern Med. 1978;138:743–6.
19. Ruedi L. Actions of vitamin A on the human and animal ear. Acta Otolaryngol. 1954;44:502.
20. Nager G. Erfahrungen mit Vitamin A in der Behandlung von Innenohrschwerhörigkeiten und Tinnitus. Pract Oto-Rhino-Laryngol. 1954;12:129.
21. Baron SH. Experiences with parenteral vitamin A therapy in deafness and tinnitus. Laryngoscope. 1951;61:530.
22. Lobell MJ. Clinical studies with parenteral vitamin A therapy in deafness. Eye Ear Nose Throat Mon. 1949;28:213.
23. Bombelli U. Il fegato nella patogenesi delle malattie otorinolaringologiche. Zitiert nach Zbl. Hals-, Nasen-Ohrenheilkd. 1959:64–5.
24. Schölmerich J. Langenberger G, Steiert B, Löhle E, Wokalek H, Tauber R, Köttgen E, Gerok W. Long term zinc substitution in patients with zinc deficiency in liver cirrhosis – results of a placebo controlled trial. Gastroenterology. 1986;90:1765(abstr.).
25. Eppinger H, Arnsteiner A. Zur Pathogenese der Polyneuritis. Z Klin Med. 1912;74:324–35.
26. Mühler E. Zur Frage der hepatogenen Polyneuritis. Dtsch. Z. Nervenheilkunde. 1960;180:176–90.
27. Dayan AD, Williams R. Demyelinating peripheral neuropathy and liver disease. Lancet. 1967;2:133–4.

28. Seneviratne KN, Peiris OA. Peripheral nerve function in chronic liver disease. J Neurol Neurosurg Psychiatry. 1970;33:609–14.
29. Kardel T, Nielsen VK. Hepatic neuropathy. Acta Neurol Scand. 1974;50:513–26.
30. Hindfelt B, Holmin T. Experimental porta-caval anastomosis and motor nerve conduction velocity in the rat. J Neurol. 1980;223:171–5.
31. Zeitlhofer J, Mamoli B, Dragosics B, Knoflach P. Electrophysiological studies in primary biliary cirrhosis. Eur Neurol. 1984;23:247–51.
32. Thomas PK, Walker JG. Xanthomatous neuropathy in primary biliary cirrhosis. Brain. 1965;88:1079–88.
33. Charron L, Peyronnard JM, Marchand L. Sensory neuropathy associated with primary biliary cirrhosis. Arch Neurol. 1980;37:84–7.
34. Jeffrey GP, Muller DP, Burroughs AK, Matthews S, Kemp C *et al.* Vitamin E deficiency and its clinical significance in adults with primary biliary cirrhosis and other forms of chronic liver disease. J Hepatol. 1987;4:307–17.
35. Arria AM, Tarter RE, Warty V, Van Thiel DH. Vitamin E deficiency and psychomotor dysfunction in adults with primary biliary cirrhosis. Am J Clin Nutr. 1990;52:383–90.
36. Munoz SJ, Heubi JE, Balistreri WF, Maddrey WC. Vitamin E deficiency in primary biliary cirrhosis: gastrointestinal malabsorption, frequency and relationship to other lipid-soluble vitamins. Hepatology. 1989;9:525–31.
37. Muller DPR, Lloyd JK, Wolff OH. Vitamin E and neurological function. Lancet. 1983;1:225–8.
38. Keeling PW, O'Day J, Ruse W, Thompson RP. Zinc deficiency and photoreceptor dysfunction in chronic liver disease. Clin Sci. 1982;62:109–11.

Section III

Liver, skin and skeleton

10
Liver and skin

M. BROTMAN

Numerous cutaneous and cutaneous appendage abnormalities are seen in patients with diseases of the liver and biliary system[1–6]. These may be classified as in Table 1. The skin lesions in each of these categories are presented in Tables 2 through 5.

NON-SPECIFIC LESIONS COMMONLY ASSOCIATED WITH HEPATOBILIARY DISEASES

Paper-money skin describes the fine, thread-like blood vessels which occur in the same distribution as spider naevi[7]. These indicate chronic liver disease.

Table 1

A.	'Non-specific' lesions commonly associated with chronic hepatobiliary diseases
B.	Lesions associated with specific disease states
C.	Systemic diseases affecting liver and skin
D.	Miscellaneous group

Table 2 'Non-specific' lesions commonly associated with hepatobiliary diseases

'Paper-money skin'	Palmar erythema
Xanthelasma	Dupuytren's contractures
Xanthomas	White nails
Icterus	White-banded nails
Spider naevi	Nail pigmentation
Gynaecomastia	Female hair distribution
Collateral vein prominence	Cutaneous pigmentation
Ecchymoses	Pruritus/lichenification
Purpura	White spots
Striae	Vitiligo

Table 3 Lesions associated with specific disease states

1. Haemochromatosis
haemosiderin deposition
melanin deposition
2. Hepatitis B
urticaria
essential mixed cryoglobulinaemia
vasculitis
erythema nodosa
periarteritis nodosa
papular acrodermatitis of childhood (Gianotti's syndrome)
3. Primary biliary cirrhosis
lichen planus
CRST syndrome
dermatomyositis
4. Chronic active hepatitis
butterfly rash
'allergic' capillaritis
acne vulgaris
splinter haemorrhages
pyoderma gangrenosum
5. Porphyria
bullae
hypertrichosis
hyper/hypopigmentation
cutaneous fragility

Table 4 Systemic diseases affecting liver and skin

Amyloidosis	Diabetes mellitus
Sarcoidosis	Syphilis
Xanthomatosis	Hereditary haemorrhagic telangiectasia
Histiocytosis	Carcinoid

Table 5 Miscellaneous

Vinyl chloride	Drug addicts
Penicillamine	Carcinoma
AIDS	

The name refers to the silk threads inserted in American dollar bills. Xanthelasma and xanthomas develop in patients with prolonged cholestasis and histologically consist of foamy cells full of cholesterol. In patients with chronic liver disease they first develop as xanthelasma around the eye, and later appear as xanthomatous nodules often on extensor surfaces and in areas of pressure.

Jaundice is due to staining of the tissues with bilirubin and possibly other pigments such as biliverdin. It is often first seen in the sclerae bound to abundant elastic tissue. With increasing severity the skin becomes progressively more pigmented.

Spider naevi are vascular lesions supplied by a central arteriole. They blanch if occluded centrally with the head of a pin and can often be well seen when pressure is applied with a glass slide. They can be pulsatile. They characteristically occur in the distribution of the superior vena cava, the face, arms and hands, and upper chest.

Gynaecomastia is one of several 'endocrine' manifestations of chronic liver disease. This can be distinguished from fat deposition by finding palpable breast tissue, often tender. This is seen in male cirrhotics, frequently associated with diminished libido and testicular atrophy. It is also commonly seen in male patients treated with spironolactone for ascites. Rather than increases in plasma oestrogens, feminization is thought to result from increased conversion of weekly androgenic steroids to oestrogens in peripheral tissues where they have a local effect. Non-alcoholic cirrhosis feminization occurs when significant portal systemic shunting occurs allowing steroidal oestrogen precursors to escape the enterohepatic circulation and undergo peripheral conversion.

Collateral vein prominence is particularly notable in the abdominal wall and may be due to collateral circulation between the left branch of the portal vein via the umbilical vein and the systemic veins. In the so-called Cruvheilier–Baumgarten syndrome with early-onset cirrhosis, a similar venous distribution may be seen in a caput medusae around the umbilicus associated with a venous hum around the umbilicus. In some patients with Budd–Chiari syndrome with both hepatic venous and inferior vena cava obstruction, dilated abdominal wall veins are seen with the flow upward.

Ecchymoses are frequently seen initially post-trauma such as at venepuncture sites and, with progression of liver disease, spontaneously. These are manifestations of the clotting disorders in liver disease, most commonly hypoprothrombinaemia.

Purpura may be generalized in patients who are thrombocytopenic. This may be seen in patients with hypersplenism and also in patients with acute pancytopenia in viral hepatitis.

Striae or stretch marks are commonly observed in patients with severe ascites or a history of such.

White spots often later develop into spider naevi. They tend to be more prominent on the arms and legs when the skin is cold. An arteriole may be found in the centre of each spot.

Vitiligo is one of the pigmentation disorders sometimes seen in patients with chronic active hepatitis (see below).

Palmar erythema most commonly affects the thenar and hypothenar eminences as well as the base of the fingers. Like spider angiomata, it probably results from endocrine imbalance. It represents an extensive collection of arteriolovenous anastomoses. These findings are not specific for cirrhosis, they appear in rheumatoid arthritis (so-called rheumatoid palms) and in pregnancy (palms of pregnancy), as well as in normals, perhaps on a hereditary basis. The condition has also been seen in patients with thyrotoxicosis and bronchial carcinoma.

Dupytren's contractures are due to progressive fibrosis of the palmar fascia and are more common in alcoholics than in control populations, particularly alcoholic cirrhotics. This lesion appears to be related to the alcohol rather than the cirrhosis.

White nails or Terry's nails[8] are commonly seen in patients with cirrhosis. The tip of the nail is pink, and in advanced cases the lunula disappears.

White-banded nails, also known as Muehrcke's lines, are transverse pale bands across the distal part of the fingernails. They were initially thought to be associated with hypoalbuminaemia, but this association is not certain. They are also seen in the nephrotic syndrome.

Nail pigmentation is infrequent, but may be seen in patients with cholestasis due to staining with bile pigments.

Clubbing[9] is seen in patients with cholestasis. Clearly this is a non-specific finding seen in many other disease states, particularly patients with chronic pulmonary disease.

Female hair distribution refers to the development of the feminine pubic hair pattern, the so-called female escutcheon. This is frequently seen in cirrhotics. Axillary hair may also become scant both in men and women. Interestingly, despite the common impression to the contrary, it is rare for male patients with cirrhosis to lose their chest hair. Commonly these patients have never had any chest hair.

Pigmentation of the skin[10] may be generalized in patients with chronic cholestasis. The pigmentation is due to melanin in the skin. Specific areas may escape pigmentation such as the so-called 'butterfly sign' on the back – an area where the patient is unable to scratch, and old scars.

Pruritus/lichenification are manifestations of cholestasis. They are often most severe in the palms and soles of the feet. The initial manifestations are scratch marks; chronic scratching may lead to marked thickening of the skin. The pathogenesis of the pruritus is not entirely clear, it was thought to be due to bile salt deposition in the skin, but this has not been confirmed[11,12].

LESIONS ASSOCIATED WITH SPECIFIC DISEASE STATES

In patients with haemochromatosis, diffuse pigmentation is most commonly brown due to melanin in the skin, leading to the term 'bronze diabetes'. In about 15% of patients the pigmentation is slate grey in colour. This may be due either to melanin in the skin or haemosiderin deposition[13]. Some patients may develop vitiligo[14].

Urticaria may be the predominant or sole feature of the transient prodromal serum-sickness-type syndrome occurring in 20–30% of patients with acute hepatitis B.

Essential mixed cryoglobulinaemia is also immune-complex-mediated – and is associated with purpura as well as arthralgia, weakness and often renal involvement.

Patients with hepatitis B may present with a variety of skin lesions. Allergic vasculitis may be associated with viral hepatitis[15], most commonly in type B hepatitis. When severe the lesions may necrose and ulcerate. They may present with an appearance characteristic of erythema nodosum, and may progress to typical periarteritis nodosa[16] with glomerulonephritis and renal failure.

Papular acrodermatitis of childhood, or so-called Gianotti-Crosti syndrome[17,18] is a profuse and diffuse eruption of deep red papules which frequently spare the trunk and may be associated with generalized lymphadenopathy. This may be seen in children who are perfectly well, but has been associated with mild, usually anicteric acute viral hepatitis B in children predominantly under 4 years of age. The evidence of acute hepatitis most commonly begins as the dermatitis starts to wane, at about the second or third week.

Lichen planus has been reported in association with both primary biliary cirrhosis and chronic active hepatitis[19,20]. The eruption has a characteristic purple or violaceous colour, tends to be symmetrical, has a predilection for the fronts of the wrists and forearms, the backs of the hands, ankles and shins, and the lumbar region. The lesions are usually intensely pruritic.

The CRST or 'crest' syndrome may be seen in patients with primary biliary cirrhosis. This syndrome comprises calcinosis (very often involving the fingertips), Raynaud's phenomenon, sclerodactyly and telangiectasia (often involving the palms). These are characteristic lesions of scleroderma, which may also be associated with primary biliary cirrhosis[21].

Dermatomyositis may also be associated with primary biliary cirrhosis. The characteristic lesion is the so-called heliotrope rash on the cheeks and over the bridge of the nose, with marked periorbital oedema and profound proximal myopathy.

Additionally, in chronic active hepatitis, several other characteristic skin lesions can be seen. Butterfly rash, most often seen in idiopathic chronic active hepatitis, is distributed as an erythematous rash on the cheeks and the bridge of the nose. 'Allergic' capillaritis[22,23] is characterized by active inflammatory papules with central crusting which gradually progress to pale depressed scars. Development of severe acne vulgaris with secondary amennorhoea and liver function abnormalities is frequently seen in young females. Splinter haemorrhages under the fingernails may be a manifestation of a generalized vasculitis. Finally, pyroderma gangrenosum may be associated with chronic active hepatitis[24].

The cutaneous manifestations of the hepatic porphyrias[25] with photosensitivity are best exemplified by the variety of lesions in porphyria cutanea tarda which include vesicles or blisters (the hallmark of the eruption), hypertrichosis, hyperpigmentation, and cutaneous fragility. Areas of prior severe blistering and erosion may result in hypopigmented scars.

SYSTEMIC DISEASES AFFECTING THE LIVER AND SKIN

In amyloidosis involvement of cutaneous blood vessels may lead to fragility resulting in pinch purpura. In sarcoidosis liver biopsy may show granulomatous lesions. The skin manifestations are variable and may include infiltrated red or purple papules or flat plaques. Xanthomatosis is characterized by deposition of lipids in the skin. As described earlier, this may be secondary to a defective metabolism of lipids as in primary biliary cirrhosis and other chronic cholestatic conditions. Similar skin lesions may also be seen in the primary hyperlipidaemias, several of which are associated with hepatic abnormalities, particularly steatosis. In generalized histiocytosis X the liver is the third most commonly involved organ after bone and skin. The liver biopsy shows granulomatous infiltrates of histiocytic cells, periportal ductular proliferation, cholestasis and little inflammation. The skin lesions[2] are discrete yellow papules and nodules, which on biopsy show characteristic cells in the dermis, particularly by electron micrococoscopy. In diabetes mellitus the liver will frequently be involved with steatosis. One characteristic skin lesion is necrobiosis lipoidica diabeticorum, occurring particularly on the lower limbs, usually relatively symmetrically. They are well-defined, slightly raised yellow plaques, often with telangiectasia, and may ulcerate. In syphilis the liver lesion may simulate acute viral hepatitis and in others show miliary granulomata. In other cases portal tract inflammation is the major lesion. The skin lesions may be quite non-specific, presenting as red papules or ulcerations. Biopsy may be necessary to make the diagnosis. In hereditary haemorrhagic telangiectasia hepatomegaly is common. Cirrhosis may occur, in some cases apparently associated with the telangiectases, in others due to viral hepatitis contracted from blood transfusions. The fibrous separations seen on liver biopsy may contain telangiectases and the venous phase of selective coeliac axis arteriography may show marked and prolonged venous blush. The carcinoid syndrome produces a violaceous rash often involving the face and neck. This syndrome occurs when liver metastases are present, although it has been reported without liver metastases in bronchial carcinoids.

MISCELLANEOUS LESIONS

Acute vinyl chloride exposure[5] may result in acute hepatic injury with isolated necrosis. More prolonged exposure can cause both hepatic fibrosis and angiosarcoma of the liver, which is multicentric. Acute exposure to vinyl chloride produces skin irritation and frost bite, including a condition known as acro-osteolysis-Raynaud's phenomenon accompanied by osteolysis of the terminal phalanges of the fingers and scleroderma-like skin changes. Penicillamine, used in the treatment of Wilson's disease and more recently in experimental trials in primary biliary cirrhosis, may produce a skin lesion indistinguishable from pemphigus vulgaris[26] in its clinical presentation, its histology and immunofluorescence changes. The eruption clears on stopping the drug, but this may take many months. Drug addicts often develop superficial thrombophlebitis at the sites of their intravenous drug injection. Examination of the skin may give immediate clues as to the source of the patient's hepatitis B or C. Intra-abdominal carcinomas, metastatic to the liver, may also metastasize to the skin. A well-known example is the so-called Sister Mary Joseph's nodule, which is a metastatis from a carcinoma of the pancreas, to the umbilicus. Finally, AIDS commonly involves the liver and biliary system. Lesions in the liver include large droplet fatty infiltration, atypical tuberculosis and other opportunistic infections, chronic active and chronic persistent hepatitis, malignant lymphomas and Kaposi's sarcoma. The bile ducts may be involved with sclerosing cholangitis and ampullary stenosis. Commonly one finds cytomegalovirus and cryptosporidia as well as atypical tuberculosis, Kaposi's sarcoma and lymphoma in ampullary and biliary tissue. The hallmark cutaneous lesion is the Kaposi's lesion.

The cutaneous manifestations of hepatobiliary disease are indeed protean. Recognition of these lesions may be extremely helpful in initiating the appropriate diagnostic studies in patients with hepatobiliary disease.

References

1. Sherlock S, Summerfield JA. Color atlas of liver disease, 2nd edn. London: Mosby Year Book; 1991.
2. duVivier A. Atlas of clinical dermatology. London: Gower Medical Publishing; 1986.
3. Sarkany I. Cutaneous manifestations of hepatobiliary disease. In: Fitzpatrick T, Elsen A, Wolff K, Freedberg I, Austen K, editors. Dermatology in general medicine, 3rd edn. New York: McGraw-Hill 1987;1947–64.
4. Zakim D, Boyer T. Hepatology a textbook of liver disease, vol. 2, 2nd edn. Philadelphia: W. B. Saunders; 1990.
5. Schiff L, Schiff E. Diseases of the liver, 6th edn. Philadelphia: J. B. Lippincott; 1987.
6. MacSween R, Anthony P, Scheuer P. Pathology of the liver, 2nd edn. New York: Churchill Livingstone; 1987.
7. Bean WB. The arterial spider and similar lesions of the skin and mucous membrane. Circulation. 1953;8:117.
8. Terry RB. White nails in hepatic cirrhosis. Lancet. 1954;1:757.
9. Reid L. Cyanosis and finger clubbing in liver disease explained? Med Trib Int Ed (Gr Brit.) 1967;2(2):25.
10. Burton JL, Kirby J. Pigmentation and biliary cirrhosis. Lancet. 1975;1:458.
11. Kirby J *et al.* Pruritic effect of bile salts. Br Med J. 1974;4:693.
12. Freedman MR, Holzbach RT, Ferguson DR. Pruritus in cholestasis: no direct causative role for bile acid retention. Am J Med. 1981;70:1011–16.
13. Chevrant-Breton J *et al.* Cutaneous manifestations of idiopathic hemochromatosis. Arch Dermatol. 1977;113:161.
14. Perdrup A, Poulsen H. Hemochromatosis and vitiligo. Arch Dermatol. 1964;90:34.
15. Popp JW, Harris TJ, Dienstag JL, Bahn AK *et al.* Cutaneous vasculitis associated with acute and chronic hepatitis. Arch Intern Med. 1981;141:623–9.
16. Goche DJ *et al.* Association between polyarteritis and Australia antigen. Lancet. 1970;2:1149.
17. Gianotti F. Papular acrodermatitis of childhood. An Australia antigen disease. Arch Dis Child. 1973;48:794.
18. San Joaquin VH, Marks MI. Gianotti disease or Gianotti–Crosti syndrome? J Paediatr. 1982;101:216.
19. Graham-Brown RAC *et al.* Lichen planus and primary biliary cirrhosis. Br J Dermatol. 1982;106:699.
20. Rebora A *et al.* Erosive lichen planus and cirrhotic hepatitis. Ital Gen Rev Dermatol. 1978;15:123.
21. Reynolds TB *et al.* Primary biliary cirrhosis with scleroderma. Raynaud's phenomenon and telangiectasis. New syndrome. Am J Med. 1971;50:302.
22. Sarkany I. Juvenile cirrhosis and allergic capillaritis of the skin. A hepato-cutaneous syndrome. Lancet. 1966;2:666–8.
23. Sarkany I. The skin lesions associated with liver disease. Prog Dermatol. 1969;4:1–6.
24. Burns DA, Sarkany I. Active chronic hepatitis and pyoderma gangrenosum: report of a case. Clin Exp Dermatol. 1979;4:465–9.
25. Berman JE, Lam Kin BC. Hepatic disease and the skin. Dermatol Clin. 1989;7:435–48.
26. Seehafer JR *et al.* Lichen planus-like lesions caused by penicillamine in primary biliary cirrhosis. Arch Dermatol. 1981;117:140.

11

Liver, joints and bone tissue

R. ZIEGLER and C. WÜSTER

INTRODUCTION

The skeleton including joints, i.e. bone tissue, cartilage and tendons comprises bradytrophic tissues. Therefore, they may be affected by disease of other organs such as the liver only if the respective disease is a chronic one. Trabecular bone has a turnover of about 4 years, compact bone of 8–9 years – the turnover of tendons may be even longer. Due to this time-course hepatopathies have to last for perhaps a year or longer until recognizable symptoms (e.g. bone loss) show up at the skeleton.

JOINTS

There is one exception to the requirement of a longer-lasting liver disease to induce joint complaints: acute viral hepatitis may be occasionally accompanied by a 'rheumatoid' syndrome which has only the significance of a symptom, but later vanishes without a persistent detriment.

In contrast, rare chronic metabolic diseases involving the liver may lead to arthropathies (see Table 1). Haemochromatosis is in 20–90% of patients accompanied by chronic osteoarthritis[1]. As in rheumatoid arthritis, the finger joints are involved but without inflammatory proliferation of the synovia leading to severe joint destruction. Bilaterally also hand, knee, and hip joints may be affected; only rarely other joints. Chondrocalcinosis (pseudogout) is quite frequently seen presenting with calcifications of menisci and disci in a symmetrical distribution. X-rays may show, besides chondrocalcinosis, cystic lesions of spongiosa, erosions of the subchondral lamella, or larger osteoarthritic defects.

Ochronosis or alkaptonuria is a rare inherited (autosomal–recessive) disease of tyrosin metabolism. Due to the defect of homogentisinase an excess

Table 1 Hepatic arthropathy

Liver disease	*Joint disease*
Infections	
Acute viral hepatitis (in 5–20%)	Arthralgia, 'rheumatoid' syndrome
Metabolic diseases	
Haemochromatosis (in 20–50%)	Osteoarthritis, chondrocalcinosis (pseudogout)
Alcaptonuria	Ochronotic arthropathy
Liver insufficiency	
Bleeding	Bleeder's joints

of homogentisinic acid is produced. This pigment is found in the urine and dyes connective tissues. Impregnation of the joint cartilage leads to accelerated degenerative arthropathy. Involved are joints near the trunk; symptoms arise at around 40 years of age from the spine. The progression of this spinal osteoarthritis is faster than in the case of mere degenerative disc disease. Furthermore, periarticular calcifications of the tendons may be seen (productive fibro-ostosis)[1]. Chronic hepatic insufficiency may be accompanied by disturbed coagulation – repeated bleedings into weight-bearing joints such as knees may lead to a clinical picture as in haemophilia.

As the observation of skeleton and joints after organ transplantation (heart, liver) only occurred recently, leading to the discovery of post-transplantation osteoporosis (see below), in the future the joints also deserve special attention. For example, after combined kidney and pancreas transplantation, severe osteopathy *and* arthropathy were described[2].

BONE TISSUE

The human skeleton is built up to its 'peak bone mass' during the first two or maximally three decades – after the 40th year there is a slow loss of 0.5–1% of bone mass per year, even in the healthy. Low peak bone mass and/or premature and/or accelerated loss due to the menopause (oestrogen deficiency) in females, or diseases impairing bone metabolism in both sexes, may lead to osteoporosis or more complex osteopathies. Figure 1 depicts factors which maintain bone: sex hormones, nutrients (especially calcium and phosphorus, protein, fluoride as a trace element, vitamin D as a pre-pro-hormone), and physical activities. Diseases may disturb sex hormone exposition, the supply of important substrates such as calcium, or may lead to immobilization (e.g. rheumatism). Furthermore, chronic inflammatory diseases may lead directly to bone loss (inflammation-mediated osteopenia, IMO[3]).

As a major digestive gland, the liver contributes (via bile) to the digestion of calcium-containing nutrients – liver diseases leading to maldigestion may impair calcium uptake. As an organ of protein turnover and formation, the

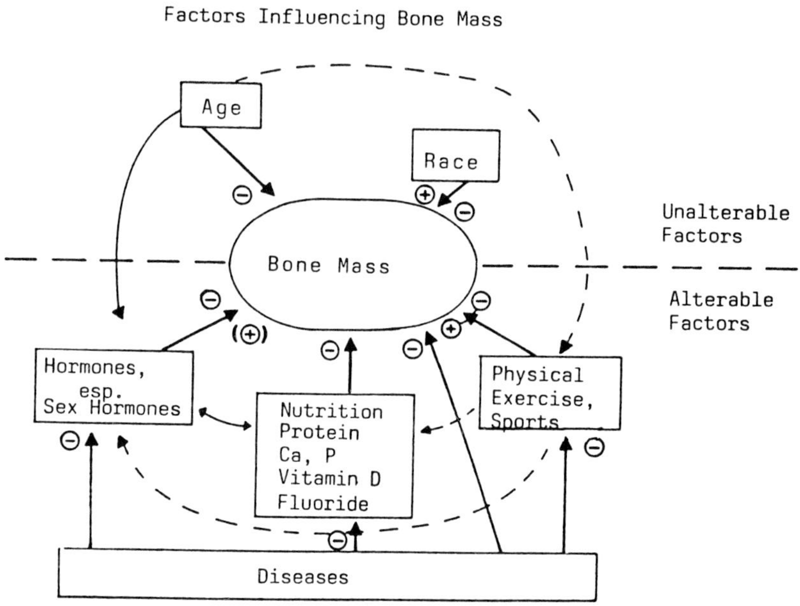

Fig. 1 Factors of importance for the development and maintenance of bone mass

insufficient liver will lead to hypoproteinaemia, which includes diminished formation of bone ground substance.

Finally, the liver is an endocrine organ which metabolizes the inactive pre-pro-hormone vitamin D to the (still not very active) first metabolite or pro-hormone 25-OH-vitamin D, calcidiol, which again enters the circulation to be metabolized to the second metabolite or so-called vitamin D hormone, i.e. 1,25-$(OH)_2$-vitamin D, calcitriol[4].

Whereas the 1α-hydroxylation of calcidiol in the kidney is already impaired during early phases of end-stage renal disease, 25-hydroxylation in the liver has a much larger functional reserve: until liver insufficiency leads to a lack of 25-OH-vitamin D, almost the whole organ has to be destroyed[4].

Table 2 summarizes which conditions or diseases of the liver could be disadvantageous for the bone.

Without a definable defect, in some predisposed individuals antiepileptic drugs induce increased hepatic microsomal P-450 enzymatic activity. The consequence is an accelerated degradation of vitamin D and calcidiol[5]. Therefore, about 10% of patients receiving these drugs develop so-called 'antiepileptic osteomalacia', which can be prevented by an adequate vitamin D supply.

In liver cirrhosis (without inducing or accompanying alcoholism) disturbances of calcium metabolism begin rather late. As already mentioned, liver insufficiency has to be almost complete before calcidiol formation is disturbed[6]. Hypoproteinaemia may be disadvantageous some time earlier – however, the restricted life expectation of these patients will make relevant

Table 2 Hepatic osteopathy

Event or disturbance in the liver	*Pathophysiological consequences*	*Disturbance of calcium homeostasis or bone metabolism*
Enzyme induction due to antiepileptic drugs	Accelerated metabolism of 25-OH-vitamin D	Osteomalacia due to antiepileptics
Liver cirrhosis (and insufficiency)	Decreased formation of 25-OH-vitamin D	Lack of 1,25-$(OH)_2$-vitamin D
	Lack of physical activity	Lack of physical stress
Alcoholic hepatopathy	Lack of calcium (beer instead of milk)	Alcoholic osteopathy (complex)
	Lack of protein	
	Disturbed metabolism of sex hormones	
Liver transplantation	Treatment with immuno-suppressive drugs (including glucocorticoids)	Post-transplantation osteopathy (complex)
	Reduced mobility	

bone diseases such as osteoporosis a rare event. Prolongation of life due to liver transplantation will require more osteoprotective efforts in the future (see below), comparable to the necessity of prevention of renal osteodystrophy after the introduction of haemodialysis and kidney transplantation years ago.

If alcoholism is involved the picture of alcoholic osteopathy is somewhat more complex: the duration of the condition may be long-lasting, a chronic lack of calcium may be induced by the lifestyle, 'beer instead of milk', often nutrition is also hypoproteinaemic, and sometimes the patients suffer from hypogonadism, which also contributes to the development of osteoporosis. It is interesting to note that (in the rat) vitamin D status influences the biological responses of the bone tissue to sex hormones[7]. This could also be relevant for humans. Presumably, alcohol also has a direct toxic effect on osteoblasts[8]; thus, the development of the disease is very complex[9] and the efficiency of therapeutic efforts depends on patient compliance and the degree of alcohol dependency.

Post-transplantation osteopathy or osteoporosis is a fairly new entity which deserves more attention[10]. During their pretransplantation observation period, the respective patients already present with lowered bone mass compared to the healthy population (Fig. 2, left column). This 'handicapped' condition may be due to their long-term disease, including suboptimal nutrition and reduced mobility. After transplantation a further bone loss takes place, which is most impressive in the patient group measured after 12 months (in our retrospective analysis). When we measured patients who were already transplanted 18 months ago or longer, their bone mass was again better. There are several explanations which need clarification in prospective studies: patients with better bone mass (as a sign of a better biological condition?) may have better life expectancy; the longer survival with the transplanted organ may improve the chance for more physical activity; the organism may be better adapted to immunosuppressive therapy. Glucocorticoids are, of course, especially a risk factor for bone[11]: they reduce

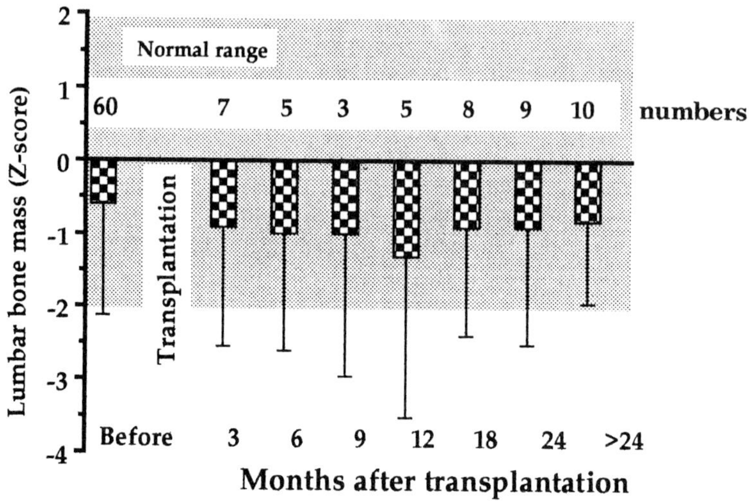

Fig. 2 Deviation of bone mass from the mean of healthy controls (*Z*-score) in patients before and after liver transplantation (lumbar spine)

calcium absorption and impair vitamin D metabolism, and they slow down bone turnover, especially by depressing new bone formation. The contribution of cyclosporin A to bone loss is not yet fully clear. Besides osteoporotic fractures only a few months after liver transplantation, osteonecrosis of the femoral head (as a typical complication of glucocorticoid treatment) is occasionally seen.

In order to prevent post-transplantation osteopathy it is necessary also to monitor the skeleton before and after transplantation. Respective recommendations have been developed[12]. Osteodensitometry and laboratory parameters serve for the patients' surveillance. Risk conditions (e.g. low bone mass) initiate preventive efforts such as substituting calcium and vitamin D. Whether antiresorptive drugs such as calcitonin or bisphosphonates are of benefit, is at present unknown. Alternative glucocorticoids with perhaps less osteoporosis-inductive potency, e.g. deflazacort[13], also need investigation. Physical exercise and (in the case of hypogonadism) hormone replacement therapy are further important tools for the prevention of this rather new type of osteoporosis. Fluoride treatment seems to be effective in increasing bone mass in transplanted patients by more than 20% of initial mass[14].

References

1. Schneider P. Gelenkerkrankungen entzündlicher und nicht-entzündlicher Komponenten (Arthropathien). In: Mathies H, Schneider P, editors. Rheumatische Krankheiten, 2nd edition. Köln: Dtsch. Ärzte-Verlag; 1987:172–86.
2. Derfus BA, Carrera GF, Komorowski RA, Ryan LM. Severe arthropathy and osteopathy following combined renal/pancreas transplantation. Transplantation. 1991;53:678–81.
3. Minne HW, Pfeilschifter J, Scharla S, Mutschelknauss S, Schwarz A, Krempien B, Ziegler R. Inflammation-mediated osteopenia in the rat: a new animal model for pathological loss of bone mass. Endocrinology. 1984;115:50–4.

4. Reichel H, Koeffler HP, Normann AW. The role of the vitamin D endocrine system in health and disease. N Engl J Med. 1989;320:980–91.
5. Hahn TJ, Birge SJ, Sharp CR, Avioli LV. Phenobarbital-induced alterations in vitamin D metabolism. J Clin Invest. 1972;51:741–8.
6. Weiss H, Rest J, Limbach HJ. Vitamin-D_3-Spiegel und Alter. Veränderungen des 1,25-Dihydroxycholecalciferol-Spiegels in verschiedenen Altersgruppen bei Normalpersonen, bei Patienten mit Osteoporose, Niereninsuffizienz und Leberzirrhose. Med Klin. 1988;83:660–6.
7. Sömjen D, Kaye AM, Harell A, Weisman Y. Modulation by vitamin D status of the responsiveness of rat bone to gonadal steroids. Endocrinology. 1989;125:1870–6.
8. Lindholm J, Steiniche T, Rasmussen E, Thamsborg G, Nielsen IO, Brockstedt-Rasmussen H, Storm T, Hyldstrup L, Schou C. Bone disorder in men with chronic alcoholism: a reversible disease? J Clin Endocrinol Metab. 1991;73:118–24.
9. Diamond T, Stiel D, Lunzer M, Wilkinson M, Roche J, Posen S. Osteoporosis and skeletal fractures in chronic liver disease. Gut. 1990;31:82–7.
10. Katz IA, Epstein S. Perspectives. Posttransplantation bone disease. J Bone Min Res. 1992;7:123–6.
11. Lukert BP, Raisz LG. Glucocorticoid-induced osteoporosis: pathogenesis and management. Ann Intern Med. 1990;112:352–64.
12. Wüster Chr. Empfehlungen zur Diagnostik und Prophylaxe einer Osteopathie nach Organtransplantationen (Herz, Lunge, Leber). Endokrinologie-Informationen. 1992;16:55–8.
13. Olgaard K, Storm T, v Wowern N, Daugaard H, Egfjord M, Lewin E, Brandi L. Glucocorticoid-induced osteoporosis in the lumbar spine, forearm, and mandible of nephrotic patients: a double-blind study on the high-dose, long-term effects of prednisone versus deflazacort. Calcif Tissue Int. 1992;50:490–7.
14. Meunier P. Effects of fluoride salts in established vertebral osteoporosis. First European Conference on Osteoporosis; 21–23 September 1992; Nice.

12

Liver and skeletal muscles: muscle wasting in cirrhosis

O. HAMBERG and H. VILSTRUP

It is a classical clinical observation that patients with severe liver disease waste muscle mass. This is recognized as a major problem, probably important for loss of quality of life and for prognosis[1]. Muscle wasting is not specific for hepatic disease but may, however, in liver patients be related to identifiable homeostatic disturbances caused by liver malfunction.

The observed muscle wasting is difficult to describe in objective terms. In liver patients most of the simple objective measures of muscle mass are hampered by oedema and other changes in body composition[2], but nonetheless almost all systematic studies support the clinical impression of significant wasting[1,3,4].

It is uncertain whether the skeletal muscles of liver patients are also deficient in respects other than mass. The frequent aetiological involvement of alcohol is important. Alcohol is acutely toxic to striated and cardiac muscle in a dose-dependent manner[5], although development of chronic alcoholic skeletal myopathia has not been convincingly documented[6]. In experimental cirrhosis in rats none of the qualitative muscle changes characteristic for alcohol feeding is encountered[7]. The predominant nerve damage in alcoholics is a distal sensory neuropathy. However, a motor nerve component is also present and may contribute towards muscle atrophy[8,9]. Patients with primary biliary cirrhosis and chronic hepatitis exhibit muscle wasting, as do patients with alcoholic liver disease[3]. Direct comparative studies on muscle biopsies and neurophysiological variables between alcoholic and non-alcoholic liver disease are not available. Immobility in patients with severe ascites or brain dysfunction may contribute to muscle wasting by reducing muscle protein synthesis[10]. These considerations prompt the assumption that the skeletal muscle changes in severe liver disease are related to the liver disease as such, and that they are primarily of a quantitative nature.

Muscle wasting is a result of an imbalance between muscle protein synthesis and breakdown. Muscle protein turnover of liver patients has not been studied directly in muscle tissues obtained by invasive biopsy techniques. The available information mostly relies on whole-body protein turnover studies. These are difficult to reconcile because of the indirect techniques with different methodological assumptions. The two most frequently used amino acid tracers are leucine and glycine, but the fate of both is disturbed by compromised liver function. These difficulties notwithstanding, most studies suggest increased muscle protein breakdown in the fasting state[11–17], at least when the rate is corrected for the decrease in lean body mass. Fasting protein synthesis is reported to be normal in most studies[11–13,16,17]. The imbalance in favour of protein breakdown is also indicated by the increased urinary loss of 3-methylhistidine[18], an indicator of myofibrillar protein breakdown, although not all of it may have been derived from skeletal muscle[19]. In one study, dealing with severely wasted patients, protein breakdown was normal but protein synthesis was decreased[20]. The decreased protein synthesis was supported by an increased net efflux from the leg of tyrosine in combination with normal efflux of 3-methyl-histidine[20]. Protein metabolism has not been investigated directly in response to food intake, but creating a fed state by giving several small meals seems not to be in favour of synthesis[11,14] as it is in normal humans[21].

Decreased protein synthesis may, obviously, be explained on the basis of decreased amino acid availability because of low protein intake. Liver patients usually eat less protein than normal subjects[22,23]. The exact cause of the anorexia that is encountered in most patients with advanced liver disease[24] has not yet been established, but several anorexic agents such as ammonia and glucagon are elevated in parallel with the severity of the liver dysfunction[25]. Furthermore, elevated plasma tryptophan levels in cirrhosis may decrease appetite via increased brain levels of serotonin. Finally, protein intake may also be decreased as a result of inexpedient medical advice.

Of interest is the fact that muscle wasting occurs in both alcoholic and non-alcoholic cirrhosis also at dietary intakes within the normal range[3,26]. This indicates that protein metabolism is disturbed in other ways than being simply attributable to decreased protein intake. This is supported by two facts. First, healthy subjects are in fact able to maintain body mass on a reduced protein intake compared with that eaten by cirrhotics and, second, cirrhotic patients do require a higher than normal protein intake to maintain neutral N-balance[27]. This may to some extent be due to a higher than normal postprandial hepatic loss of amino nitrogen as urea nitrogen. In cirrhosis urea synthesis is less efficiently down-regulated by carbohydrates so that fewer amino acids remain available for tissue build-up in the patients[28].

Insulin and amino acids are main regulators of protein metabolism[29]. Amino acids stimulate protein synthesis and insulin potentiates the effect. Insulin in the presence of low amino acid concentration has no effect, whereas insulin by itself is a more potent inhibitor of protein breakdown than are amino acids[30–33]. In liver patients, marked hyperinsulinaemia is a consistent finding, attributed to decreased hepatic degradation and pancreatic hypersecretion. Blood total amino acid concentration tends to be increased[34,35] due to decreased hepatic conversion, frequently to some extent counteracted by low protein intake. The stimulation of whole-body protein synthesis by insulin has been reported to be normal, as has the inhibition of protein breakdown by insulin[16]. As expected, however, both insulin and amino acid concentrations tended to be higher among the liver patients, in keeping with the possibility of decreased sensitivity of both protein synthesis and breakdown to amino acids and insulin. Relative insulin resistance of glucose disposal is a well-known phenomenon in liver disease, and steady-state infusion experiments confirm the existence of the same problem as to amino acid disposal[36–38].

The increased levels of cytokines, e.g. tumour necrosis factor[39,40], may also affect the balance between muscle protein synthesis and breakdown in a direction of a net loss.

The cause of insulin resistance with regard to disposal of amino acids as well as of glucose is unknown, but may be related to the sustained hyperinsulinaemia and receptor exhaustion[41]. It is also conceivable that the resistance with regard to protein synthesis is to some extent due to inadequate composition of the blood free amino acid pool, particularly in the fasting state with low branched-chain amino acids. This does not explain the hyperinsulinaemia itself, which may be initiated by a decreased glucose uptake by the cirrhotic liver as suggested indirectly by some data[42]. At the moment, however, no direct measurements by the hepatic vein catheterization technique are available.

Increased protein breakdown with utilization of amino acids for gluconeogenesis in liver patients may be due to their accelerated transition to fasting metabolism with early recruitment of alternative fuels[43,44]. A major reason for this peculiarity seems to be deficient non-oxidative glucose disposal[41], taken to reflect decreased storage of glycogen in skeletal muscles[45] and liver[43], as also described as a primary event in other hyperinsulinaemic states such as type II diabetes. The defect hepatic glycogen storage necessitates mobilization of amino acids from muscles as gluconeogenic precursors for maintenance of hepatic glucose production. Accordingly, the gluconeogenic contribution to hepatic glucose production has been reported to be markedly increased in cirrhotic patients[43].

Glucose uptake by muscular tissues is decreased in experimental anhepatic situations, and is normalized by inclusion of a liver, or by addition of precipitated liver extract[46,47]. This suggests the existence of a blood-borne non-precipitable liver factor that promotes non-oxidative glucose metabolism, and is lacking in patients with failing liver function. This factor has not yet been identified, but there are several likely candidates among active peptides, for example insulin-like growth factor 1, which is decreased in patients with cirrhosis[48].

This hypothetical chain of established events connects failing liver function with muscle wasting, and may be initiated by the liver via deficient synthesis or release of this liver factor, and by deficient handling of glucose and insulin (Fig. 1).

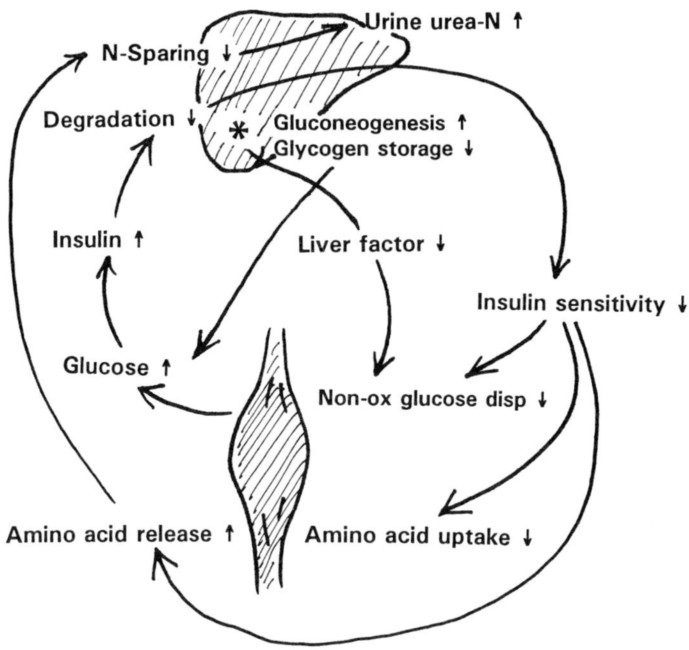

Fig. 1 Hypothetical chains of events connecting failing liver function with muscle wasting. The events as such are well-documented phenomena (cf. text and references). It is assumed that lack of hepatic synthesis of an unidentified factor that promotes muscle glucose uptake plays an important role, together with hyperinsulinaemia and ensuring insulin resistance with regard to glucose and protein/amino acid metabolism. Other key events are decreased non-oxidative glucose disposal in muscles and liver, accelerated mobilization of amino acids from muscles during fasting, and deficient sparing by carbohydrates of hepatic nitrogen elimination as urea

The most obvious possibility of clinical intervention is hyperalimentation. Lean body mass may be improved by strenuous and long-standing dietary regimens[49]. Branched-chain amino acid supplement does not influence protein metabolism[50] or nutritional state[51]. Likewise, short-term total parenteral nutrition is not able to reverse the negative arteriovenous amino acid gradient across the leg in cirrhotic patients[52]. It is probably worthwhile to secure a protein and energy intake in the upper range of normal and to divide daily intake into several meals to avoid the accelerated fasting[53]. Tailored amino acid supplementation is motivated only in patients with hepatic encephalopathy who cannot otherwise tolerate desirable protein intake.

The effect of systematic physical exercise and training combined with protein supplement has not been reported.

At the moment there is no well-founded suggestion as to rational therapy of the muscle wasting of liver patients. Identification and supplementation of the mentioned liver factor is awaited. Until then, crippling muscle wasting contributes to the indications for liver transplantation.

References

1. Mendenhall CL, Anderson S, Weesner RE *et al.* Protein–calorie malnutrition associated with alcoholic hepatitis. Am J Med. 1984;76:211–17.
2. Kondrup J, Nielsen K, Hamberg O. Nutritional therapy in patients with liver cirrhosis. Eur J Clin Nutr. 1992;46:239–46.
3. Morgan MY. Enteral nutrition in chronic liver disease. Acta Chir Scand. 1981;507 (suppl):81–90.
4. Bunout D, Gattas V, Iturriaga H *et al.* Nutritional status of alcoholic patients: its possible relationship to alcoholic liver damage. Am J Clin Nutr. 1983;38:469–73.
5. Urbano-Marquez A, Estruch R, Navarro-Lopez F *et al.* The effects of alcoholism on skeletal and cardiac muscle. N Engl J Med. 1989;320:409–15.
6. Del Villar Negro A, Merino Angulo J, Rivera-Pomar JM. Skeletal muscle changes in chronic alcoholic patients. A conventional, histochemical, ultrastructural and morphometric study. Acta Neurol Scand. 1984;70:185–96.
7. Preedy VR, Gove CD, Panos MZ *et al.* Liver histology, blood biochemistry and RNA, DNA and subcellular protein composition of various skeletal muscles of rats with experimental cirrhosis: implications for alcoholic muscle disease. Alcohol & Alcoholism 1990;25:641–9.
8. Guiheneuc P, Bathien N. Two patterns of results on polyneuropathies investigated with the H reflux. Correlation between proximal and distal conduction velocities. J Neurol Sci. 1976;30:83–94.
9. Liberson WT, Chong YC, Fried P. Terminal latencies in the superior gluteal nerve compared to those in distal peroneal and tibial nerves. Electromyography Clin Neurophysiol. 1979;19:15–26.
10. Gibson JNA, Halliday D, Morrison WL *et al.* Decrease in human quadriceps muscle protein turnover consequent upon leg immobilisation. Clin Sci. 1987;72:503–9.
11. Millikan WJ, Jr, Henderson JM, Galloway JR *et al. In vivo* measurement of leucine metabolism with stable isotopes in normal subjects and in those with cirrhosis fed conventional and branched-chain amino acid-enriched diets. Surgery. 1985;98:405–12.
12. Mullen KD, Denne SC, McCullough AJ *et al.* Leucine metabolism in stable cirrhosis. Hepatology. 1986;6:622–30.
13. Shanbhogue RLK, Bristrian BR, Laksham K *et al.* Whole body leucine, phenylalanine, and tyrosine kinetics in end-stage liver disease before and after hepatic transplantation. Metabolism. 1987;36:1047–53.
14. Swart GR, van den Berg JWO, Wattimena JLD *et al.* Elevated protein requirements in cirrhosis of the liver investigated by whole body protein turnover studies. Clin Sci. 1988;75:101–7.
15. Kohno M, Fuji T, Hirayama C. N-15 Glycine metabolism in normal and cirrhotic subjects. Biochem Med Metab Biol. 1990;43:201–13.
16. Petrides AS, Luzi L, Reuben A *et al.* Effect of insulin and plasma amino acid concentration on leucine metabolism in cirrhosis. Hepatology. 1991;14:432–41.
17. McCullough AJ, Mullen KD, Kalhan SC. Body cell mass and leucine metabolism in cirrhosis. Gastroenterology. 1992;102:1325–33.
18. Zoli M, Marchesini G, Dondi C *et al.* Myofibrillar protein catabolic rates in cirrhotic patients with and without muscle wasting. Clin. Sci. 1982;62:683–6.
19. Emery PW, Cotellessa L, Holness M *et al.* Different patterns of protein turnover in skeletal and gastrointestinal smooth muscle and the production of N-methylhistidine during fasting in the rat. Bio Sci Rep. 1986;6:143–53.
20. Morrison WL, Bouchier IAD, Gibson JNA, Rennie MJ. Skeletal muscle and whole-body protein turnover in cirrhosis. Clin Sci. 1990;78:613–19.
21. Motil KJ, Matthews DE, Bier D *et al.* Whole-body leucine and lysine metabolism: response to dietary protein intake in young men. Am J Physiol. 1981;240:E712–21.
22. Mendenhall C, Bongiovanni G, Goldberg S *et al.* VA Cooperative study on alcoholic hepatitis. III. Changes in protein-calorie malnutrition associated with 30 days of hospitalization with and without enteral nutritional therapy. J PEN. 1985;9:590–6.
23. Hamberg O, Nielsen K, Vilstrup H. Effects of an increase in protein intake on hepatic efficacy for urea synthesis in healthy subjects and in patients with cirrhosis. J Hepatol. 1992;14:237–43.

24. Achord JL. Malnutrition and the role of nutritional support in alcoholic liver disease. Am J Gastroenterol. 1987;82:1–7.
25. Smith-Laing G, Orskov H, Gore MBR, Sherlock S. Hyperglucagonaemia in cirrhosis. Diabetologia. 1980;19:103–8.
26. Nielsen K, Kondrup J, Martinsen L *et al.* Nutritional assessment and adequacy of dietary intake in hospitalized patients with alcoholic liver cirrhosis. Br J Nutr. (in press).
27. Swart GR, van den Berg JWO, van Vuure JK *et al.* Minimum protein requirements in liver cirrhosis determined by nitrogen balance measurements at three levels of protein intake. Clin Nutr. 1989;8:329–36.
28. Hamberg O, Vilstrup H. Cirrhosis impairs hepatic contribution to the nitrogen sparing effect of glucose. Clin Nutr. 1991(suppl 2);10:19–20.
29. Bennet WM, Rennie MJ. Protein anabolic actions of insulin in the human body. Diabet Med. 1991;8:199–207.
30. Tessari P, Inchiostro S, Biolo G *et al.* Differential effects of hyperinsulinemia and hyperaminoacidemia on leucine-carbon metabolism *in vivo*. J Clin Invest. 1987;79:1062–9.
31. Castellino P, Luzi L, Simonson DC *et al.* Effect of insulin and plasma amino acid concentrations on leucine metabolism in man. J Clin Invest. 1987;80:1784–93.
32. Gelfand RA, Barett EJ. Effect of physiologic hyperinsulinemia on skeletal muscle protein synthesis and breakdown in man. J Clin Invest. 1987;80:1–6.
33. Pacy PJ, Nair KS, Ford C, Halliday D. Failure of insulin infusion to stimulate fractional muscle protein synthesis in type 1 diabetic patients. Diabetes. 1989;38:618–24.
34. Vilstrup H. Synthesis of urea after stimulation with amino acids: relation to liver function. Gut. 1980;21:990–5.
35. Marchesini G, Bianchi GP, Zoli M *et al.* Plasma amino acid response to protein ingestion in patients with liver cirrhosis. Gastroenterology. 1983;85:283–90.
36. Vilstrup H, Bucher D, Krag B, Damgård SE. Elimination of infused amino acids from plasma of control subjects and of patients with cirrhosis of the liver. Eur J Clin Invest. 1982;12:197–202.
37. Ferenci P, Bratusch-Marrain P, Waldhausl WK *et al.* Impaired plasma amino-acid clearance in patients with cirrhosis of the liver and portocaval shunt: its relation to insulin resistance. Eur J Clin Invest. 1984;14:255–61.
38. Marchesini G, Bianchi GP, Vilstrup H *et al.* Plasma clearances of branched-chain amino acids in control subjects and in patients with cirrhosis. J Hepatol. 1987;4:108–17.
39. Tilg H, Wilmer A, Vogel W *et al.* Serum levels of cytokines in chronic liver diseases. Gastroenterology. 1992;103:264–74.
40. Sheron N, Bird G, Goka J *et al.* Elevated plasma interleukine-6 and increased severity and mortality in alcoholic hepatitis. Clin Exp Immunol. 1991;84:449–53.
41. Petrides AS, Groop LC, Riely CA, DeFronzo RA. Effect of physiologic hyperinsulinemia on glucose and lipid metabolism in cirrhosis. J Clin Invest. 1991;88:561–70.
42. Leatherdale BA, Chase J, Rogers J *et al.* Forearm glucose uptake in cirrhosis and its relationship to glucose tolerance. Clin Sci. 1980;59:191–8.
43. Owen OE, Reichle FA, Mozzoli MA *et al.* Hepatic, gut, and renal substrate flux rates in patients with hepatic cirrhosis. J Clin Invest. 1981;68:240–52.
44. Owen OE, Trapp VE, Reichard GA *et al.* Nature and quantity of fuels consumed in patients with alcoholic cirrhosis. J Clin Invest. 1983;72:1821–32.
45. Kruszynska Y, Williams N, Perry M, Home P. The relationship between insulin sensitivity and skeletal muscle enzyme activities in hepatic cirrhosis. Hepatology. 1988;8:1615–19.
46. Lang S, Goldstein MS, Levine R. Influence of the liver on uptake of glucose by extrahepatic tissues. Am J Physiol. 1954;177:447–50.
47. Petersen KF, Tygstrup N. A liver factor increase glucose uptake in rat hindquarter. J Hepatol. 1991;13(suppl 2):S59.
48. Hattori N, Kurahahci H, Ikekubo K *et al.* Serum growth hormone-binding protein, insulin-like growth factor-I, and growth hormone in patients with liver cirrhosis. Metabolism. 1992;41:377–81.
49. Nielsen K, Kondrup J, Martinsen L *et al.* Protein requirement and retention in malnourished patients with liver cirrhosis. Clin Nutr. 1992(suppl);11:91.
50. Weber FL Jr, Bagby BS, Licate L, Kelsen SG. Effects of branched-chain amino acids on nitrogen metabolism in patients with cirrhosis. Hepatology. 1990;11:942–950.

51. Marchesini G, Dioguardi FS, Bianchi GP *et al.* Long-term oral branched-chain amino acid treatment in chronic hepatic encephalopathy. A randomized, double-blind, casein-controlled study. J Hepatol. 1990;11:92–101.
52. Gladisch R, Leweling H, Mase E *et al.* Peripheral exchange of amino acids (AA) postabsorptively and during total parenteral nutrition (TPN) in patients with liver cirrhosis. J Hepatol. 1990;10(suppl 1):S8.
53. Swart GR, Zillikens MC, van Wuure JK, van den Berg JWO. Effect of a late evening meal on nitrogen balance in patients with cirrhosis of the liver. Br Med J. 1989;299:1202–3.

Section IV
Liver and kidney

13

Physiological basis of interactions between liver and kidney

L. M. BLENDIS

One of the major complications of chronic liver disease is sodium retention with the development of ascites and oedema. However, several important points should be considered when examining liver and kidney interactions physiologically. At any point in time only a minority of patients with cirrhosis have ascites. Ascites is much commoner in some types of cirrhosis, such as alcoholic micronodular cirrhosis, than others, such as primary biliary cirrhosis. Finally, certain manoeuvres can reverse the sodium rentention without altering the liver function. Therefore, perhaps the most important question is: what is the major hepatic affector site for initiating the sodium-retaining lesion?

One of the earliest and most reproducible animal models for sodium retention was the chronic caval dog in which the lumen of the inferior vena cava (IVC) above the hepatic veins was constricted to about 60% of its cross-sectional area, following which the dog developed ascites by 48 h[1] (Fig. 1). If the IVC was constricted below the hepatic veins no ascites developed[2]. The effect of this model was to cause acute hepatic congestion and postsinusoidal portal hypertension. Orloff and co-workers[3] refined the model by graded ligation of the hepatic veins in the dog. When a certain portal pressure was reached, the dogs began to retain sodium[3]. Again, the histology was that of hepatic congestion. The problem with both models was how much the reduced venous return and hence cardiac output, resulting in a low output state, contributed to the sodium retention[4]. The ideal animal model for defining the role of raised hepatic sinusoidal pressure in causing sodium retention would be one of acute reversible portal hypertension, whilst maintaining cardiac output, arterial pressure, renal blood flow (RBF) and glomerular filtration rate (GFR) constant. This was achieved using Orloff's method of hepatic vein ligation and constriction of the remaining superior

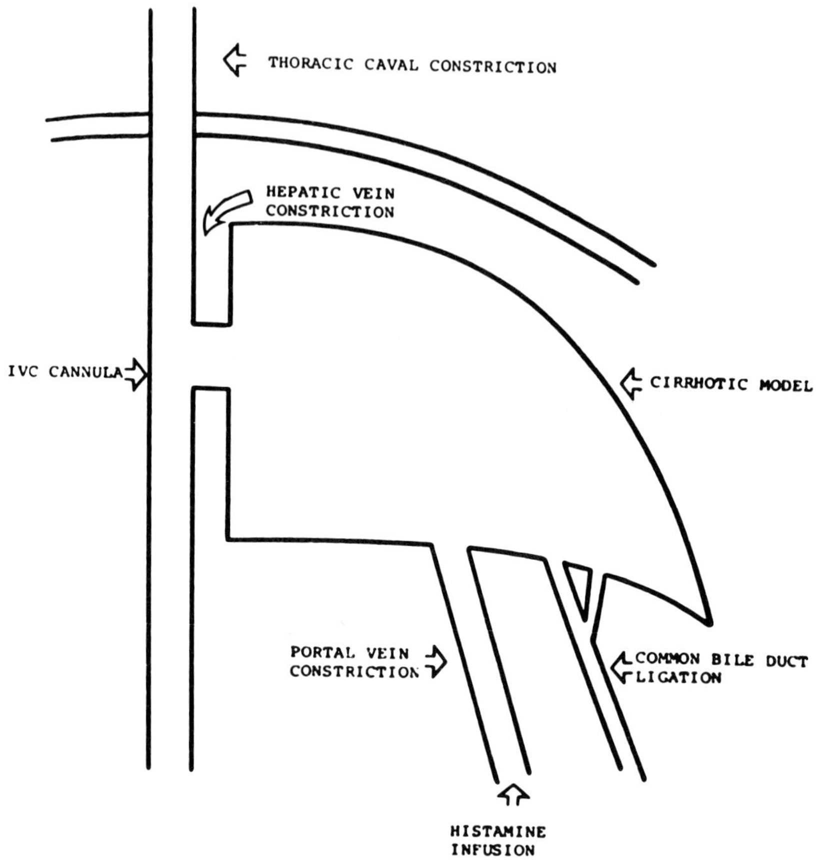

Fig. 1 Diagram of animal models used to explore hepatorenal interactions

hepatic vein, by means of an adjustable loop in the dog, whilst maintaining systemic and renal haemodynamics constant, by a graduated infusion of canine plasma[5]. In this way sinusoidal pressure was increased by 50% for 90 min. During this period in the group of eight dogs, urine volume and urine sodium output decreased by 60% (Fig. 2). At the end of the period the constriction on the superior hepatic vein was loosened, portal pressure returned to control levels, together with urine and sodium output. Cardiac output, renal blood flow and GFR remained unchanged throughout (Fig. 2.)

The liver histology in these dogs was normal. The study was repeated in another seven dogs, except that the portal vein was constricted, resulting in an identical 50% rise, this time in presinusoidal portal pressure, but there were no urinary changes. Other acute models which have produced similar results include histamine infusion into the portal vein[6].

In contrast, the problem with chronic portal hypertension models is that they develop cirrhosis. Therefore, in these models there are two possible factors: sinusoidal portal hypertension and abnormal liver function[7]. To

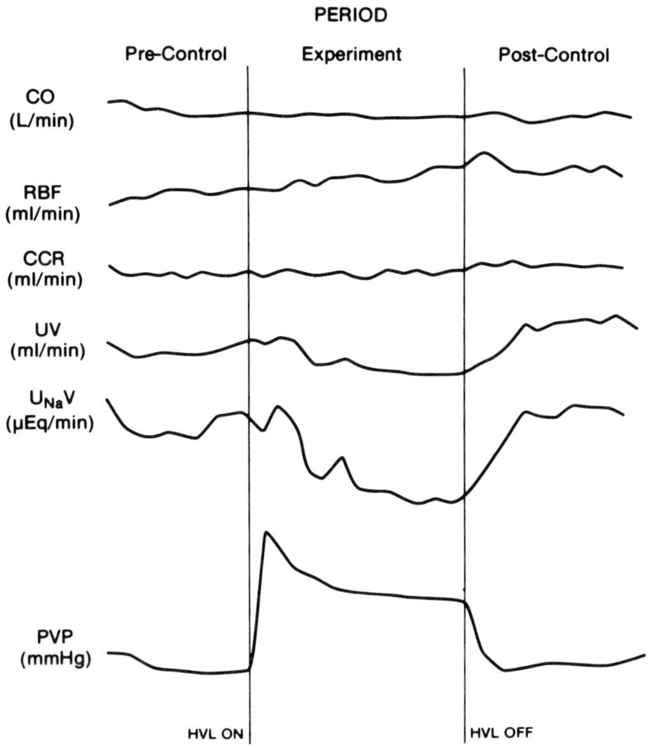

Fig. 2 A graphic illustration of the changes in a typical experiment of controlled, partial hepatic vein constriction. To be noted are the absence of changes in systemic and renal haemodynamics with acute portal hypertension induced by this method. In contrast, decreases in urine volume and sodium output are seen. (Reprinted from ref. 5, with permission of *Hepatology*)

dissect these factors, Levy and co-workers used the chronic bile duct ligated dog model which had previously been shown to result in salt and water retention[8].

In these cirrhotic dogs, in which portal hypertension had been reversed by a side to side portacaval shunt, no sodium retention occurred. Such dogs then escaped from the sodium retention effect of mineralocorticoids. In contrast, if these shunts became blocked the dogs once again retained sodium when given mineralocorticoids and failed to 'escape' from the effects.

Is there evidence of such a mechanism in humans? In a recent study, Warner and co-workers[9] found that non-ascitic cirrhotic patients were able to remain in sodium balance when challenged with 100 mmol sodium diet, by significant compensatory elevations of plasma atrial natriuretic peptide (pANP) levels compared to controls.

In these non-ascitic patients the elevated pANP levels were highly significantly correlated with sinusoidal pressures, which were all below 15 mmHg. This suggested that the elevated pressure was an important factor in causing sodium retention, resulting in an increase in intravascular and atrial volume with the resultant stimulation of ANP[10]. In two reviews of large numbers of non-ascitic and ascitic patients undergoing portal pressure measurements, it was shown that all cirrhotic patients with sinusoidal pressures below 8 mmHg were ascites-free on ultrasound[11,12]. Thus, it appears that there may be a critical threshold level of sinusoidal pressure, below which renal sodium retention is not encountered, but above which it is, resulting in the compensatory stimulation of ANP secretion. However, at some variable point, changes emanating from the splanchnic vascular compartment, as a result of the sinusoidal portal hypertension, overwhelm the compensatory increases in pANP resulting in sodium and fluid retention, with the formation of ascites. Portal hypertension continues to play a role at least initially, since a significant correlation was found between sinusoidal pressure and sodium excretion in patients with 'early' ascites[12] (Fig. 3).

The next important question is: 'What is the signal to the kidney to retain sodium?' The possibilities include hormonal, neuronal reflex or haemodynamic changes. Thus far, no sodium-retaining hormone has been described that is stimulated by a rise in hepatic sinusoidal pressure. The known sodium-retaining hormones, such as the renin–angiotensin–aldosterone system, have been shown to be normal or depressed in pre-ascitic cirrhotic patients[13], suggesting early volume expansion due to sodium retention. The possibility of a hepatorenal neuronal axis has been raised by a number of investigators. First, Kostreva and co-workers[14] suggested the presence of hepatic baroreceptors sensing intrahepatic hypertension and sending a non-volume-dependent signal to the kidney via the sympathetic nervous system.

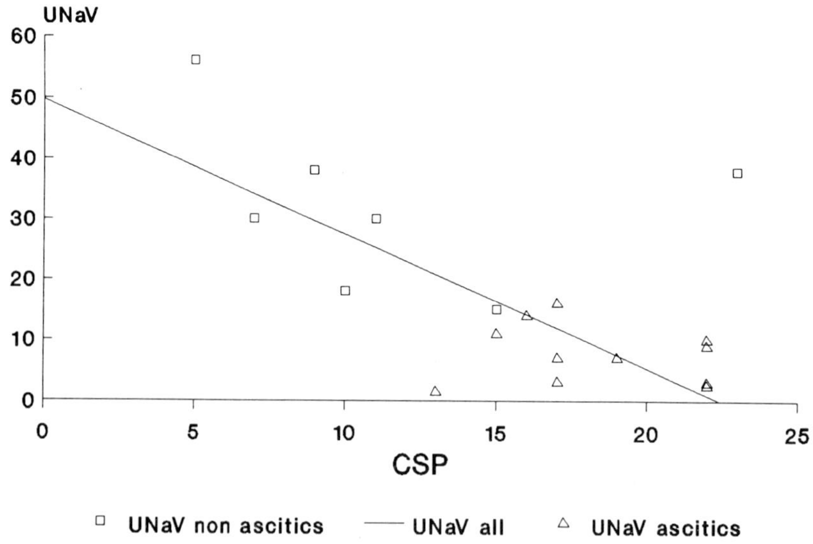

Fig. 3 Correlation between corrected sinusoidal pressure (CSP) and 24 h urinary sodium excretion (UNAV) in ascitic and 'early' ascitic patients; $r = -0.61$; $p < 0.01$ (reprinted with permission of Elsevier, publishers of *Journal of Hepatology*)

Then, in a recent study, Levy and Wexler[15] showed that hepatic denervation resulted in a modification of the sodium retention in the cirrhotic dog. On the renal side Koepke *et al.*[16] have shown that renal sympathetic denervation improves the responsiveness of the kidney in the cirrhotic rat to exogenous ANP.

An alternative theory involves circulatory changes as a result of portal hypertension. There is now universal acceptance that portal hypertension is associated with a hyperdynamic splanchnic circulation with vasodilation and increased portal venous inflow.[17] One theory suggests that, as a result, there is generalized vasodilation with decreasing effective arterial filling, leading to sodium retention[18]. However, a recent study in the rat with partial portal vein stenosis showed that the immediate effects of portal hypertension were a fall in systemic vascular resistance and a rise in cardiac output, followed days later by an increase in sodium space and finally an increase in superior mesenteric artery blood flow[19].

There is mounting evidence that portal hypertension may exert its renal effect by causing alterations in the systemic circulation, such as systemic hypotension, blunted cardiovascular responsiveness[20], and an abnormal hypertensive pressor response to change in posture[21]. In a recent study in cirrhotic rats, Bomzon *et al.*[22] confirmed the inverted hypertensive response. In addition, they found a diminished hypotensive response in precirrhotic portal hypertensive rats, confirming in a chronic model that portal hypertension *per se* in the absence of cirrhosis affects the autonomic control of the systemic vasculature.

Thus, when a compensated cirrhotic patient changes from an upright to a supine position, this results in a greater increase in cardiac output and ANP, and a decrease in peripheral vascular resistance, indicating an adaptation to overfilling[22]. Such data suggest that the elevated cardiac output and decreased arterial blood pressure are the circulatory response to, and thus consequence of, circulatory overfilling, rather than the cause. Further evidence for overfilling by studies in which such patients undergo head-out water immersion showed that they have a greater increase in pANP and an exaggerated natriuretic response[24] (Fig. 4).

In summary, there is mounting evidence that sinusoidal portal hypertension *per se* is the initial affector mechanism for renal sodium retention, rather than cirrhosis or impairment of liver function. However, the mechanism(s) by which the kidney receives the message or the interaction pathway remains uncertain, and an area of continued exciting basic and clinical investigation.

ACKNOWLEDGEMENTS

I thank our clinical research fellows over the past 15 years, and Ms Nancy Law and the nursing staff of the Clinical Investigation Unit, who through their efforts in performing the careful metabolic studies have made this chapter possible.

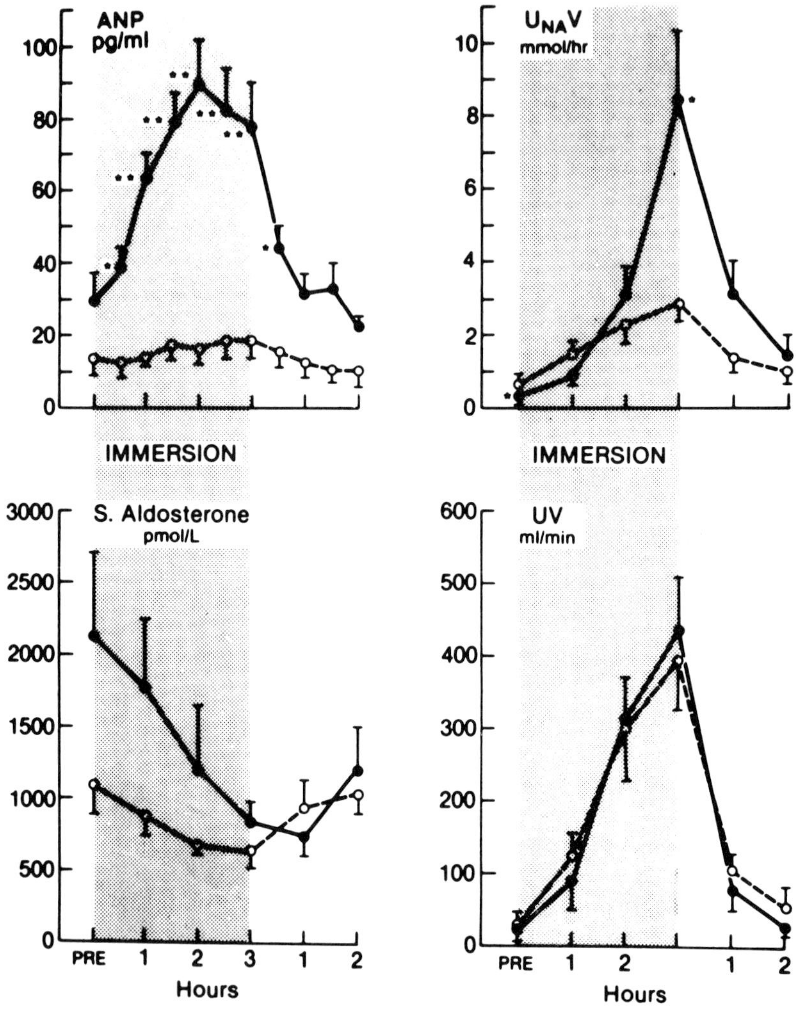

Fig. 4 Effect of 3 h of water immersion on atrial natriuretic peptide (ANP), serum aldosterone, urinary sodium excretion ($U_{NA}V$) and urinary volume (UV) in five normal volunteers, represented by open circles connected by broken line and five cirrhotics, represented by closed circles connected by solid lines. Significant values between controls and cirrhotics; $*p < 0.05$, $**p < 0.01$ (reprinted with permission of *Clinical and Investigative Medicine*)

References

1. Davis JO, Howell DS. Mechanisms of fluid and electrolyte retention in experimental preparations in dogs. Circ Res. 1953;1:171–6.
2. Levinsky NG, Lalone RC. Sodium excretion during acute saline loading in dogs with vena caval constriction. J Clin Invest. 1965;44:565–70.

3. Orloff MJ, Baddeley RM, Ross TH. Experimental ascites, production of hepatic outflow block and ascites with a hepatic vein choker. Ann Surg. 1965;161:258–62.
4. Anderson RJ, Cronin RE, McDonald KM, Schrier RW. Mechanisms of portal hypertension induced alterations in renal hemodynamics, renal water excretion and renin secretion. J Clin Invest. 1976;58:964–70.
5. Campbell V, Greig PD, Cranford J, Langer B, Silverman M, Blendis LM. A comparison of acute reversible pre and post sinusoidal portal hypertension on salt and water retention in the dog. Hepatology. 1982;2:54–8.
6. Levy M. Renal function in dogs with acute hepatic venous outflow block. Am J Physiol. 1974;227:1074–83.
7. Unikowsky B, Wexler MJ, Levy M. Dogs with experimental cirrhosis of the liver, but without intrahepatic hypertension do not retain sodium or form ascites. J Clin Invest. 1983;72:1594–604.
8. Better OS, Massry SG. Effect of chronic bile duct obstruction on renal handling of salt and water. J Clin Invest. 1972;551:402–11.
9. Warner LC, Campbell PJ, Morali GA, Logan AG, Skorecki KL, Blendis LM. The response of atrial natriuretic factor and sodium excretion to dietary sodium challenges in patients with chronic liver disease. Hepatology. 1990;12:460–6.
10. Sagnella GA, Markandu ND, Shore AC, MacGregor GA. Effects of changes in dietary sodium intake and saline infusion on immunoreactive atrial natriuretic peptide in human plasma. Lancet. 1985;2:1208–11.
11. Rector WG. Portal hypertension; a permissive factor only in the development of ascites and variceal bleeding. Liver. 1986;72:1594–604.
12. Morali GA, Sniderman KW, Deitel KM, Tobe S, Witte-Sullivan H, Simon M, Heathcote J, Blendis LM. Is sinusoidal portal hypertension a necessary factor for the development of hepatic ascites? J Hepatol. 1992; in press.
13. Bernardi M, Trevisani F, Santini C, DePalma R, Gasbarrini G. Aldosterone related blood volume expansion in cirrhosis before and during the early phase of ascites formation. Gut. 1983;24:761–6.
14. Kostreva DR, Castaner A, Kampine JP. Reflex effects of hepatic baroreceptors on renal and cardiac sympathetic nerve activity. Am J Physiol. 1980;238:R390–4.
15. Levy M, Wexler MJ. Hepatic denervation alters first phase urinary sodium excretion in dogs with cirrhosis. Am J Physiol. 1987;253:F664–71.
16. Koepke JP, Jones S, Dibona GF. Renal nerves mediate blunted natriuresis to atrial natriuretic peptide in cirrhotic rats. Am J Physiol. 1987;252:R1019–23.
17. Vorobioff J, Bredfeldt JE, Groszmann RJ. Hemodynamic circulation in portal hypertensive rat model. Am J Physiol. 1983;244:G52–7.
18. Schrier RW, Arroyo V, Bernardi M, Epstein M, Henriksen JH, Rodes J. Peripheral arterial vasodilation hypothesis; a proposal for the initiation of renal sodium and water retention in cirrhosis. Hepatology. 1988;8:1151–7.
19. Albillos A, Colombato LA, Groszmann RJ. Vasodilatation and sodium retention in prehepatic portal hypertension. Gastroenterology. 1992;102:931–5.
20. MacGilchrist AJ, Sumner D, Reid JL. Impaired pressor reactivity in cirrhosis; evidence for a peripheral vascular defect. Hepatology. 1991;13:689–94.
21. Bernardi M, Trevisani F, Santini C, Zolli G, Baraldini M, Ligabue A, Gasbarrini G. Plasma norepinephrine, weak neurotransmitters and renin activity during active tilting in liver cirrhosis; relationship with cardiovascular homeostasis and renal function. Hepatology. 1983;3:56–64.
22. Bomzon A, Weinbroum A, Blendis LM. Pressor response to a postural change in cirrhosis; an experimental study in the CCl_4 treated rat. Clin Sci. 1992;82:147–56.
23. Bernardi M, DiMarco C, Trevisani F, De Collibus C, Fornale L, Baraldini M, Andreone A *et al.* The hemodynamic status of preascitic cirrhosis; an evaluation under steady state conditions and after postural change. Hepatology. 1992;16:341–6.
24. Campbell PJ, Leung WM, Logan AG, Debowski TE, Blendis LM, Skorecki KL. Hyper-responsiveness to water immersion in sodium retaining cirrhotics; the role of atrial natriuretic factor. Clin Invest Med. 1988;11:392–5.

14

Pathogenesis of hepatorenal syndrome

D. HÄUSSINGER and F. LANG

INTRODUCTION

The hepatorenal syndrome can be defined as unexplained renal failure occurring in patients with liver disease in the absence of clinical, laboratory or anatomical evidence of other known causes of renal failure[1]. It is characterized by avid sodium and water retention, resulting in oliguria with a urine being typically almost sodium-free and retaining the capacity to concentrate, at least in early stages. The biochemical characteristics of urine in these patients are indistinguishable from those found in patients with prerenal azotaemia. Thus, in many instances renal failure due to hepatorenal syndrome can only be differentiated from prerenal azotaemia by the lack of improvement following volume expansion. There is considerable agreement that hepatorenal syndrome is functional in nature: kidneys transplanted from a patient who died with hepatorenal syndrome regain their normal function in the recipient[2] and orthotopic liver transplantation in a patient with hepatorenal syndrome restores kidney function[3]. However, so far the search for a unique pathophysiological mechanism causing hepatorenal syndrome has failed. Rather, a multitude of mechanisms join in bringing about this fatal complication. Several excellent reviews have appeared previously on this topic[1,4,5]; this chapter puts emphasis on a potential pathogenetic role of recently discovered hepatorenal interactions, namely a serotoninergic hepatorenal reflex and a putative liver-borne diuretic factor, and their potential role in the pathogenesis of hepatorenal syndrome.

GENERAL CONSIDERATIONS

In hepatorenal syndrome, renal blood flow, GFR and urinary sodium and water output are decreased with largely maintained functional integrity of the tubuli. The reduction of renal perfusion predominantly involves the kidney cortex. Renal arteriography disclosed marked beading and tortuosity of the interlobar and proximal arcuate arteries and an absence of distinct cortical nephrograms and vascular filling of the cortical vessels. These vascular abnormalities were found to subside when the kidneys were examined angiographically post mortem[6]. Different pathogenetic mechanisms are thought to contribute to these haemodynamic abnormalities, finally producing hepatorenal syndrome, a clinical syndrome of marked variability regarding both clinical presentation and course. Among them alterations of systemic haemodynamics, an imbalance between intrarenal vasoconstrictors and vasodilators, but also direct effects of the liver on kidney function, such as activation of a hepatorenal reflex and the role of a 'liver-borne diuretic factor' need to be discussed.

ALTERATIONS OF SYSTEMIC HAEMODYNAMICS

The part of circulating volume that is effective in stimulating volume receptors has been termed 'effective plasma volume', although the precise volume receptors involved are still elusive. It appears that decreased effective plasma volume in cirrhotics provides one stimulus for sodium and water retention in these patients by activation of the renin–angiotensin–aldosterone system and stimulation of vasopressin secretion. Although this compensation leads to a progressive increase in extracellular fluid, it may not normalize effective plasma volume because of fluid sequestration into other compartments such as the peritoneal cavity. This sequestration may be augmented by a high intrasinusoidal pressure and hypoalbuminaemia; i.e. parameters governing the Starling forces. Thus, sodium and water retention in the cirrhotic is rendered ineffective in terms of normalizing 'effective plasma volume': renal water and sodium retention continue because the resulting fluid overload bypasses the normal feedback control mechanisms.

The pathogenesis of decreased 'effective plasma volume' in cirrhosis is multifactorial; besides fluid sequestration systemic vasodilation appears to be especially important. Vasodilation can be attributed to a diminished clearance of substance P or vasoactive intestinal peptide by the diseased liver[7,8] and, probably more relevant, to bacterial endotoxin overflow into systemic circulation via portosystemic collaterals[9–11]. Indeed, high concentrations of circulating endotoxin are found in cirrhotics even without clinical evidence for infection[10,11]. Endotoxin stimulates the formation of cytokines, such as tumour necrosis factor, interferons and interleukins, which act to induce nitric oxide synthase in vascular endothelia and many other cell types (for review see ref. 12). This inducible form of nitric oxide synthase, once expressed, remains active for many hours, producing the highly potent vasodilator nitric oxide from arginine. Indeed, the hyperdynamic circulation in cirrhosis which is associated with hypotension and systemic vasodilation, can at least in part be attributed to an increased nitric oxide production[13,14]. Expression of the inducible form of nitric oxide synthase can be blocked by dexamethasone[15,16]; this may explain the reported stimulation of diuresis in some patients with liver disease by glucocorticoid administration[17]. Systemic vasodilation results in an activation of the sympathetic tone and cardiac output in order to maintain systemic blood pressure. Such a compensation, however, can be compromised not only under conditions of excessive peripheral nitric oxide production, but also by an impaired cardiac output due to myocardial dysfunction (e.g. alcoholic cardiomyopathy) and fluid sequestration (oedema and ascites formation) due to hypoalbuminaemia and increased intrasinusoidal pressure. This may explain why development of ascites and systemic hypotension was found to be associated with either increased or decreased or unaltered cardiac output[18]. Tense ascites may also compromise the venous blood return through the inferior vena cava, favouring oedema formation[5].

Much discussion has been devoted to the question of whether fluid sequestration is primary or secondary to renal sodium and water retention. It is likely that both mechanisms may operate in parallel or in sequence, because neither the classical 'underfilling' nor the 'overflow' theory can account exclusively for all observed derangements of volume regulation in liver cirrhosis[19]. Clearly, 'underfilling' of the vascular bed (i.e. a decreased 'effective plasma volume') will stimulate renal sodium and water retention, but there is also unequivocal evidence from animal experiments that renal sodium and water retention precedes the formation of ascites even in the absence of measurable alterations of systemic haemodynamics[20,21]. However, the possibility that initial water and sodium retention may have occurred in response to a subtle, non-measurable volume deficit was not excluded[21]. Interestingly, the 'early phase sodium retention' was abolished by hepatic denervation[20], pointing to an important role of neurohumoral mechanisms in mediating this renal response; i.e. mechanisms distinct from a simple 'underfilling' of the vascular bed (see later).

One consequence of diminished 'effective plasma volume' is activation of the sympathetic nervous system in order to maintain adequate tissue perfusion. Both arterial blood pressure and intravascular volume are sensed by high- and low-pressure baroreceptors, respectively, the latter acting as volume sensors in the cardiac atria. In addition, activation of the sympathetic nervous system may also be triggered by an increased intrasinusoidal pressure and/or liver cell swelling[19,22–24]. Activation of the sympathetic nervous tone and activation of sympathetic renal nerves produces a decrease in renal blood flow and glomerular filtration rate and stimulates sodium reabsorption[25,26]. Because a variety of in part unrelated signals (arterial blood pressure, venous filling, intrasinusoidal pressure, possibly also liver cell volume) can modify sympathetic nervous tone, the lack of correlation between cardiac output and renal perfusion found in cirrhotics[18,27] may no longer be surprising. In line with an important role of sympathetic hyperactivity in the pathogenesis of sodium retention, ascites formation and functional renal failure in cirrhosis is also the finding that noradrenaline plasma concentrations are normal in compensated cirrhosis but rise markedly in the ascitic cirrhotic and even more when hepatorenal syndrome develops[28,29]. Increased plasma noradrenaline levels are due to increased noradrenaline release but not to an impaired degradation[30–32]. Interestingly, in contrast to normal individuals there is a net output of noradrenaline by the kidney in cirrhotic patients[30–32], suggesting an increased activity of the renal sympathetic nervous system.

IMBALANCE BETWEEN RENAL VASOCONSTRICTORS AND VASODILATORS

Apart from the activation of the sympathetic nervous system, many other mediators have been implicated for bringing about renal vasoconstriction and sodium retention in hepatorenal syndrome (for reviews see refs 1, 5, 19 and 29), such as the renin–angiotensin–aldosterone system, an imbalance between vasodilating and vasoconstricting eicosanoids, alterations of the kallikrein–kinin system, altered concentrations of endotoxin, platelet-activating factor, atrial natriuretic peptide, antidiuretic hormone and vasoactive intestinal peptide. Some of these changes may be seen to result from an increased sympathetic nervous tone, but impaired hepatic elimination of some of these vasoactive agents may contribute, and in some instances the alterations may reflect epiphenomena without a major pathogenetic relevance for the development of hepatorenal syndrome. For a detailed discussion the reader is referred to refs 1, 5, 19 and 29. The plasma and urine concentrations of cysteinyl leukotrienes are enhanced in cirrhotic patients with hepatorenal syndrome[33,34] and these compounds elicit preglomerular vasoconstriction, a decrease in renal blood flow and glomerular filtration rate[35,36]. Whether enhanced leukotriene excretion in hepatorenal syndrome is due to an increased leukotriene formation inside the kidney, or merely reflects the inability of the liver to eliminate these potent mediators of inflammation, is unclear. Enhanced concentrations of vasoconstrictive thromboxanes are encountered in patients with advanced liver disease, but inhibition of thromboxane synthesis was without consistent beneficial effect on renal function[37]. The vasoconstricting action of sympathetic nerves, leukotrienes and thromboxanes is opposed by vasodilating prostaglandins[38] and it appears that hepatorenal syndrome is less frequent in patients with advanced liver cirrhosis exhibiting a high urinary prostaglandin excretion (for review see ref. 29). In line with this, inhibition of prostaglandin synthesis by indomethacin has been found to cause a rapid deterioration in renal function in advanced liver disease.

DIRECT REGULATION OF RENAL FUNCTION BY THE LIVER

Recent animal studies suggest that the liver directly regulates renal function via both a hepatorenal reflex and one or more humoral factors. Although not yet proven, both mechanisms could participate in the pathogenesis of hepatorenal syndrome: theoretically hepatorenal syndrome could be in part due to an enhanced hepatorenal reflex activity and/or a decreased release of the hypothetical liver-borne diuretic factors from the diseased liver. These phenomena could also explain the early phase of renal sodium and water retention preceding detectable alterations of systemic haemodynamics.

The serotoninergic hepatorenal reflex

The hepatorenal reflex can be elicited in the rat by infusion of glutamine into the superior mesenteric vein at a rate (2 μmol/min) which increases the portal glutamine concentration[23,24] by about 0.5 mmol/l. As shown in Fig. 1, mesenteric infusion of glutamine markedly decreases glomerular filtration rate (GFR) and urinary output, as well as sodium excretion. These changes are paralleled by a slight increase of systemic blood pressure (by 3 ± 1 mmHg) and a proportional decrease of *p*-aminohippurate (PAH) clearance by 67 ± 14%, such that the ratio of PAH clearance/GFR was not affected by mesenteric glutamine administration. Thus, the observed effects are not due to alterations of systemic haemodynamics, and apparently a decrease in renal blood flow is responsible for the fall of GFR. The effect of mesenteric glutamine on renal function was reversible following glutamine withdrawal

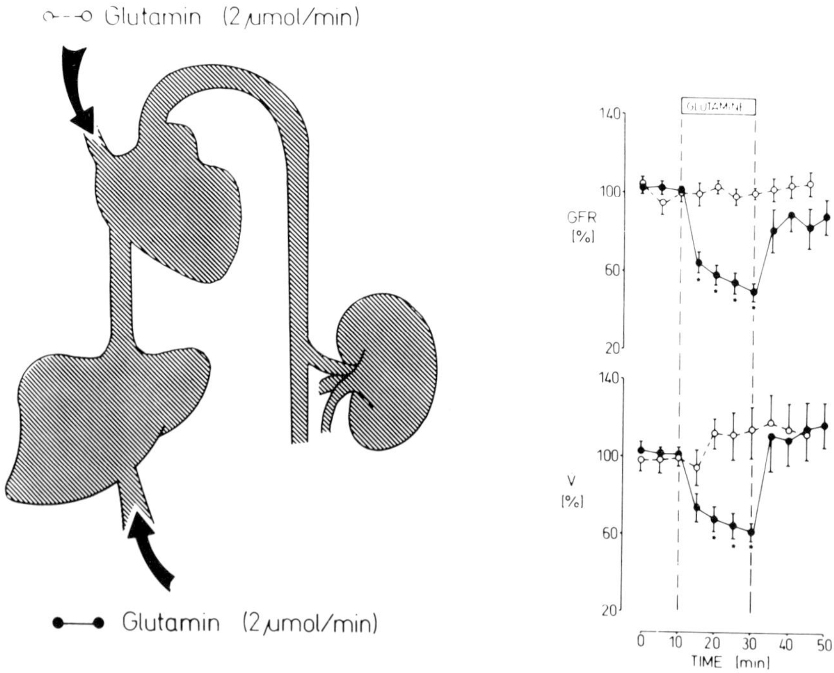

Fig. 1 Effect of glutamine on renal GFR and urinary flow rate (V). Glutamine (2 μmol/min) was delivered either to the superior mesenteric vein (●; $n = 16$) or to a jugular vein (○; $n = 9$). Values are expressed as percentages of the respective values before infusion of glutamine; i.e. 1.42 ± 0.10 ml/min for GFR and 2.32 ± 0.23 μl/min for urine flow. Values are given as means ± SEM. *Denotes significant differences ($p < 0.05$) between the effects of jugular and mesenteric glutamine infusion. From ref. 23

and was not observed when identical amounts of glutamine were infused into the jugular vein (Fig. 1). This latter finding rules out the possibility that systemic effects of the infused glutamine were responsible for the effect on the kidneys, and rather suggests a specific effect of glutamine on the liver. It should be emphasized that the difference between mesenteric and jugular infusion of glutamine largely resides in the concentration of glutamine reaching the liver, because extensive studies on the regulation of glutamine metabolism in perfused rat liver have shown that only about 5% of the glutamine dose administered to the mesenteric vein will be removed during a single liver passage[39–41].

The effect of mesenteric glutamine on renal function was fully blocked after either hepatic denervation, spinal transection at the cervicothoracic junction or periarterial renal denervation[23]. In line with this, unilateral periarterial kidney denervation blocks the hypofiltrative effect of mesenteric glutamine on GFR in the denervated, but not in the intact kidney (Fig. 2). The effect of mesenteric glutamine on GFR is abolished in the presence of the serotonin receptor antagonist methysergide and can be mimicked by infusion of serotonin into the mesenteric vein[24]. Hepatic vagotomy also

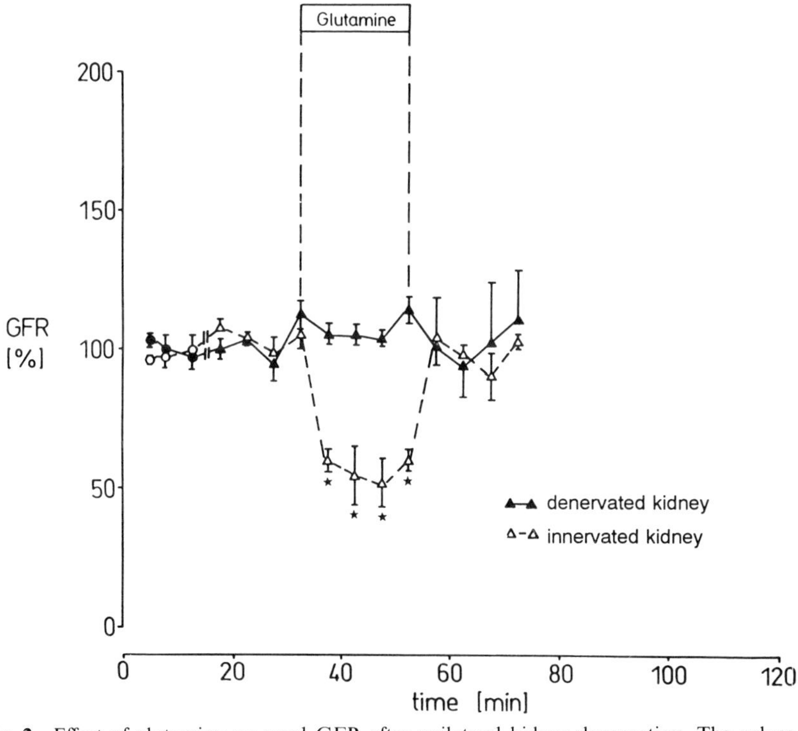

Fig. 2 Effect of glutamine on renal GFR after unilateral kidney denervation. The values of the denervated kidney (▲) are compared with those of the contralateral intact kidney (△). Glutamine (2 μmol/min) was delivered to the superior mesenteric vein. Values are expressed as percentages of the respective values before glutamine infusion. *Denotes significant differences ($p < 0.05$) between the response of the intact and the denervated kidney following mesenteric glutamine infusion

blunts the effect of mesenteric serotonin infusion on GFR[24]. We interpret these data in terms of a serotoninergic transmission of the hepatorenal reflex in the liver (Fig. 3).

The mechanism by which mesenteric glutamine activates the hepatorenal reflex is not fully known. The most likely, but causally not yet proven, mechanism is that the hepatorenal reflex is triggered by glutamine-induced liver cell swelling, rather than by the formation of a metabolite derived from the infused amino acid in the liver. Glutamine induces liver cell swelling up to 12% due to concentrative uptake of the amino acid into hepatocytes[42] and liver cell volume changes were recently recognized as an important determinant for metabolic liver cell function (for reviews see refs 43 and 44). Glutamine-induced hepatocyte swelling occurs within 2–3 min; the effect is already maximal at portal glutamine concentrations of about 2 mmol/l and is half-maximal[45] at about 0.7 mmol/l. Thus, raising the portal glutamine concentration from 0.5 to about 1 mmol/l, as done in the experiments depicted in Fig. 1, will increase liver cell volume by about 4%. In line with the idea that glutamine-induced liver cell swelling activates the hepatorenal reflex is the finding that the reflex is also activated upon infusion of serine, which also swells liver cells[45], whereas mesenteric infusion of glutamate, which does

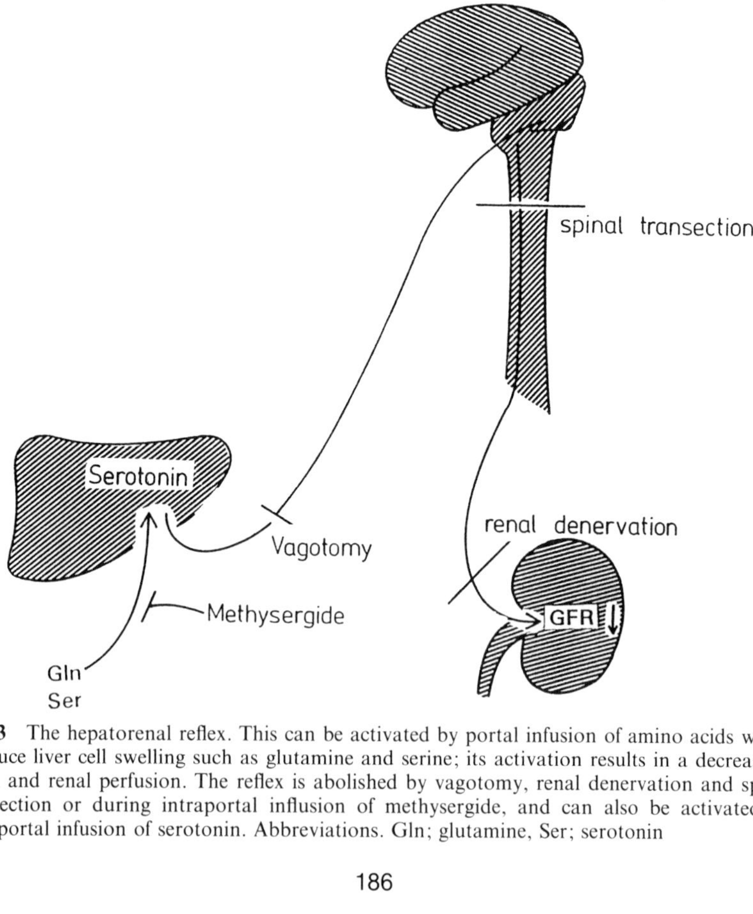

Fig. 3 The hepatorenal reflex. This can be activated by portal infusion of amino acids which produce liver cell swelling such as glutamine and serine; its activation results in a decrease of GFR and renal perfusion. The reflex is abolished by vagotomy, renal denervation and spinal transection or during intraportal influsion of methysergide, and can also be activated by intraportal infusion of serotonin. Abbreviations. Gln; glutamine, Ser; serotonin

not lead to cell swelling[45], has virtually no effect on renal function[23]. The mechanism by which cell swelling exerts the serotoninergic response remains to be elucidated. In this respect, however, it is of interest that the metabolism of a variety of amino acids was found to change following cell swelling[42,46]. Liver cell swelling could exert its effect on the reflex activity by raising the intrasinusoidal pressure or by other forms of mechanical stress on yet undefined sensing structures. Although glutamine-induced cell swelling in the isolated perfused rat liver is not accompanied by a detectable increase of portal perfusion pressure, this may well occur *in vivo*. Renal nerve activity was recently shown to be enhanced upon an increase of intrasinusoidal pressure; an effect which was abolished following hepatic denervation[22].

The hepatorenal reflex appears to be silent under most physiological conditions, since intraportal infusion of methysergide does not *per se* alter GFR appreciably[24]. The reflex, however, may be triggered by increased intrasinusoidal pressure, which may occur in response to a variety of stimuli or noxes causing liver cell swelling. For example, cell injury frequently leads to cell swelling, due to impairment of Na^+/K^+ ATPase (for reviews see refs 43 and 47) and cell swelling following liver hypoxia could then increase the intrasinusoidal pressure and thereby trigger the reflex. Conjugated bile acids have recently been shown to induce liver cell swelling[48]. Thus, one might speculate to what extent cholestasis could contribute to the triggering of the hepatorenal reflex. Some experimental data are indeed consistent with enhanced renal nerve activity in liver disease. Renal denervation reverses the sodium retention in experimental liver cirrhosis and experimental cardiac insufficiency[49–51]; both conditions are associated with an enhanced intrasinusoidal pressure. Thus, it is likely that the deterioration of renal function under these conditions is at least in part a result of enhanced renal nerve activity. In line with this, the early phase of sodium retention, which precedes the overt formation of ascites and haemodynamic changes in cirrhotic dogs, is prevented by hepatic denervation[20]. This suggests that activation of the hepatorenal reflex could play a role in initiating the disturbance of volume homeostasis, before alterations of systemic haemodynamics become detectable. Such a view is also augmented by the finding that in patients with hepatorenal syndrome lumbar sympathetic blockade proved to be effective in increasing GFR and urine flow[51].

The hypothetical liver-borne diuretic factor

There is accumulating evidence that the liver can release one or more humoral principles with diuretic activity. Such a hypothetical liver-borne diuretic factor (LBDF) is probably released by the liver following perivascular nerve stimulation and portal administration of glucagon[23,52–54].

When glucagon is infused into the mesenteric vein of rats at rates (1 ng/min) roughly mimicking its postprandial release *in vivo*, there is an increase of GFR and urinary flow, which does not occur when the same amount of hormone is infused into the jugular vein[23] (Fig. 4). Only higher infusion

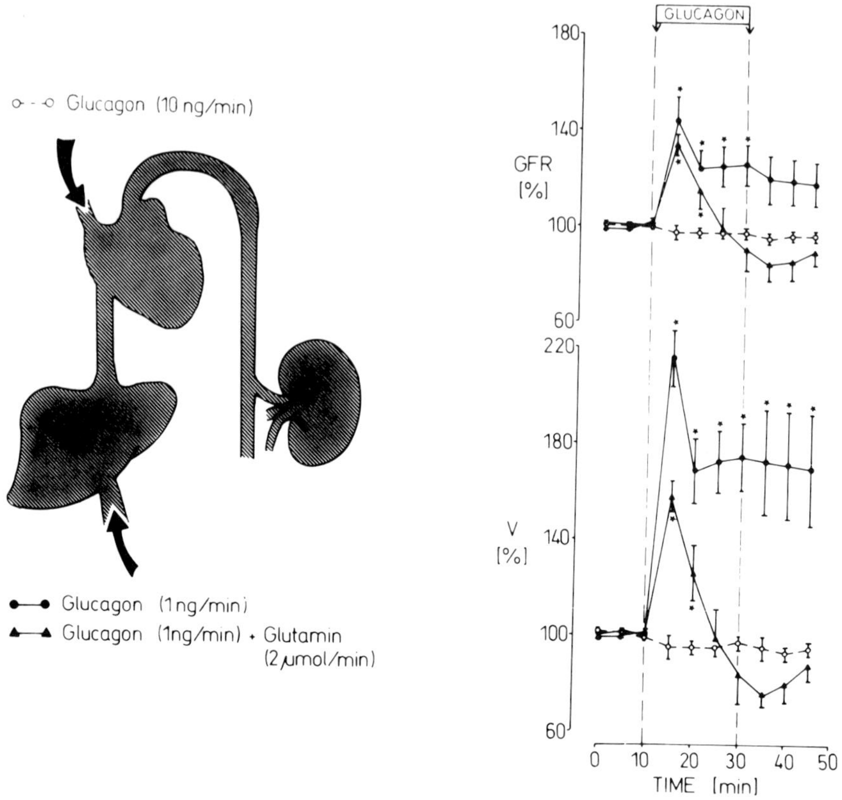

Fig. 4 Effect of glucagon on renal GFR and urinary flow rate (V). Glucagon (1 ng/min) was delivered to the superior mesenteric vein alone (●; $n = 7$), to the superior mesenteric vein together with glutamine (2 µmol/min) (▲; $n = 7$) or to a jugular vein alone (○; $n = 4$). Values are expressed as percentages of the respective values before effector infusion. *Denotes significant differences ($p < 0.05$) between the effects of mesenteric and jugular glucagon infusion. From ref. 23

rates (10 ng/min) into the jugular vein proved to enhance GFR, probably acting again via the liver. Likewise portal administration of glucagon in the dog increased GFR[53]. Glucagon was recently shown to induce liver cell shrinkage[55,56] and to reverse glutamine-induced cell swelling[23]. Indeed, glucagon prevents the decrease of GFR following mesenteric glutamine administration (Fig. 4). Although these data might suggest that glucagon-induced cell shrinkage could block the hepatorenal reflex, its action appears to involve a putative LBDF, because the hyperfiltrative effect of mesenteric glucagon is not abolished after hepatic denervation or transection of the spinal cord (unpublished result).

The existence of a hormone released by the liver with a diuretic action was postulated by Uranga as early as 1969[57]. This so-called 'glomerulopressin' is released by amphibian livers and is found in the blood of volume-expanded rabbits[58] and glucagon-treated dogs[59]. It is at present unclear whether the glomerulopressin is identical to the LBDF accounting for our observations.

The involvement of LBDF and/or glomerulopressin in the pathophysiology of hepatorenal syndrome is at present purely hypothetical. However, it was hypothesized that failure of the liver to produce the putative 'glomerulopressin' in cirrhosis may be involved in the pathogenesis of hepatorenal syndrome[60]. For example, in this condition the untoward effect of the hepatorenal reflex may not be counteracted by the simultaneous release of the hyperfiltrative hormones.

CONCLUSIONS AND PERSPECTIVES

The pathogenesis of hepatorenal syndrome is complex and several mechanisms combine to decrease renal blood flow, GFR and urinary output. Our view on the interplay of major pathogenetic events is schematically depicted in Fig. 5. Peripheral vasodilation and (probably later) fluid sequestration in the cirrhotic leads to a decrease of effective plasma volume triggering compensatory responses, such as activation of the sympathetic nervous system and the renin–angiotensin–aldosterone system. This results in fluid and water retention by the kidney. However, this compensation is rendered ineffective, because the fluid retained is sequestered due to hypoproteinaemia and portal hypertension (ascites, oedema) and will not increase effective plasma volume, which is the underlying stimulus for fluid retention. Hepatocyte swelling producing mechanical stress on cellular structures in the sinusoid and/or an increase of the intrasinusoidal blood pressure may be a rather early event, which activates the hepatorenal reflex and consequently renal

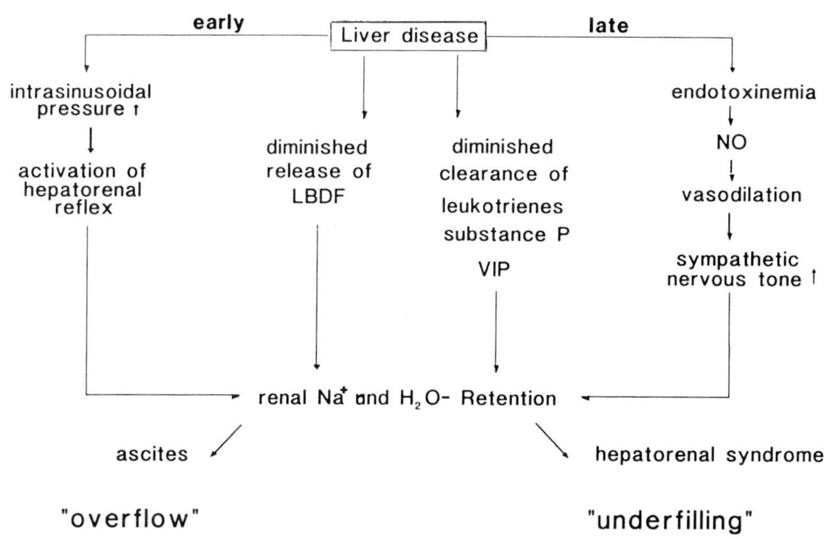

Fig. 5 Tentative hypothesis on the pathogenesis of hepatorenal syndrome. For details see text

sodium and fluid retention, even before overt ascites develops. Simultaneously, the release of LBDF from the diseased liver may be blunted, augmenting the renal response. Disturbances in the local or systemic production of various eicosanoids can aggravate renal hypoperfusion. Many questions remain open. They relate to the exact pharmacology of the serotoninergic hepatorenal reflex, the characterization of LBDF and the role of NO in regulating tissue-specific perfusion. Further studies are required to delineate the interplay between cell volume, reflex activation and LBDF release under physiological conditions and their interplay with other effectors on volume homeostasis. It is hoped that this short chapter will stimulate further research in this area.

References

1. Epstein M. Hepatorenal syndrome. In: Epstein M (editor). The kidney in liver disease. Baltimore: Williams & Wilkins; 1988:89–118.
2. Koppel MH, Coburn JW, Mims MM, Goldstein H, Boyle JD, Rubini ME. Transplantation of cadaveric kidneys from patients with hepatorenal syndrome. Evidence for the functional nature of renal failure in advanced liver disease. N Engl J Med. 1969;280:1367–71.
3. Iwatsuki S, Popovtzer MM, Corman JL, Ishikawa M, Putnam CW, Katz FH, Starzl TE. Recovery from hepatorenal syndrome after orthotopic liver transplantation. N Engl J Med. 1973;289:1155–9.
4. Schrier RW, Arroyo V, Bernardi M, Epstein M, Henrikson JH, Rhodes J. Peripheral arterial vasodilatation hypothesis: a proposal for the initiation of renal sodium and water retention in cirrhosis. Hepatology. 1988;8:1151–7.
5. Levy M. Hepatorenal syndrome. In: Seldin DW, Giebisch G, editors. The kidney: physiology and pathophysiology. New York: Raven Press; 1992:3305–26.
6. Epstein M, Berk DP, Hollenberg NK, Adams DF, Chalmers TC, Abrams HL, Merrill JP. Renal failure in the patient with cirrhosis. The role of active vasoconstriction. Am J Med. 1970;49:175–85.
7. Hörtnagl H, Singer EA, Lenz K, Kleinberger G, Lochs H. Substance P is markedly increased in plasma of patients with hepatic coma. Lancet. 1984;ii:480–3.
8. Lenz K, Hörtnagl H, Druml W, Grimm A, Laggner B, Schneeweiss Z, Kleinberger G. Beneficial effect of 8-ornithine-vasopressin on renal dysfunction in decompensated cirrhosis. Gut. 1989;30:90–6.
9. Bourgoignie JJ, Valle GA. Endotoxin and renal dysfunction in liver disease. In: Epstein M, editor. The kidney in liver disease. Baltimore: Williams & Wilkins; 1988:486–507.
10. Lumsden AB, Henderson JM, Kutner MH. Endotoxin levels measured by a chromatographic assay in portal, hepatic and peripheral blood in patients with cirrhosis. Hepatology. 1988;8:232–6.
11. Yomota M, Kambayashi J, Tanaka T, Tsujinaka T, Sakon M, Mori T. A simple turbometric time assay of the endotoxin in plasma. J Biochem Biophys Meth. 1989;18:97–104.
12. Moncada S, Palmer RMJ, Higgs EA. Nitric oxide: physiology, pathophysiology and pharmacology. Pharmacol Rev. 1991;43:109–42.
13. Vallance P, Moncada S. Hyperdynamic circulation in cirrhosis: a role for nitric oxide? Lancet. 1991;337:776–8.
14. Pizcueta MP, Bosch J, Whittle BJR, Moncada S. Effects of inhibiting nitric oxide biosynthesis on the systemic and splanchnic circulation of rats with portal hypertension. Br J Pharmacol. 1992;105:184–90.
15. O'Connor KJ, Moncada S. Glucocorticoids inhibit the induction of nitric oxide synthase and the related cell damage in adenocarcinoma cells. Biochim Biophys Acta. 1991;1097:227–31.
16. Palmer RMJ, Bridge L, Foxwell NA, Moncada S. The role of nitric oxide in endothelial cell damage and its inhibition by glucocorticoids. Br J Pharmacol. 1992;105:11–12.
17. Lintrup J, Friis T, Nissen NI. Comparative studies on the diuretic and biochemical effects of prednisolone and spironolactone in hepatic cirrhosis. J Lab Clin Med. 1966;94:520–36.

18. Epstein B, Schneider N, Befeler B. Relationship of systemic and intrarenal hemodynamics in cirrhosis. J Lab Clin Med. 1977;89:1175–87.
19. Better OS, Schrier RW. Disturbed volume homeostasis in patients with cirrhosis of the liver. Kidney Int. 1983;23:303–11.
20. Levy M, Wexler MJ. Renal sodium retention and ascites in dogs with experimental cirrhosis but without portal hypertension or increased splanchnic vascular capacity. J Lab Clin Med. 1978;94:3305–536.
21. Levy M, Allotey JBK. Temporal relationship between urinary salt retention and altered systemic hemodynamics in dogs with experimental cirrhosis. J Lab Clin Med. 1978;92:560–9.
22. Kostreva D, Cataner A, Kampine J. Reflex effects of hepatic baroreceptors on renal and cardiac sympathetic nerve activity. Am J Physiol. 1980;238:R390–4.
23. Lang F, Tschernko E, Schulze E, Öttl I, Ritter M, Völkl H, Hallbrucker C, Häussinger D. Hepatorenal reflex regulating kidney function. Hepatology. 1991;14:590–4.
24. Lang F, Öttl I, Freudenschuß K, Honeder M, Tschernko E, Häussinger D. Serotoninergic hepatorenal reflex regulating renal glomerular filtration rate. Pflügers Arch Physiol. 1991;419:111–13.
25. Bichet DG, Van Putten VJ, Schrier RW. Potential role of increased sympathetic activity in impaired sodium and water excretion in cirrhosis. N Engl J Med. 1982;397:1552–7.
26. Reid IA, Morris BJ, Ganong WF. The renin angiotensin system. Ann Rev Physiol. 1978;40:377–10.
27. Ring-Larsen H, Hesse B, Stigsby B. Effect of porto-systemic anastomosis on renal hemodynamics in cirrhosis. Gut. 1976;17:865–70.
28. Arroyo V, Gaya J, Deulofeu R, Rimola A, Perez-Ayuso RM, Rivera F, Rodes J. Sympathetic nervous activity, renin-angiotensin system and renal excretion of prostaglandin E_2 in cirrhosis. Relationship to functional renal failure and sodium and water excretion. Eur J Clin Invest. 1983;13:271–8.
29. Arroyo V, Ginés P, Jiménez W, Rodés J. Ascites, renal failure and electrolyte disorders in cirrhosis. Pathogenesis, diagnosis and treatment. In: McIntyre N, Benhamou JP, Bircher J, Rizzetto M, Rodés J, editors. Oxford textbook of hepatology. Oxford: Oxford Medical Publishers; 1991:429–70.
30. Henriksen J, Christensen N, Ring-Larsen H. Noradrenaline and adrenaline concentrations in various vascular beds in patients with cirrhosis. Relation to hemodynamics. Clin Physiol. 1981;1:293–304.
31. Henriksen J, Ring-Larsen H, Kanstrup IL, Christensen NJ. Splanchnic and renal elimination and release of catecholamines in cirrhosis. Evidence of enhanced sympathetic nervous activity in patients with decompensated cirrhosis. Gut. 1984;25:1034–43.
32. Willet I, Esler M, Burke F, Leonard P, Dudley F. Total and renal sympathetic nervous system activity in alcoholic cirrhosis. J Hepatol. 1985;1:639–48.
33. Huber M, Kästner S, Schölmerich J, Gerok W, Keppler D. Analysis of cysteinyl leukotrienes in human urine: enhanced excretion in patients with liver cirrhosis and hepatorenal syndrome. Eur J Clin Invest. 1989;19:53–60.
34. Keppler D. Stoffwechsel und Analyse von Leukotrienen *in vivo*. Klin Wochenschr. 1988;66:9997–1004.
35. Badr KF, Brenner BM, Ichikawa I. Effects of leukotriene D_4 on glomerular dynamics in the rat. Am J Physiol. 1987;253:F239–43.
36. Gulbins E, Parekh N, Rauterberg EW, Schlottmann K, Steinhausen M. Cysteinyl leukotriene actions on the microcirculation of the normal and split hydronephrotic rat kidney. Eur J Clin Invest. 1991;21:184–96.
37. Zipser RD, Kronborg I, Rector W, Reynolds T, Daskalopoulos G. Therapeutic trial of thromboxane synthesis inhibition in the hepatorenal syndrome. Gastroenterology. 1984;87:1228–32.
38. Epstein M, Lifschitz M. Renal eicosanoids as determinants of renal function in liver disease. Hepatology. 1987;7:1359–67.
39. Häussinger D, Gerok W, Sies H. Regulation of flux through glutaminase and glutamine synthetase in isolated perfused rat liver. Biochim Biophys Acta. 1983;755:272–8.
40. Häussinger D. Hepatocyte heterogeneity in glutamine and ammonia metabolism and the role of an intercellular glutamine cycle during ureogenesis in perfused rat liver. Eur J Biochem. 1983;133:269–75.

41. Häussinger D, Sies H. Effect of phenylephrine on glutamate and glutamine metabolism in isolated perfused rat liver. Biochem J. 1984;221:651–8.
42. Häussinger D, Lang F, Bauers K, Gerok W. Interactions between glutamine metabolism and cell volume regulation in perfused rat liver. Eur J Biochem. 1990;188:689–95.
43. Häussinger D, Lang F. Cell volume in the regulation of hepatic function: a mechanism for metabolic control. Biochim Biophys Acta. 1991;1071:331–50.
44. Häussinger D. The hepatocellular hydratation state: a regulator of liver cell function. Hepatol Rapid Lit Rev. 1992;22:V–VIII.
45. Wettstein M, vom Dahl S, Lang F, Gerok W, Häussinger D. Cell volume regulatory responses of isolated perfused rat liver: the effect of amino acids. Biol Chem Hoppe-Seyler. 1990;371:493–501.
46. Häussinger D, Lang F. Osmolarity regulates hepatic nitrogen metabolism. J Cell Biochem. 1990;43:355–61.
47. Lang F, Völkl H, Häussinger D. General principles in cell volume regulation. Comp Physiol. 1990;4:1–25.
48. Häussinger D, Hallbrucker C, Saha N, Lang F, Gerok W. Cell volume is a major determinant of bile acid excretion. Biochem J. 1992;288:681–9.
49. DiBona GF, Herman PJ, Sawin LL. Neural control of renal function in edema-forming ascites. Am J Physiol. 1988;254:R1017–24.
50. Koepke JP, Jones S, DiBona GF. Renal nerves mediate blunted natriuresis to atrial natriuretic peptide in cirrhotic rats. Am J Physiol. 1987;252:R1019–23.
51. Solis-Herruzo JA, Duran A, Favela V, Castellano G, Madrid JL, Munoz-Yague MT, Morillas JD, Estenoz J. Effects of lumbar sympathetic block on kidney function in cirrhotic patients with hepatorenal syndrome. J Hepatol. 1987;5:167–73.
52. Lang F, Öttl I, Tschernko E, Häussinger D. Influence of hepatic α-adrenergic innervation on renal glomerular filtration rate. Pflügers Arch. 1992; submitted.
53. Premen AJ. Importance of the liver during glucagon-mediated increases in canine renal hemodynamics. Am J Physiol. 1985;249:F319–22.
54. Lang F, Tschernko E, Häussigner D. Hepatic regulation of renal function. Exp Physiol. 1992;77:663–73.
55. Hallbrucker C, vom Dahl S, Lang F, Gerok W, Häussinger D. Modification of liver cell volume by insulin and glucagon. Pflügers Arch. 1991;418:519–21.
56. vom Dahl S, Hallbrucker C, Lang F, Häussinger D. Regulation of liver cell volume by hormones. Biochem J. 1992;280:105–9.
57. Uranga J. The hepatic production of a glomerular pressure substance in the toad (*Bufo arenarum*). Gen Comp Endocrinol. 1969;13:179–84.
58. Uranga J, Fuenzalida R. Effect of glomerulopressin and a rabbit glomerulopressin-like substance in the rat. Horm Metab Res. 1975;7:180–4.
59. Uranga J, Fuenzalida R, Rapoport AL, del Castillo E. Effect of glucagon and glomerulopressin on the renal function of the dog. Horm Metab Res. 1979;11:275–9.
60. Alvestrand A, Bergström J. Glomerular hyperfiltration after protein ingestion, during glucagon infusion and in insulin-dependent diabetes is induced by a liver hormone: deficient production of this hormone in hepatic failure causes hepatorenal syndrome. Lancet. 1984;1:195–7.

15

Hepatorenal syndrome: differential diagnosis and therapy

P. GENTILINI

INTRODUCTION

Patients affected by liver cirrhosis are usually admitted to the hospital because of complications. The most frequent complication is represented by ascites. According to what has previously been reported by several authors, it is necessary first to perform a diagnostic paracentesis, then to monitor the patients with the aim of assessing liver and renal function and electrolyte balance. In decompensated patients an observation period of 1 week, during which they maintain bed rest and a sodium-restricted diet, allows one to obtain:

1. information on the characteristics of the ascitic fluid;
2. data on liver and renal function;
3. in some cases (about 10–15%), a complete recovery from ascites, possibly adding low doses of human albumin.

In patients who do not respond to this simple regimen it is necessary to add diuretics in a sequential manner according to an overall accepted protocol[1].

During diuretic treatment we can obtain:

1. indications on the minimum dosage useful in obtaining negative sodium balance and stable equilibrium of body weight;
2. progressive selection of cases at risk: those patients who respond less and less to sequential diuretic treatment.

On the basis of this careful therapeutic approach we are able to identify a number of patients, examined during the first admission (about 6%), who present a progressively weaker response to diuretics and plasma expanders and, further, show typical signs of refractory ascites[1]. This clinical situation corresponds to a large abdominal fluid accumulation which cannot be removed through diuretic treatment, or if it is removed, is accompanied by the occurrence of severe side-effects[2,3]

Although a definition for refractory ascites should take into consideration other elements, for example the compliance of patients to a sodium- and water-restricted diet and a bed rest regimen, the use of human albumin or other plasma expanders, and finally the correct approach to sequential treatment with diuretics, the definition reported above seems to be accepted worldwide. It is also necessary, however, to consider the relationship between refractory ascites and the possible occurrence of renal function impairment (RFI), given that most cases with refractory ascites and renal dysfunction eventually present an open hepatorenal syndrome (HRS).

Considering the two different stages of RFI, as shown in Table 1, a significant decrease in renal clearances has been observed in patients affected by active chronic hepatitis and more often in liver cirrhosis[4,5]. However, not all patients with refractory ascites present the typical signs of overt HRS, rather every patient with tense or refractory ascites generally shows signs of RFI (the first stage of HRS) on the basis of their condition or, more often, after diuretic treatment and hospital admission[6,7].

Even if HRS occurs in fulminant hepatic failure, alcoholic hepatitis or liver cancer[8,9], the majority of patients with refractory ascites and HRS have advanced liver cirrhosis. In almost every patient with decompensated cirrhosis there is the possibility of a progressive decrease in renal clearances, especially in older patients, without a close relationship to the behaviour of the renal prostaglandin system or the severity of liver disease[10,11].

Sometimes the onset of HRS can be very fast, and in this case it seems more appropriate to define this syndrome as an unexpected and unforeseen situation of renal failure which occurs without any evidence of known causes for acute renal failure[10,12,13].

In this setting it seems essential to consider the effective arterial blood volume (EABV), the circulating volume which stimulates volume arterial receptors. In patients with refractory ascites, and particularly with HRS, the

Table 1 Stages of renal functional impairment in patients with liver cirrhosis

Stage I or latent HRS	*Stage II or overt HRS*
Serum creatinine <1.5	Serum creatinine >1.5
BUN <0.5	BUN >0.5
Reduction (>50%) in renal clearances (RPF and GFR)	More marked reduction in renal clearances
Deficit in free water clearance	Oliguria (<250 ml/day)
Sodium retention (positive balance)	Urinary sodium <10 mEq/l
Renal haemodynamic alterations:	U/P osmolality ratio >1
Cortical hypoperfusion	U/P creatinine ratio >30
Arteriovenous shunts	More marked renal haemodynamic alterations
Improvement after plasma expansion (?)	No improvement after plasma expansion

level of EABV seems decreased because of the disturbance of the Starling forces regulating the fluid balance within the extracellular fluid compartment, especially in hepatosplanchnic microcirculation, and the decrease in total peripheral resistances[10,14]. This phenomenon plays an important role in stimulating general vasoactive systems such as the sympathetic nervous system (SNS) and the renin–angiotensin–aldosterone system (RAA), and in determining abnormal sodium and water retention.

The infusion of large amounts of plasma expanders in patients with refractory ascites and HRS is usually not effective in inducing recovery, but only gives the possibility of distinction between HRS and pseudo-hepatorenal syndrome or prerenal azotaemia[10,13]. In fact, patients with advanced liver cirrhosis are generally susceptible to prerenal arotaemia and acute renal failure, with a rapid decrease in the glomerular filtration rate (GFR) due to severe renal hypoperfusion[13,15]. Because of the latter, there is a reduction in urea more than in creatinine clearance, even if the plasma urea level increases less because of its decreased hepatic synthesis[13]. Only these patients, with prerenal acute failure, show a good response to plasma expanders.

The permanent decreased EABV in advanced liver cirrhosis may play a fundamental role in increasing sodium reabsorption at the renal tubule, and at the same time predisposing to HRS[6,16,17].

DIFFERENTIAL DIAGNOSIS

In an attempt to seek a correct diagnosis it is necessary, above all, to consider acute tubular necrosis (ATN) and then postrenal acute renal failure (PRARF), generally due to obstructive uropathy (papillary necrosis, bleeding in urinary tract) sometimes observed in patients with liver cirrhosis[13]. The comparative examination can be performed considering some clinical and biochemical characteristics, as shown in Table 2.

Some clinical observations seem to support the hypothesis that HRS represents a particular RFI, which becomes more and more evident, leading to the stage of no return, also on the basis of histological modifications. In fact, renal biopsies performed in these patients sometimes showed only mild, not significant, glomerular and tubular modifications[6,7,18] (Fig. 1), but in other cases histological alterations, including tubular damage and leucocyte infiltration in vasa-recta[19–21] were evident (Figs 2 and 3). These histological findings, and the report of some rapid manifestations of HRS, explain why in some circumstances the distinction between suddenly deteriorating chronic RFI and ATN can be very difficult.

Since the principal distinction between HRS and ATN, from a pathophysiological point of view, is based on the presence, or lack of, histological alterations in patients where it is difficult to perform renal biopsy, it is possible to consider data in favour of and against the functional nature of HRS (Tables 3 and 4).

Table 2 Characteristics and signs of acute renal failure in patients with liver cirrhosis

Parameters	*PA*	*HRS*	*ATN*	*PRARF*
Liver disease	Often severe	Severe	Variable, eventually jaundiced	Severe, generally alcoholic
Precipitating factors	Diuretics, diarrhoea, bleeding	None	Nephrotoxic drugs, shock	Papillary necrosis, bleeding in urinary tract
Onset	Days	Days or weeks	Hours	Hours
Urine volume	Oliguria	Oliguria	Generally oliguria	Oliguria
Urine sodium concentration	< 10 mEq/l	< 10 mEq/l	Generally < 10 mEq/l	> 30 mEq/l
U/P osmolality ratio	> 1	> 1	1	1
U/P creatinine ratio	< 30	> 30	< 20	< 30
Urine sediment	Normal	Generally normal	Debris, casts	Variable
Central venous pressure	< 5 cmH_2O	– 10 cmH_2O	– 10 cmH_2O	– 10 cmH_2O
Response to plasma expanders	Good	None, Preventive?	None	None
Prognosis	Good	Poor	Variable	Variable

PA: Prerenal azotaemia; HRS: heptorenal syndrome; ATN: acute tubular necrosis; PRARF: postrenal acute renal failure

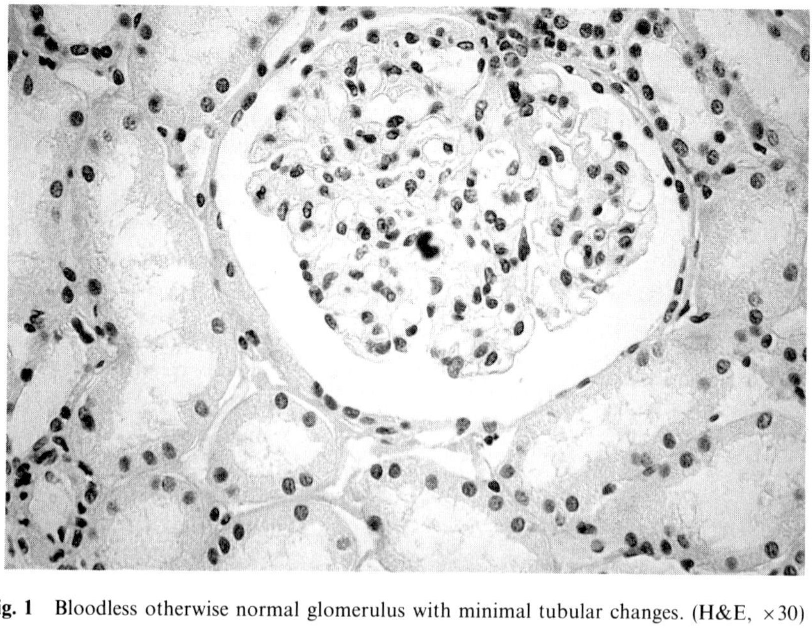

Fig. 1 Bloodless otherwise normal glomerulus with minimal tubular changes. (H&E, ×30)

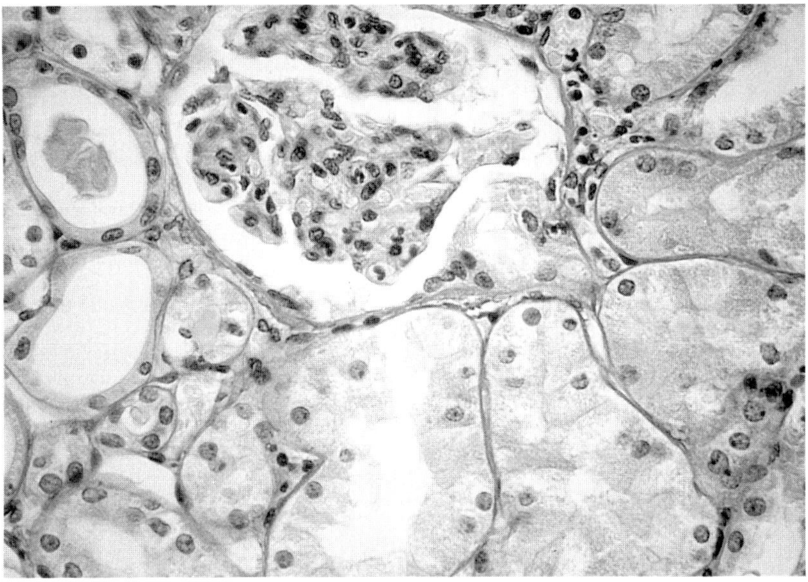

Fig. 2 Tubular epithelial lesions and pigmented casts. Suggestive of acute tubular necrosis (H&E ×30)

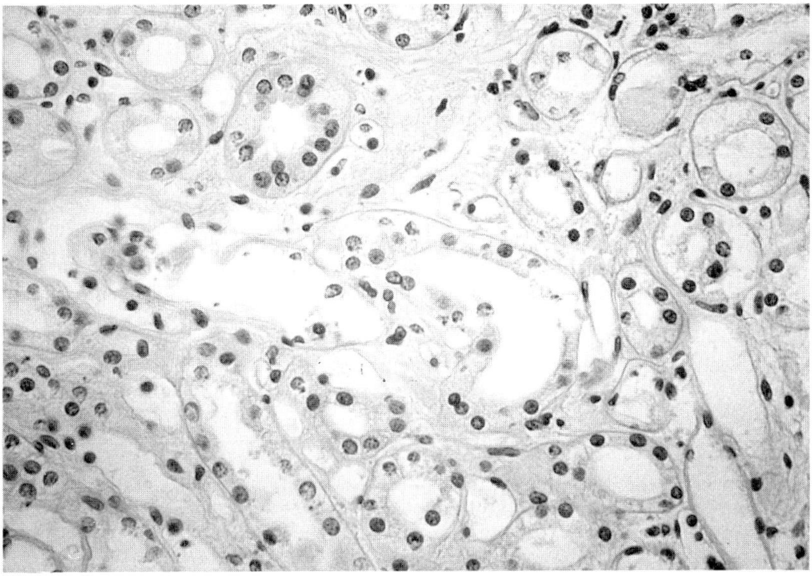

Fig. 3 Various types of tubular cell lesion up to denudation of basal membrane. Finding again suggestive of acute tubular necrosis (H&E ×30)

Table 3 Data suggesting the functional nature of the HRS

A. Alterations of renal haemodynamics and function already occurring in some patients with chronic active hepatitis, without any influences on the course of the disease[4]
B. Rare spontaneous recovery[22], occurring after a well-documented improvement in liver function[10]
C. Absence of active sediment in urine
D. Reduction in GFR generally less severe than in ATN
E. Apparent integrity of tubular function, as indicated by high active sodium and free water reabsorption[10,13]
F. Presence of haemodynamic alterations, theoretically reversible, with a greater reduction of blood flow in extrasplanchnic area in patients with the HRS than in those without the HRS[23]
G. Absence of interstitial oedema and other specific morphological alterations in renal biopsy taken *in vivo*
H. Peculiarity of HRS, even if severe and irreversible, as a reflection of a broader fatal event and not as the most important determinant of the patient's survival[10]
I. Typical angiographic pattern (marked beading and tortuosity of the interlobar and proximal arcuate arteries, absence of filling of the cortical vessels and of a distinct cortical nephrogram)
J. Normalization of the arteriographic alterations in post-mortem angiography in patients who die with the HRS, suggesting the functional nature of renal cortical vasoconstriction
K. Return towards normal function of the kidneys obtained from patients with the HRS when transplanted to other subjects[25]
L. Recovery from the HRS of patients undergoing liver transplantation[26–28]

Table 4 Data suggesting the organic nature of the HRS

A. Irreversible in most cases
B. Poor response to treatment
C. Rapid worsening, even if death occurs due to other causes (i.e. sepsis, pneumonia, gastrointestinal bleeding)
D. Slow improvement of renal function when the patient with the HRS undergoes liver transplantation[26] and/or the patient's kidneys are transplanted to new recipients[25,29]
E. Functional similarities between the HRS and ATN characterized by increased tubular sodium reabsorption, particularly ATN due to burns, sepsis and radio-opaque contrast material administration[30]
F. Functional similarities between ATN and the HRS, in which urinary sodium concentration tends to increase in the final stage (Fig. 4)
G. Absence of evident tubular damage in several cases of typical ATN[31–33]
H. Histological alterations sometimes reported in the HRS[21,34] similar to those observed in ATN[35–37], such as infiltration of mononuclear cells in the vasa recta, increased number of mesangial cells and mild tubular cell damage, as in some of our observations (Figs 2 and 3)
I. Lack of improvement in renal haemodynamic changes after portosystemic shunting, despite a reduction of portal pressure and an improvement in cardiac output[10,38]
J. Similarities in renal arteriographic findings between patients with compensated cirrhosis[4,39] and those with ATN[40], showing constriction of arcuate segmented arteries and arterioles
K. Lack of therapeutic effect of the blockade of the renin–angiotensin–aldosterone system in patients with ATN[41–43] as well as in patients with decompensated cirrhosis[44]
L. Final events for both ATN and the HRS represented by arterial vasoconstriction in the renal cortex in presence of a modified blood flow to the medulla and a progressive decrease in GFR[45,46].

HYPOTHESIS

In patients affected by liver cirrhosis and refractory ascites, HRS can occur without an evident relationship with the severity of liver disease or fluid accumulation; however it is very rare to observe real HRS without refractory ascites. In those unusual cases, mostly due to acute liver injury or hepatic cancer, the same pathogenetic mechanisms have been suggested[8,9,47,48].

Considering that the functional and histological alterations reported in patients affected by HRS or ATN are sometimes similar, and given that the cause of acute renal failure in liver cirrhosis can be represented by ATN or HRS, with prevalence of the former[6,10], it is likely that these phenomena may be closely related[20].

In fact, patients with liver cirrhosis who show signs of ATN due to administration of aminoglycosides, or spontaneously during shock, excrete urine with low sodium content, similar to those with real HRS[49]. In these cases tubular damage may be heterogeneous and tubuli, where urine could be rich in sodium, may be obstructed and dilated, thus not contributing to the formation of final urine and to its contents of sodium and lysozyme[21].

The hyperreabsorption of sodium during HRS may be explained on the basis of:

1. a high number of intact tubuli, or
2. the backleak theory, according to which the glomerular filtrate, because of damage of tubular cells, is largely reabsorbed[32,50].

In this case the decreased creatinine or inulin excretion by patients with cirrhosis and acute renal failure, is not necessarily based on the lack of glomerular filtration, but rather on tubular damage[50]. In fact, in experimental acute renal failure, glomerular filtration remains unchanged[51,52]. Further, glomerular filtration often seems maintained by increased production of angiotensin II, playing a protective role in humans during cirrhosis, both with and without ascites[44].

However, an imbalance of vasoactive substances and the prevalence of the vasoconstricting ones have been reported in HRS. In fact, low levels of prostaglandins (PGs) and a high level of angiotensin II, TxA_2 and vasopressin have been observed in this situation[53–56].

RFI, characterized by a significant decrease in renal clearances, can be shown not only during liver cirrhosis, but also during chronic active hepatitis and other liver diseases with and without intrahepatic cholestasis[4,57]. These phenomena may represent the preclinical stage of HRS, while the second stage is characterized by the spontaneous increase in serum creatinine and BUN, a urine to plasma osmolality ratio greater than 1, and by a rapid decline in urinary sodium excretion and in the urinary flow rate (< 250 ml/day) (Table 1). During the second stage, usually irreversible and with a poor prognosis (almost all patients die within 3 weeks)[6], histological alterations, similar to those reported in patients with ATN, can be observed. Moreover, cases with HRS can go on to develop typical ATN with modifications of the urine, which becomes isotonic and sodium-rich as in some of our observations (Fig. 4)[13,21].

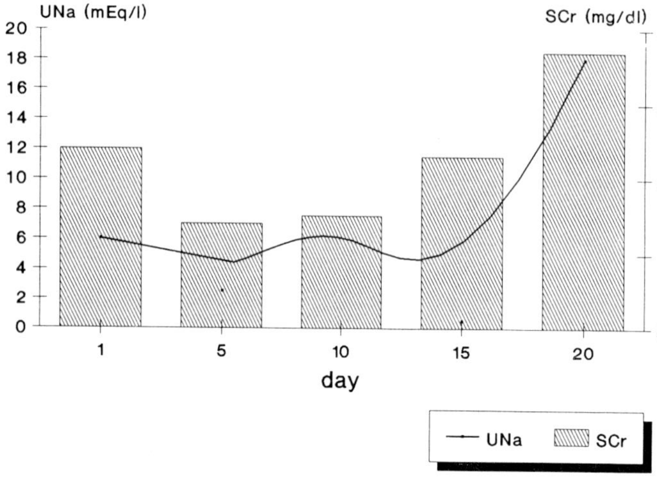

Fig. 4 Serum creatinine and urinary sodium excretion in a patient with terminal hepatorenal syndrome

Thus, it is possible to suggest that the initially lengthy period of RFI, often demonstrable with specific functional tests, is based only on functional renal alterations, while the second and shorter period may be principally based on superimposed morphological alterations, although with markedly different expression. During the first period there are several modifications in the general and renal systems, with progressive alterations of the RAA system, the SNS, and an increased production of vasopressin, kinins and arachidonic acid metabolites. Every system seems to play a protective role, given that the block in production of each substance generally induces a quick decrease in renal function, often mediated by decreased systemic arterial pressure[44,58].

During the second stage of renal dysfunction, and particularly in those with HRS, exhaustion of the renal autacoid system can be demonstrated through the maintenance of relatively prevalent vasoconstrictive substances such as TxA_2 and angiotensin II[55,56]. In this setting some mild or more severe tubular damage may occur, explaining the general irreversibility of HRS observed.

TREATMENT OF REFRACTORY ASCITES AND HRS

General procedures

Because this syndrome can be precipitated by the use of diuretics and, once established, it is almost invariably irreversible, prevention is obviously the best approach, especially in delaying its occurrence[10]. Moreover, it is mandatory to make a definitive diagnosis in order to exclude ATN and acute prerenal azotaemia (Table 2), which may be successfully treated. In this

Table 5 Treatment of hepatorenal syndrome

1. General procedures
2. Conservative care
3. Experimental medical therapy
4. Invasive procedures:
repeated paracentesis
dialysis
LeVeen shunt
intrahepatic stent
surgical shunts
liver transplantation

context it is necessary to keep in mind that abuse of some drugs (NSAIDs, lactulose, lactitol, β-blockers) or a non-judicious paracentesis can worsen renal function in cirrhotic patients[10]. It is also necessary to prevent digestive bleeding, metabolic disorders and the occurrence of spontaneous bacterial peritonitis. This latter phenomenon, occurring in up to 10% of ascitic patients admitted to the hospital[59,60], can make standard therapeutic measures ineffective.

Conservative care

The second requisite, in order to obtain a better survival rate in patients with decompensated cirrhosis, is represented by applying accurate sequential treatment, using the lowest possible dosage of diuretics and avoiding side-effects[1]. At the same time, the general measures indicated for the initial approach towards patients with ascites (bed rest and a sodium-restricted diet with infusion of low doses of human albumin) may maintain a fair hydroelectrolyte balance. A sodium-restricted diet of about 40 mEq per day may counteract the positive sodium balance; the sodium restriction is useful in reducing drug requirement[61,62]. Further restrictions are usually unnecessary and may worsen anorexia and malnutrition often shown by these patients[63]. Bed rest reduces the degree of activation of the RAA system and SNS[60], avoiding a more severe renal cortex vasoconstriction, a fall in GFR and an increase in sodium reabsorption[64]. Furthermore, bed rest increases response to diuretics[65].

The restriction of water intake is necessary in case of hyponatraemia, hypo-osmolality and reduction of free water clearance[66,67]. Large amounts of plasma expanders in advanced liver cirrhosis can ensure a rapid improvement in both prerenal azotaemia and in ATN[10]. Albumin infusion may, by itself, improve haemodynamics and renal sensitivity to diuretics in all patients with decompensated cirrhosis[68], and is also useful in patients with hyponatraemia[69]. On the other hand, in the general approach towards patients with refractory ascites, an aggressive diuretic therapy could precipitate a functional renal impairment in open HRS.

The first diuretic used in the treatment of decompensated cirrhosis is an aldosterone antagonist (spironolactone or potassium canrenoate), which is effective for a long period of time in non-azotaemic patients with hyperaldosteronism and ascites even relatively refractory[63,70,71]. When this drug is no longer effective on its own it is necessary to add a loop diuretic[1].

Furosemide is still one of the safest and most important loop diuretics[72,73], but has little effect in patients with refractory ascites and/or HRS. Its effectiveness in patients with tense ascites depends on the individual's albumin serum level and the capability of excreting the drug via the organic acid transport pathway of the proximal tubule[74–76].

Furosemide, when used alone, is effective in inducing a good diuretic response in only 50% of patients with cirrhosis and ascites[71,77], and may produce severe hypokalaemia for the increased potassium delivery by the distal nephron[78]. On the contrary, the combined use of spironolactone and furosemide potentiates the natriuretic effect of these drugs and decreases the incidence of potassium derangements. When ascites is removed (with a body weight loss of less than 500 g per day), the diuretic treatment must be maintained at the lowest possible dosage.

In refractory ascites, other diuretics such as ethacrynic acid, bumetamide, piretamide and distal diuretics (spironolactone, potassium canrenoate, triamterene, amyloride, benzothiazides) are also ineffective[79,80].

In some cases with tense ascites the use of torasemide, a new and more potent loop diuretic, can ameliorate sodium and water excretion and delay the onset of refractory ascites[75,81].

Experimental therapy

Experimental medical therapy, in order to restore diuresis in patients with tense ascites, can be performed especially in those patients who show good renal function but respond less and less to diuretics.

Even if strong activation of the RAA system and SNS have been thought to be responsible for the vasoconstriction of the renal outer cortex and decrease in GFR leading to HRS[82–84], the administration of α-adrenergic blocking agents such as phentolamine, phenoxybenzamine and clonidine has shown no therapeutic effect[24,85,86]; β-blockers such as propranolol are also without effect[87,88]. Moreover, angiotensin II antagonists such as saralazine, or ACE inhibitors such as captopril, rather than being useful, can induce arterial hypotension followed by a significant decrease in renal function and water and sodium excretion[89,90]. Recent evidence from our laboratory indicates that a low dose of captopril (12.5 mg) impairs renal function and sodium excretion without affecting arterial pressure[44].

Autacoid systems are also thought to be involved in the pathogenesis of RFI. The prostaglandins and kinins system, when activated, may play a protective role in patients with decompensated cirrhosis[56,91,92]. In fact the suppression of cyclo-oxygenase activity leads to a rapid decrease in renal function and sodium excretion[93,94]. The same systems appear exhausted in

HRS, where residual production of TxA_2 prevails and determines final vasoconstriction together with other vasoconstrictive substances (angiotensin II, catecholamines, and perhaps leukotrienes and PAF)[55,75,92,95].

On the basis of the above-mentioned functional modifications, TxA_2 synthase inhibitors such as daroxiben and OKY 046 have been administered, but the effect on sodium and renal function was modest or absent[96,97]. OKY 046, however, was useful in partially restoring the furosemide renal sensitivity of patients with tense ascites, suggesting that increased TxA_2 synthesis may reduce the furosemide-induced diuresis[98].

More recently, treatment with ONO 3708, a TxA_2 receptor antagonist, led to a significant improvement in free water clearance in patients with decompensated cirrhosis without HRS[99]. Until now, no other experimental attempts have been performed in humans to obtain renal improvement through modification of the intrarenal production and release of vasodilating kinins, vasoconstricting leukotrienes and PAF, which have been found increased in urine and blood of patients with HRS[95,100].

Experimental administration of a PAF antagonist, BN 52021, in animals, induced an increase in peripheral vascular resistance, a decrease in cardiac output and a slight or mild increase in arterial pressure, but had no significant effect on renal function[101].

Considering that systemic hypotension is one of the principal causes of renal impairment, dopamine, a metabolic precursor of norepinephrine and epinephrine, was administered to patients with ascites but only with a transient and modest effect[102]. An inconstant effect was also observed with octopressin, a synthetic analogue of vasopressin, which was able to induce renal vasodilation and peripheral vasoconstriction[103,104].

Lenz *et al.*[105,106] recently reported good results with short-term administration of 8-ornithin vasopressin in patients with decompensated cirrhosis. This treatment determined an improvement in renal function and water and sodium excretion, counteracting the hyperdynamic state typical of these patients.

The atrial natriuretic factor (ANF) and other substances such as the natriuretic hormone (or hypothalamic factor) and the brain natriuretic peptide have been shown to be increased in patients with liver cirrhosis[107–113]. Since the activity of these molecules may be counteracted by antinatriuretic factors, as suggested by Blendis *et al.*[114], the administration of ANF has been tried. With intravenous infusion of ANF we showed that about 50% of decompensated cirrhotics respond to the treatment, while the non-responders showed the highest plasma levels of renin and aldosterone, suggesting that greater activation of the SNS and RAA system may induce resistance to the natriuretic effects of ANF[108].

Invasive procedures

Evacuative paracentesis of about 5 litres per day with contemporaneous infusion of 40 g of human albumin or total paracentesis accompanied by administration of 6 g of albumin per litre of ascitic fluid removed, represents one of the most effective and safest procedures able to remove ascites, even in patients with refractory ascites. Repeated paracentesis with albumin infusions are generally well tolerated and usually do not modify plasma volume, cardiac output, renal function and ability to excrete water load, plasma levels of ADH, norepinephrine and aldosterone and plasma renin activity; further, they are able to shorten hospital stay and may improve prognosis[115–118]. However, the effects of paracentesis on patients with HRS remain uncertain and some personal results are anedoctal.

Other authors have proposed, for the treatment of ascites, the reinfusion of ascitic fluid into a peripheral vein or directly into the abdominal cavity after filtration and concentration. The first method was proposed some years ago[119]: a special machine (*Rhodiascit*) aspirates the ascitic fluid, concentrates it by ultrafiltration and then reinfuses it through a catheter into a vein, saving proteins. The second method is called *dialytic ultrafiltration with reinfusion of ascites intraperitoneally* (*DURAP*). These procedures are almost free of side-effects such as hypovolaemia, electrolyte imbalance and arterial hypotension[120–122], while, in order to prevent disseminated intravascular coagulation, an antiplatelet treatment with aspirin and dypiridamole has recently been proposed[123]. These procedures, however, do not seem to give better results in patients with tense ascites and HRS than other procedures.

Peritoneal dialysis has been tried in the treatment of acute prerenal failure[124], but even in those cases there are several difficulties represented mainly by the continuous accumulation of ascitic fluid, coagulative problems, need for surgical placement of the catheter and insufficient rate of clearance[13].

Moreover, the use of continuous arterovenous haemofiltration in patients with RFI and/or hepatic encephalopathy has been suggested. This treatment is not dangerous and does not provoke changes in intracranial pressure[125], but the results seem inconclusive so far, especially in patients with HRS.

Haemodialysis has been considered useful in determining the removal of creatinine, urea and other arotaemic molecules from blood, and the accumulation of sodium and water at the same time. This treatment generally leads to hypotension which, *per se*, is capable of inducing a worsening of renal function especially in patients with cardiovascular instability, bleeding tendency or sepsis[13]. Anecdotal reports describe favourable results in some patients with RFI submitted to dialysis alone[126], or in combination with other therapeutic procedures[127,128]. Therefore, haemodialysis can play an important role in the treatment of patients with acute renal failure, especially prerenal, and impending hepatic transplantation[6,129].

With the aim of removing ascitic fluid with permanent recuperation, LeVeen *et al.* (1974) proposed the surgical placement of a catheter connecting the peritoneal cavity to the jugular vein[130]. This catheter, provided with a unidirectional valve, ensures an intermittent flow of fluid depending on the increase of abdominal pressure, generally leading to a fast and permanent disappearance of ascites and to the restoration of normal activity of the SNS and the RAA system, and the improvement of renal function and sodium excretion, even in patients with RFI[131–133]. However, even if the procedure is normally well tolerated and enables several patients to return to an almost normal sodium diet with only small doses of diuretics, it is often associated with severe side-effects such as heart failure, oesophageal bleeding, sepsis, disseminated intravascular coagulation or obstruction of the catheter itself[134–137]. The insertion of a titanium tip at the end of the catheter may reduce the risk of thrombosis of the jugular and superior cava veins, but does not represent a definitive success.

The same can be said for other types of prothesis: the Denver and the Cordis–Hakim shunts, for example, provide some technical modifications of the valves, but generally do not offer any significant advantage if compared to the LeVeen shunt[138,139]. Recent controlled trials compared the LeVeen shunt to repeated paracentesis and to other surgical shunts but did not demonstrate a better efficacy of this procedure: the shunt does not affect the survival of these patients and the prognosis seems especially related to the grade of hepatic imbalance[140,141].

To date, it is reasonable to recommend the LeVeen implant in haemodynamically stable patients without hypovolaemia and with a good hepatic function, who may provide the best results[13,63].

Transjugular intrahepatic portosystemic stent–shunt (*TIPS*) insertion, originally proposed as a new non-operative decompressing treatment of variceal haemorrage[142], has recently been used in patients with refractory ascites and HRS[143]: the results of a pilot study show that this procedure may represent an effective treatment for this disease, reducing or removing ascites and improving renal function. In addition, all patients studied improved in nutritional status and Child's class, probably for reduced congestion of the intestinal vascular system.

Side-to-side portacaval or distal splenorenal surgical shunts, commonly performed in the 1950s and 1960s, generally led to the rapid disappearance of portal hypertension and ascites[144–146], but the occurrence of hepatic encephalopathy and, in several cases, a lack of recovery from renal failure[38], suggest that these more invasive surgical procedures may still be performed in well-selected patients, generally in good condition and with preserved liver function.

Since common clinical experience shows that patients with HRS always present poor prognosis, that the treatment of this complication is without definitive effect and sometimes may also induce iatrogenic damage[13,147], the only definitive treatment is represented by liver transplantation. This particularly invasive surgical treatment is normally considered for younger patients, especially with non-infective chronic liver disease[148,149]. Gonwa *et al.*[27] have recently reported long-term and good survival in patients affected by liver cirrhosis and HRS who, after transplantation, return to acceptable renal function. Considering renal function, it is possible to select patients for transplantation on the basis of the following parameters:

1. decreasing creatinine clearance,
2. very low urinary sodium excretion,
3. presence of refractory ascites,
4. lack of response to prolonged plasma expansion,
5. imbalance in arachidonic metabolites in urine with prevalence of TxB_2[150].

ACKNOWLEDGEMENTS

This work was supported by grants from Consiglio Nazionale delle Ricerche (Rome, Italy), and Ministero Italiano dell'Università e della Ricerca Scientifica e Tecnologica (MURST)-Progetto Nazionale Cirrosi Epatica ed Epatiti Virali (Rome, Italy). Financial support was also provided by Fondazione Italiana per lo Studio del Fegato (Italian Liver Foundation, Florence, Italy).

References

1. Gentilini P, La Villa G, Laffi G, Buzzelli G, Pinzani M, Cominelli F, Moscarella S, Birardi A. Sodium retention in cirrhosis: aspects of pathophysiology and treatment. Front Gastrointest Res. 1986;9:203–18.
2. Arroyo V, Epstein M, Gallus G, Gentilini P, Ring-Larsen H, Salerno F. Refractory ascites in cirrhosis: mechanism and treatment. Gastroenterol Int. 1989;2(4):195–207.
3. Gentilini P, Laffi G, La Villa G, Marra F, Pinzani M, Carloni V, Foschi M, Casini Raggi V. Refractory ascites. Gastroenterol Int. 1992; in press.
4. Gentilini P, Laffi G, Buzzelli G, Stefani P, Scarpelli P, Paladini S, Smorlesi C, La Villa G, Forti G. Functional renal alterations in chronic liver disease. Digestion. 1980;20:73–8.
5. Gentilini P, Laffi G, La Villa G, Pinzani M, Buzzelli G, Pampana A, Smorlesi C, Moscarella S, Birardi A. Pathogenetic mechanisms in renal function impairment in cirrhotics. Front Gastrointest Res. 1984;8:235–45.
6. Papper S. Hepatorenal syndrome. In: Epstein M, editor. The kidney in liver disease, 2nd edn. New York: Elsevier; 1983:87–106.
7. Epstein M. Hepatorenal syndrome. In: Berk JE, editor. Bockus Gastroenterology, 4th edn. Philadelphia: WB Saunders; 1985:3138–49.
8. Ritt DJ, Whelan G, Werner DJ, Eigenbrodt EH, Schenker S, Combes B. Acute hepatic necrosis with stupor or coma. Medicine. 1969;48:151–72.
9. Vesin P, Roberti A, Viguie RR. Defaillance renale fonctionelle terminale chez des malades atteints de cancer du foie, primitif ou secondaire. Sem Hop Paris. 1965;26:1216 20.
10. Epstein M. Hepatorenal syndrome. In: Epstein M, editor. The kidney in liver disease, 3rd edn. Baltimore: Williams & Wilkins; 1988:89–118.
11. Gentilini P, Laffi G, La Villa G, Cominelli F, Buzzelli G. Aging and liver cirrhosis. Reduced response to diuretic treatment of ascites. In: Courtois Y, Faucheux B, Forette B, Knook DL, Treton JA, editors. Modern trends in aging research. Colloque INSERM, London: John Libbey Eurotext, 1986;147:185–91.
12. Papadakis M, Arieff AI. Unpredictability of clinical evaluation of renal function in cirrhosis: a prospective study. Am J Med. 1987;82:945–52.
13. Lopez-Novoa JM, Diez J. Acute renal failure in liver disease: clinical, diagnostic, and therapeutic aspects. In: Cameron S, Davison AM, Grunfeld JP, Kerr D, Ritz E, editors. Oxford textbook of clinical nephrology. Oxford University Press; 1992;2:1098–109.
14. Cohn JN. Renal hemodynamic alterations in liver disease. In: Suki WN, Eknoyan G, editors. The kidney in systemic disease, 2nd edn. NewYork: John Wiley & Sons; 1981:509–19.
15. Kelleher SP, Berl T. Acute renal failure associated to hypovolemia. In: Brenner BM, Lazarus JM, editors. Acute renal failure, 2nd edn. New York: Churchill-Livingstone; 1988:233–50.
16. Witte CL, Witte MH, Dumont AE. Lymph imbalance in the genesis and perpetuation of the ascites syndrome in hepatic cirrhosis. Gastroenterology. 1980;78:1059–66.
17. Better OS, Schrier RW. Disturbed volume homeostasis in patients with cirrhosis of the liver. Kidney Int. 1983;23:303–11.
18. Shear L, Kleinerman J, Gabuzda GJ. Renal failure in patients with cirrhosis of the liver. Clinical and pathological characteristics. Am J Med. 1965;39:184–98.
19. Mandal AK, Lansing M, Fahmy A. Acute tubular necrosis in hepatorenal syndrome: an electron microscopic study. Am J Kidney Dis. 1982;2:368–74.

20. Solez K. Pathogenesis of acute renal failure. Int Rev Exp Pathol. 1983;24:277–333.
21. Wilkinson SP, Hirst D, Day DW, Williams R. Spectrum of renal tubular damage in renal failure secondary to cirrhosis and fulminant hepatic failure. J Clin Pathol. 1978;31:101–7.
22. Clark F, O'Leary JP. Survival associated with hepatorenal syndrome. Southern Med J. 1979;72:87–92.
23. Fernandez-Seara J, Prieto J, Quiroga J, Zozaya JM, Cobos MA, Rodriguez-Eire JL, Garcia-Plaza A, Leal J. Systemic and regional hemodynamics in patients with liver cirrhosis and ascites with and without functional renal failure. Gastroenterology. 1989;97(5):1304–12.
24. Epstein M, Berk DP, Hollenberg NK, Adams DF, Chalmers TC, Abrams HL, Merrill JP. Renal failure in the patient with cirrhosis. The role of active vasoconstriction. Am J Med. 1970;49:175–85.
25. Koppel MH, Coburn JW, Mims MM, Goldstein H, Boyle JD, Rubini ME. Transplantation of cadaveric kidneys from patients with hepatorenal syndrome. Evidence for the functional nature of renal failure in advanced liver disease. N Engl J Med. 1969;280:1367–71.
26. Iwatsuki S, Popovtzer MM, Corman JL, Ishikawa M, Putnam CW, Katz FH, Starzl TE. Recovery from hepatorenal syndrome after orthotopic liver transplantation. N Engl J Med. 1973;289:1155–9.
27. Gonwa TA, Morris CA, Goldstein RM, Husberg BS, Klintmalm GB. Long-term survival and renal function following liver transplantation in patients with and without hepatorenal syndrome. Experience in 300 patients. Transplantation. 1991;51(2):428–30.
28. Chmielewski C. Case study: end stage liver failure patient managed with CAVH pretransplant. Anna J. 1991;18(6):583–4.
29. McDonald FD, Brennan LA, Turcotte JG. Severe hypertension and elevated plasma renin activity following transplantation of 'hepatorenal donor' kidneys into anephric recipients. Am J Med. 1973;54:39.
30. Linton AL, Eliahou H, Solez K. Acute renal failure. A continuing enigma. Renal Failure. 1987;10:29–37.
31. Olsen S. Renal histopathology in various forms of acute anuria in man. Kidney Int. 1976;10:S2–8.
32. Solez K, Morel-Maroger L, Sraer JD. The morphology of 'acute tubular necrosis' in man: analysis of 57 renal biopsies and a comparison with the glycerol model. Medicine. 1979;58:362–76.
33. Olson S, Solez K. Pathogenesis of acute renal failure in light of new morphological data. Clin Nephrol. 1987;27:271–7.
34. Wilkinson SP. Hepatorenal disorders. New York: Marcel Dekker; 1982.
35. Solez K. Acute renal failure ('acute tubular necrosis', infarction, and cortical necrosis). In: Heptinstall RH, editor. Pathology of the kidney, 3rd edn. Boston: Little Brown; 1983:1069–148.
36. Solez K, Kramer EC, Fox JA, Heptinstall RH. Medullary plasma flow and intravascular leucocyte accumulation in acute renal failure. Kidney Int. 1974;6:24–37.
37. Solez K, Kramer EC, Heptinstall RH. The pathology of acute renal failure. Leucocyte accumulation in the vasa recta. Am J Pathol. 1974;73:31a.
38. Ring-Larsen H, Hesse B, Stigsby B. Effect of portal-systemic anastomosis on renal hemodynamics in cirrhosis. Gut. 1976;17:865–70.
39. Kew MC, Varma RR, Williams HS, Brunt PW, Hourigan KJ, Sherlock S. Renal and intrarenal blood flow in cirrhosis of the liver. Lancet. 1971;2:504–10.
40. Hollenberg NK, Adams DF. Vascular factors in the pathogenesis of acute renal failure in man. In: Friedman EA, Eliahou HE, editors. Proceedings of conference on acute renal failure. DHEW publication (NIH) no. 74-608. Washington, DC: Department of Health, Education and Welfare;1974:209–29.
41. Ishikawa I, Hollenberg NK. Pharmacologic interruption of the renin-angiotensin system in myohemoglobinuric acute renal failure. Kidney Int. 1976;10:S183–90.
42. Mason J, Kain H, Shingar T, Welsch J. The early phase of experimental acute renal failure. V. The influence of suppressing the renin-angiotensin system. Pflugers Arch. 1979;380:233–43.
43. Oken DF, Cotes SC, Flamenbaum W, Powell-Jackson JD, Lever AF. Active and passive immunization to angiotensin in experimental acute renal failure. Kidney Int. 1975;7:12–18.
44. Gentilini P, Romanelli RG, La Villa G, Maggiore Q, Pesciullesi E, Cappelli G, Casini Raggi V, Foschi M, Marra F, Pinzani M, Buzzelli G, Laffi G. Effects of low dose captopril

on renal hemodynamics and function in patients with cirrhosis of the liver. Gastroenterology. 1993;104:588–94.
45. Hollenberg NK, Adams DF, Oken DE, Abrams HL, Merrill JP. Acute renal failure due to nephrotoxins. Renal hemodynamic and angiographic studies in man. N Engl J Med. 1970;282:1329–34.
46. Epstein M. Renal functional abnormalities in cirrhosis: pathophysiology and management. In: Zakim D, Boyer TD, editors. Hepatology: a textbook of liver disease. Philadelphia: WB Saunders; 1982:446–64.
47. Wilkinson SP, Davies MH, Portmann B. Renal failure in otherwise uncomplicated acute viral hepatitis. Br Med J. 1978;2:338–41.
48. Ring-Larsen H. Associated renal failure. In: Williams R, editor. Liver failure. Edinburgh: Churchill-Livingstone; 1986:72–92.
49. Diamond JR, Yoburn DC. Nonoliguric acute renal failure associated with a low fractional excretion of sodium. Ann Intern Med. 1982;96:596.
50. Conger JD, Briner VA, Schrier RW. Acute renal failure: pathogenesis, diagnosis and management. In: Schrier RW, editor. Renal and electrolyte disorders, 4th edn. Boston: Little Brown; 1992:495–537.
51. Barenberg RL, Solomon S, Papper S, Anderson R. Clearance and micropuncture study of renal function in mercuric chloride-treated rats. J Lab Clin Med. 1968;72:473.
52. Flamenbaum W, McDonald FD, Di Bona GF, Oken DE. Micropuncture study of renal tubular factors in low-dose mercury poisoning. Nephron. 1971;8:221–34.
53. Lianos EA, Alavi N, Tobin M, Venuto R, Bentzel CJ. Angiotensin induced sodium excretion patterns in cirrhosis: role of renal prostaglandins. Kidney Int. 1982;21:70–7.
54. Zipser RD, Radvan GH, Duke R, Little TE. Exaggerated urinary thromboxane B_2 and diminished prostaglandin E_2 in hepatorenal syndrome. Clin Res. 1982;30:108A.
55. Zipser RD, Radvan GH, Kronborg KJ, Duke R, Little TE. Urinary thromboxane B_2 and prostaglandin E_2 in the hepatorenal syndrome: evidence for increased vasoconstrictor and decreased vasodilated factors. Gastroenterology. 1983;84:697–703.
56. Laffi G, La Villa G, Pinzani M, Ciabattoni G, Patrignani P, Mannelli M, Cominelli F, Gentilini P. Altered renal and platelet arachidonic acid metabolism in cirrhosis. Gastroenterology. 1986;90:274–82.
57. Gentilini P, Laffi G, Buzzelli G, Cappelli G, Stefani P, Smorlesi C, La Villa G, Mazzanti R. Functional renal alterations in intrahepatic cholestasis. In: Gentilini P, Popper H, Sherlock S, editors. Problems in intrahepatic cholestasis. Basel: Karger; 1979:125–31.
58. Arroyo V, Bosch J, Mauri M, Rivera F, Navarro-Lopez F, Rodes J. Effects of angiotensin II blockade on systemic and hepatic hemodynamics and on the renin angiotensin aldosterone system in cirrhosis with ascites. Eur J Clin Invest. 1981;11:221–9.
59. Runyon BA. Spontaneous bacterial peritonitis: an explosion of information. Hepatology. 1988;8:171–5.
60. Hoefs JC. Diagnostic paracentesis: a potent clinical tool. Gastroentrology. 1990;98:230–6.
61. Reynolds TB, Lieberman FL, Goodman AR. Advantages of treatment of ascites without sodium restriction and without complete removal of excess fluid. Gut. 1978;19(6):549–53.
62. Gauthier A, Levy VG, Quinton A, Michel H, Rueff B, Descos L, Durbec JP, Fermanian J, Lancrenon S. Salt or no salt in the treatment of cirrhotic ascites: a randomized study. Gut. 1986;27(6):705–9.
63. Arroyo V, Gines P, Jimenez W, Rodes J. Ascites, renal failure and electrolyte disorders in cirrhosis. Pathogenesis, diagnosis and treatment. In: McIntyre N, Benhamou JP, Bircher J, Rizzetto M, Rodes J, editors. Oxford textbook of clinical hepatology. Oxford University Press; 1991;2:429–70.
64. Bernardi M, Santini C, Trevisani F, Baraldini M, Ligabue A, Gasbarrini G. Renal function impairment induced by change in posture in patients with cirrhosis and ascites. Gut. 1985;26:629–35.
65. Ring-Larsen H, Henriksen JH, Wilken C, Clausen, Pals, Christensen NJ. Diuretic treatment in decompensated cirrhosis and congestive heart failure: effect of posture. Br Med J. 1986;292(6532):1351–3.
66. Pockros PD, Reynolds TB. Rapid diuresis in patients with ascites from chronic liver disease: the importance of peripheral oedema. Gastroenterology. 1986;90:1827.
67. Arroyo V, Rodes J, Gutierrez-Lizarraga MA, Revert L. Prognostic value of spontaneous

hyponatremia in cirrhosis with ascites. Am J Dig Dis. 1976;21:249–56.
68. Reynolds TB, Lieberman FL, Redeker AG. Functional renal failure with cirrhosis. The effect of plasma expansion therapy. Medicine. 1967;46(2):191–6.
69. McCormick PA, Mistry P, Kaye G, Burroughs AK, McIntyre N. Intravenous albumin infusion is an effective therapy for hyponatremia in cirrhotic patients with ascites. Gut. 1990;31:204–7.
70. Liddle GW. Aldosterone antagonists and triamterene. Ann NY Acad Sci. 1966;139:466–70.
71. Perez-Ayuso RM, Arroyo V, Planas R, Gaya J, Bory F, Rimola A, Rivera R, Rodes J. Randomized comparative study of efficacy of furosemide versus spironolactone in nonazotemic cirrhosis with ascites. Relationship between the diuretic response and the activity of the renin–aldosterone system. Gastroenterology. 1983;84:961–8.
72. Burg MB. Tubular chloride transport and the mode of action of some diuretics. Kidney Int. 1976;9:189–97.
73. Williamson HE. Furosemide and ethacrinic acid. J Clin Pharmacol. 1977;17:633–72.
74. Odlind B. Relation between tubular secretion and effects of five loop diuretics. J Pharmacol Exp Ther. 1979;211:238–44.
75. Gentilini P, Laffi G. Renal functional impairment and sodium retention in liver cirrhosis. Digestion. 1989;43:1–32.
76. Pinzani M, Laffi G, Meacci E, La Villa G, Cominelli F, Gentilini P. Implication of thromboxane A_2 in furosemide-induced sodium and water diuresis in cirrhosis with ascites. Ital J Gastroenterol. 1987;19:307.
77. Moult PJ, Lunzer MR, Trash DB, Sherlock S. Use of bumetamide in the treatment of ascites due to liver disease. Gut. 1974;15(12):988–92.
78. Good DW, Wright FW. Luminal influences on potassium secretion: sodium concentration and fluid flow rate. Am J Physiol. 1979;236:F192.
79. Galambos JT. Cirrhosis. Philadelphia: Saunders; 1979.
80. Arroyo V, Rimola A, Rodes J. Pathogenesis and treatment of ascites. In: Thomas HC, Jones EA, editors. Recent advances in hepatology, vol. 2. Edinburgh: Churchill-Livingstone; 1986:155–74.
81. Laffi G, Marra F, Buzzelli GP, Azzena G, Meacci E, De Feo ML, La Villa G, Gentilini P. Comparison of the effects of torasemide and furosemide in nonazotemic cirrhotic patients with ascites: a randomized, double-blind study. Hepatology. 1991;13(b):1101–5.
82. Maxwell MH, Breed ES, Schwartz IL. Renal venous pressure in chronic congestive heart failure. J Clin Invest. 1950;29:342–8.
83. Bichet D, Van Putten V, Schrier RW. Potential role of sympathetic activity in the sodium and water excretion in cirrhotic patients. N Engl J Med. 1982;307:1552–7.
84. Ring-Larsen H, Henriksen JH. Pathogenesis of ascites formation and hepatorenal syndrome: humoral and hemodynamic factors. Semin Liver Dis. 1986;6:341–52.
85. Baldus WP. Etiology and management of renal failure in cirrhosis and portal hypertension. Ann NY Acad Sci. 1969;170:267.
86. Roulot D, Moreau R, Gaudin C, Bacq Y, Braillon A, Hadengue A, Frohly P, Lebrec D. Long-term sympathetic and hemodynamic responses to clonidine in patients with cirrhosis and ascites. Gastroenterology. 1992;102:1309–18.
87. Wilkinson SP, Smith IK, Clarke M. Intrarenal distribution of plasma flow in cirrhosis as measured by transit renography: relationship with plasma renin activity and sodium and water excretion. Clin Sci Mol Med. 1977;52:469–75.
88. Meacci E, La Villa G, Laffi G, Cominelli F, Di Donato M, Dabizzi P, Albani F, Gentilini P. Systemic haemodynamics, renal and platelet function during propranolol administration in patients with compensated cirrhosis. Liver. 1987;7:110–15.
89. Pariente EA, Bataille C, Bercoff E, Lebrec D. Acute effects of captopril on systemic and renal hemodynamics and on renal function in cirrhotic patients with ascites. Gastroenterology. 1985;88:1255–9.
90. Daskalopoulos G, Pinzani M, Murray N, Hirschberg R, Zipser RD. Effects of captopril on renal function patients with cirrhosis and ascites. J Hepatol. 1987;4:330–6.
91. Zipser RD, Hoefs JC, Speckart PF, Zia PK, Horton R. Prostaglandins: modulators of renal function and pressor resistance in chronic liver disease. J Clin Endocrinol Metab. 1979;48:895–900.
92. Laffi G, Smorlesi C, La Villa G, Pinzani M, Pampana S, Mazzanti R, Buzzelli GP, Gentilini

P. The possible role of prostaglandins in renal impairment in patients with chronic liver disease. Ital J Gastroenterol. 1983;15:256–8.
93. Boyer TD, Zia PK, Reynolds TB. Effect of indomethacin and prostaglandin A_1 on renal function and plasma renin activity in alcoholic liver disease. Gastroenterology. 1979;77:215–22.
94. Laffi G, Daskalopoulos G, Kronborg I, Hsuet W, Gentilini P, Zipser RD. Effects of sulindac and ibuprofen in patients with cirrhosis and ascites. An explanation for the renal-sparing effect of sulindac. Gastroenterology. 1986;90:182–7.
95. Huber M, Kastner S, Scholmerich J, Gerok W, Keppler D. Analysis of cysteinyl leukotrienes in human urine: enhanced excretion in patients with liver cirrhosis and hepatorenal syndrome. Eur J Clin Invest. 1989;19:53–60.
96. Gentilini P, Laffi G, Meacci E, La Villa G, Cominelli F, Pinzani M, Buzzelli GP. Effects of OKY 046, a thromboxane-synthase inhibitor, on renal function in nonazotemic cirrhotic patients with ascites. Gastroenterology. 1988;94:1470–7.
97. Zipser RD, Kronberg IJ, Rector W, Reynolds TB, Daskalopoulos G. Therapeutic trial of thromboxane synthesis inhibition in the hepatorenal syndrome. Gastroenterology. 1984;87:1228–32.
98. Pinzani M, Laffi G, Meacci E, La Villa G, Cominelli F, Gentilini P. Intrarenal thromboxane A_2 generation reduces the furosemide-induced sodium and water diuresis in cirrhosis with ascites. Gastroenterology. 1988;95:1081–7.
99. Gentilini P, Laffi G, Marra F, Azzena G, Fognani G. Selective thromboxane A_2 receptor antagonism increases free-water clearance in cirrhotic patients with ascites. Hepatology. 1989;10:717(A).
100. Caramelo C, Fernandez-Gallardo S, Santos JC, Inarrea P, Sanchez-Crespo M, Lopez-Novoa JM, Hernando L. Increased levels of platelet-activating factor in blood from patients with cirrhosis of the liver. Eur J Clin Invest. 1987;17:7–11.
101. Villamediana LM, Sanz E, Fernandez-Gallardo S, Caramelo C, Sanchez-Crespo M, Braquet P, Lopez-Novoa JM. Effects of the platelet-activating factor antagonist BN 52021 on the hemodynamics of rats with experimental cirrhosis of the liver. Life Sci. 1986;39:201–5.
102. Barnardo DE, Baldus WP, Maher FT. Effects of dopamine on renal function in patients with cirrhosis. Gastroenterology. 1970;58:524–31.
103. Cohn JN, Tristani FE, Khatri LM. Renal vasodilator therapy in the hepatorenal syndrome. Med Ann (DC). 1970;39:1–7.
104. Kew MC, Varma RR, Sampson DJ. The effect of octapressin on renal and intrarenal blood flow in cirrhosis of the liver. Gut. 1972;13:293–6.
105. Lenz K, Hortnagl H, Druml W, Grimm G, Laggner A, Schneeweiss B, Kleinberger G. Beneficial effect of 8-ornithin vasopressin on renal dysfunction in decompensated cirrhosis. Gut. 1989;30:90–6.
106. Lenz K, Hortnagl H, Druml W, Reither H, Schmid R, Schneeweiss B, Laggner A, Grimm G, Gerbes AL. Ornipressin in the treatment of functional renal failure in decompensated liver cirrhosis. Effects on renal hemodynamics and atrial natriuretic factor. Gastroenterology. 1991;101(4):1060–7.
107. Gerbes AL, Arendt RM, Paumgartner G. Atrial natriuretic factor. Possible implications in liver disease. J Hepatol. 1987;5:123–32.
108. Laffi G, Pinzani M, Meacci E, La Villa G, Renzi D, Baldi E, Cominelli F, Marra F, Gentilini P. Renal hemodynamic and natriuretic effects of human atrial natriuretic factor infusion in cirrhosis with ascites. Gastroenterology. 1989;96:167–77.
109. Fernandez-Cruz A, Marco J, Caudraro LM. Plasma levels of atrial natriuretic peptide in cirrhotic patients. Lancet. 1985;2:1439–40.
110. Renner F, Hartter E, Pidlich J. Atrial natriuretic peptide, hepatic cirrhosis and ascites (abstract). Basel: VII International Basel Liver Week; 1986.
111. Epstein M. Pathogenesis of renal sodium handling in cirrhosis. Am J Nephrol. 1983;3:297–309.
112. La Villa G, Asbert M, Jimenez W, Gines P, Claria J, Lopez C, Planas R, Llach J, Gaya J, Rivera F, Gentilini P, Arroyo V, Rodes J. Natriuretic hormone activity in the urine of cirrhotic patients. Hepatology. 1990;12(3):467–75.
113. La Villa G, Romanelli RG, Casini Raggi V, Tosti-Guerra C, De Feo ML, Marra F, Laffi G, Gentilini P. Plasma levels of brain natriuretic peptide in patients with cirrhosis. Hepatology. 1992;16(1):in press.
114. Blendis LM, Legaut L, Morali G, Warner LC, Logan AG, Skorecki KL. The role of ANF

in ascites. In: Gentilini P, Arias IM, Arroyo V, Schrier RW, editors. Liver disease and renal complications. New York: Raven Press; 1990;263–75.
115. Gordon ME. The acute effects of abdominal paracentesis in Laennec's cirrhosis upon exchanges of electroloytes and water, renal function and haemodynamics. Am J Gastroenterol. 1960;33:15–37.
116. Quintero E, Gines P, Arroyo V, Rimola A, Bory F, Planes R, Viver J, Cabrera J, Rodes J. Paracentesis versus diuretics in the treatment of cirrhotics with tense ascites. Lancet. 1985;1:611–12.
117. Kao HW, Rakov NE, Sabage S, Reynolds TB. The effect of large volume paracentesis on plasma volume – a cause of hypovolemia? Hepatology. 1985;5:403–7.
118. Gines P, Tito L, Arroyo V, Planas R, Panes L, Viver J, Torres M, Humbert P, Rimola A, Llach J, Badalamenti S, Jimenez W, Gaya J, Rodes J. Randomized comparative study of therapeutic paracentesis with and without intravenous albumin in cirrhosis. Gastroenterology. 1988;94:1493–502.
119. Levi VG, Opolon P, Pauleau N, Caroli J. Treatment of ascites by reinfusion of concentrated peritoneal fluid – review of 318 procedures in 210 patients. Postgrad Med J. 1975;51:564–6.
120. Adler AJ, Feldman J, Friedman EA, Berlyne GM. Use of extracorporeal ascites dialysis in combined hepatic and renal failure. Nephron. 1982;30:31–5.
121. Raju SF, Achord JL. The effects of dialytic ultrafiltration and peritoneal reinfusion in the management of diuretic resistant ascites. Am J Gastroenterol. 1984;79:308–12.
122. Landini S, Coli U, Fracasso A, Morachiello P, Righetto F, Scanferla F, Genchi R, Bazzato G. Spontaneous ascites filtration and reinfusion (SAFR) in cirrhotic patients. Int J Artif Organs. 1985;8:277–80.
123. Tang HH, Salem HH, Wood LJ, Dudley FJ. Coagulopathy during ascites reinfusion: prevention by antiplatelet therapy. Gastroenterology. 1992;102:1334–9.
124. Ring-Larsen H, Clausen E, Ranek L. Peritoneal dialysis in hyponatremia due to liver failure. Scand J Gastroenterol. 1973;8:33–40.
125. Davenport A, Will EJ, Davison AM, Swindells S, Cohen AT, Miloszewski KJ, Losowsky MS. Changes in intracranial pressure during haemofiltration in oliguric patients with grade IV hepatic encephalopathy. Nephron. 1986;53:142–6.
126. Keller F, Wagner K, Lenz T, Pommer W, Hahn G, Molzahnm M, Krause PH. Hemodialysis in hepatorenal syndrome. Report of two cases. Gut. 1985;26:208–11.
127. Kearns PJ, Polhemus RJ, Oakes D, Rabkin R. Hepatorenal syndrome managed with hemodialysis then reversed by peritovenous shunting. J Clin Gastroenterol. 1985;7:341–3.
128. Landini S, Coli U, Lucatello S, Fracasso A, Morachiello P, Toffoletto P, Bazzato G. Plasma exchange and dialysis. Combined treatment in acute renal insufficiency secondary to severe hepatopathies. Minerva Nefrol. 1981;28:179–86.
129. Ellis D, Avner ED. Renal failure and dialysis therapy in children with hepatic failure in the perioperative period of orthotopic liver transplantation. Clin Nephrol. 1986;25:295–303.
130. LeVeen HH, Christoudias G, Moon JP, Luft R, Falk G, Grossberg S. Peritoneovenous shunting for ascites. Ann Surg. 1974;180:580–90.
131. Berkowitz HD, Mullen JL, Miller LD, Rosato EF. Improved renal function and inhibition of renin and aldosterone secretion following peritoneo-venous (LeVeen) shunt. Surgery. 1978;84:120–6.
132. Blendis LM, Greig PD, Langer B, Baigrie RS, Ruse J, Taylor BR. The renal and hemodynamic effects of the peritoneovenous shunt for intractable ascites. Gastroenterology. 1979;77:250–7.
133. Epstein M. Peritoneo-venous shunt in the management of ascites and the hepatorenal syndrome. Gastroenterology. 1982;82:790–9.
134. Bernhoft RA, Pellegrini CA, Way LW. Peritoneovenous shunt for refractory ascites. Operative complications and long-term results. Arch Surg. 1982;117:631–5.
135. Darsee JR, Fulenwider JT, Rikkers LF, Ansley JD, Nordlinger BF, Ivey G, Heymsfield SB. Hemodynamics of LeVeen shunt pulmonary edema. Ann Surg. 1981;194:189–92.
136. Markey W, Payne JA, Straus A. Hemorrhage from esophageal varices after placement of the LeVeen shunt. Gastroenterology. 1979;77:341–3.
137. Ragni MV, Lewis H, Spero JA. Ascites-induced LeVeen shunt coagulopathy. Ann Surg. 1983;198:91–5.
138. LeVeen HH, Vujic I, D'Ovidio NG, Hutto RB. Peritoneovenous shunt occlusion. Etiology,

diagnosis, therapy. Ann Surg. 1984;200:212–23.

139. Fulenwider JT, Galambos JD, Smith RB III, Henderson JM, Warren WD. LeVeen vs Denver peritoneovenous shunts for intractable ascites of cirrhosis. A randomized, prospective trial. Arch Surg. 1986;121:351–5.
140. Stanley MM, Ochi S, Lee KK, Nemchausky BA, Greenlee HB, Allen MJ, Baum RA, Gadacz TR, Camara DS. The Veterans Administration Cooperative Study on Treatment of Alcoholic Cirrhosis with Ascites. Peritovenous shunting as compared with medical treatment in patients with alcoholic cirrhosis and massive ascites. N Engl J Med. 1989;321:1632–8.
141. Gines P, Arroyo V, Vargas V, Planas R, Casafont F, Panes J, Hoyos M, Viladomiu L, Rimola A, Morillas R, Salmeron JM, Gines A, Esteban R, Rodes J. Paracentesis with intravenous infusion of albumin as compared with peritoneovenous shunting in cirrhosis with refractory ascites. N Engl J Med. 1991;325(12):829–35.
142. Rossle M, Noldge G, Pararnau JM, Haag K, Sellinger M, Wenz W, Gerok W. Transjugular intrahepatic portosystemic stent–shunt (TIPS): experience with an improved technique. Hepatology. 1991;14:96A.
143. Ochs A, Sellinger M, Haag K, Noeldge G, Kirste G, Gerok W, Rossle M. Transjugular intrahepatic portosystemic stent–shunt (TIPS) for treatment of refractory ascites and hepatorenal syndrome: results of a pilot study. Gastroenterology. 1992;102(4):863A.
144. McDermott WV Jr. The treatment of cirrhotic ascites by combined hepatic and portal decompression. N Engl J Med. 1958;259;899–901.
145. Welch HF, Welch GS, Carter JH. Prognosis after surgical treatment of ascites: results after side-to-side shunt in 40 patients. Surgery. 1964;56:75–82.
146. Franco D, Vons C, Smadja C. Resultats des derivations portales dans le traitement de l'ascite irreducible de la cirrhose. Minerva Med. 1987;78:689–91.
147. Epstein M, Norsk P. Renin–angiotensin system in liver disease. In Epstein M, editor. The kidney in liver disease, 3rd edn. Baltimore: Williams & Wilkins; 1988:331–55.
148. Horisawa M, Reynolds TB. Exchange transfusion in hepatorenal syndrome with liver cirrhosis disease. Arch Intern Med. 1976;136:1135–7.
149. Rimola A, Gavaler JS, Shade RR, el-Lankany S, Starzl TE, Van Thiel DH. Effects of renal impairment on liver transplantation. Gastroenterology. 1987;93:148–56.
150. Gentilini P, Laffi G, La Villa G. Hepatorenal syndrome and liver transplantation. Transplant Proc. 1985;17:(suppl 2):127–8.

16

Interrelation between liver and kidney disease

E. H. STRØM, F. GUDAT and M. J. MIHATSCH

INTRODUCTION

Diseases involving the kidneys and liver will in this presentation be separated into three groups (Table 1): (a) diseases and conditions with simultaneous manifestation in the liver and kidney, (b) liver diseases following primary kidney diseases, and (c) renal diseases following primary liver diseases.

Table 1 Liver and kidney diseases

A. Diseases with simultaneous manifestations in the liver and kidney:
hereditary metabolic diseases
malformation syndromes
toxic conditions
infectious diseases
circulatory shock
amyloidosis
diseases in drug abuse
B. Liver disease following primary renal disease:
in renal carcinoma
after renal transplantation
C. Renal disease following primary liver disease (Table 2)

DISEASES WITH SIMULTANEOUS MANIFESTATIONS IN THE LIVER AND KIDNEY

A wide range of diseases involve the kidney and the liver at the same time[1].

1. *Hereditary metabolic diseases* can affect the liver and kidney in several ways. In glycogenosis type 1 (von Gierke's disease) there is an enzyme defect in the renal tubular cells as well as in the hepatocytes. This results in hepatomegaly and enlarged kidneys accompanied by abnormalities in renal tubular function. This condition is often known as the hepatorenal form of glycogen storage disease.

   In the newly recognized carbohydrate-deficient glycoprotein (CDG) syndrome, where there is a defect in glycoprotein metabolism, renal microcysts and liver fibrosis commonly appear[2].

   In primary oxalosis the hepatic enzyme defect gives rise to renal oxalate deposition and kidney failure, though the liver itself is little affected by disease. This condition is one of the very few diseases where patients can benefit from combined liver and kidney transplantation.
2. Renal and hepatic abnormalities can be found in several *malformation syndromes*. A combination of renal cysts, liver cysts and/or liver fibrosis is a common finding in the autosomal recessively inherited type of polycystic kidney disease (ARPKD). However, it occurs infrequently in the autosomal dominantly inherited type (ADPKD). In the ARPKD renal failure may develop together with portal hypertension. In nephronophtisis liver fibrosis may also be found.
3. Several compounds with *toxic effect* on both organs may give rise to acute renal and liver failure, as seen in poisoning with carbon tetrachloride and various fungi. Intravenous therapy in childhood with high-dose sorbitol or fructose may cause polyuric renal failure with acute yellow liver atrophy[3]. Possible pathogenetic mechanisms are direct dose-related damage of the kidney and liver or a toxic effect through hyperosmolality.
4. *Infectious multiorgan failure* with renal and liver involvement can develop not only in several bacterial infections, but also in parasitic infections, as in malaria. In Weil's leptospirosis an acute interstitial nephritis may occur.
5. *Circulatory shock* may cause acute renal failure through acute tubular necrosis, and this may be seen together with centrilobular liver necrosis and liver failure.
6. Intravenous *drug abusers* may have multifactorial coexistent liver and kidney diseases as a result of infection with human immunodeficiency virus (HIV), hepatitis B and C virus or from the drug itself. An HIV-associated nephropathy has recently been described, consisting of glomerular, tubular and interstitial lesions. This condition may also be found in patients who have not developed AIDS or AIDS-related complex[4]. It is clinically characterized by nephrotic syndrome and rapidly progressive renal failure.
7. Primary and secondary *amyloidosis* may appear in the liver and kidney simultaneously. Secondary amyloidosis may be a complication of long-term heroin abuse, especially in people who inject the drug subcutaneously[5].

LIVER DISEASE FOLLOWING PRIMARY RENAL DISEASE

Liver disease consequent to kidney disease is rather infrequent. *Renal cell carcinoma* may very seldom precipitate liver dysfunction (Stauffer's syndrome), characterized by non-tender hepatomegaly without jaundice with increased serum alkaline phosphatase and bilirubin as well as hypoprothrombinaemia[6]. Histological examination of the liver reveals non-specific reactive hepatitis with Kupffer cell hyperplasia. Following nephrectomy the clinical and morphological features return to normal. Secondary amyloidosis of the liver may occasionally be seen in renal cell carcinoma also.

Following *renal transplantation* and dialysis liver disease is reported with an incidence of up to 50% (for references, see ref. 7). Viral disease was found to be most important. However, the incidence of post-transplant hepatitis declined sharply after vaccination against hepatitis B virus. Adverse drug reactions in the liver in renal transplanted patients treated with azathioprine are reported, although the degree to which the drug is toxic to the liver is still controversial[8].

RENAL DISEASE FOLLOWING PRIMARY LIVER DISEASE (Table 2)

Hepatorenal syndrome

End-stage liver disease and fulminant hepatic failure of any aetiology may be complicated by the hepatorenal syndrome in which an oliguric renal failure occurs in the absence of clinical and laboratory evidence of other causes of renal dysfunction. Considered to be a functional disorder, the pathogenetic mechanisms are still poorly understood. Morphological changes in the kidney explaining the renal failure are generally lacking. However, a large proportion of patients with chronic liver disease have glomerular changes which could contribute to the haemodynamic abnormalities taking place in this syndrome. Histological signs of acute tubular necrosis can be observed (Fig. 1), at least in severe cases[9]. Iwatsuki *et al.*[10] reported recovery of renal function after liver transplantation, and cadaveric kidneys from patients with the hepatorenal

Table 2 Renal disease following primary liver disease

1. Hepatorenal syndrome
2. Hepatic glomerulosclerosis
3. Glomerulonephritis in viral hepatitis:
   (a) in chronic HBV/HCV hepatitis
   (b) in acute hepatitis (serum sickness disease)
4. Systemic disease in HBV/HCV infection:
   (a) panarteritis nodosa
   (b) mixed-type cryoglobulinaemia
5. IgA nephropathy (IgA nephritis)
6. Renal disease after liver transplantation

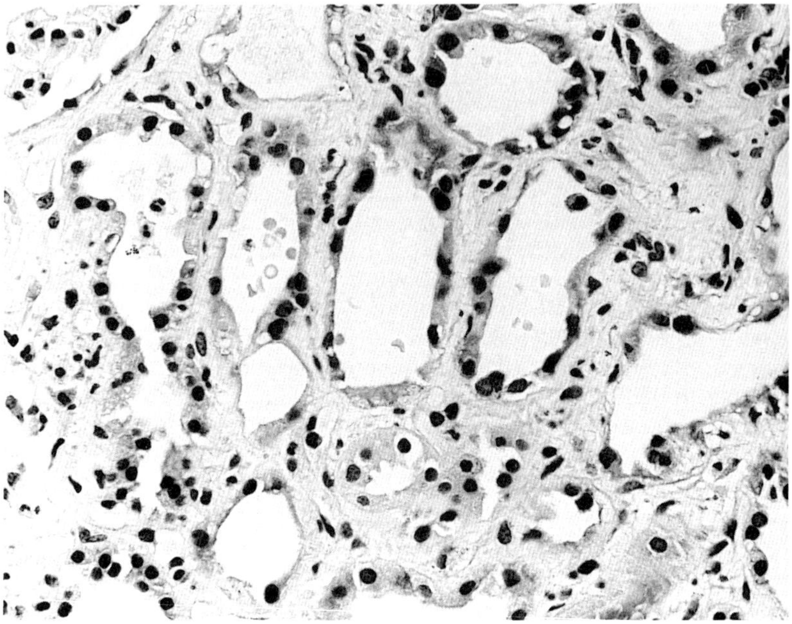

Fig. 1 Hepatorenal syndrome. Acute tubular necrosis with tubular dilatation and interstitial oedema (H&E, ×350)

syndrome have successfully been used for transplantation[11]. Both these observations are in favour of a functional or reversible damage in the kidneys in the hepatorenal syndrome.

Hepatic glomerulosclerosis

In chronic liver diseases sclerotic glomeruli with mesangial matrix increase, capillary wall thickening, in severe cases similar to diabetic glomerulosclerosis, were observed. This entity most likely also encompassed some forms of proliferative glomerular conditions of immune complex type, such as IgA nephropathy, to be described below. We feel the term hepatic glomerulosclerosis should be restricted to a condition where the glomerular mesangium shows unspecific widening or sclerosis with no or minimal cellular proliferation without immune deposits other than occasional IgM and C3. Furthermore, thickening and reduplication of the glomerular basement membrane with mesangial or subendothelial deposition of numerous small (500–1000 nm) lucent zones containing small clusters of dense, granular material[12] may be found (Fig. 2). These findings are not specific for hepatic glomerulosclerosis, they are also found in kidneys from patients with the hereditary lecithin cholesterol acyltransferase deficiency[13].

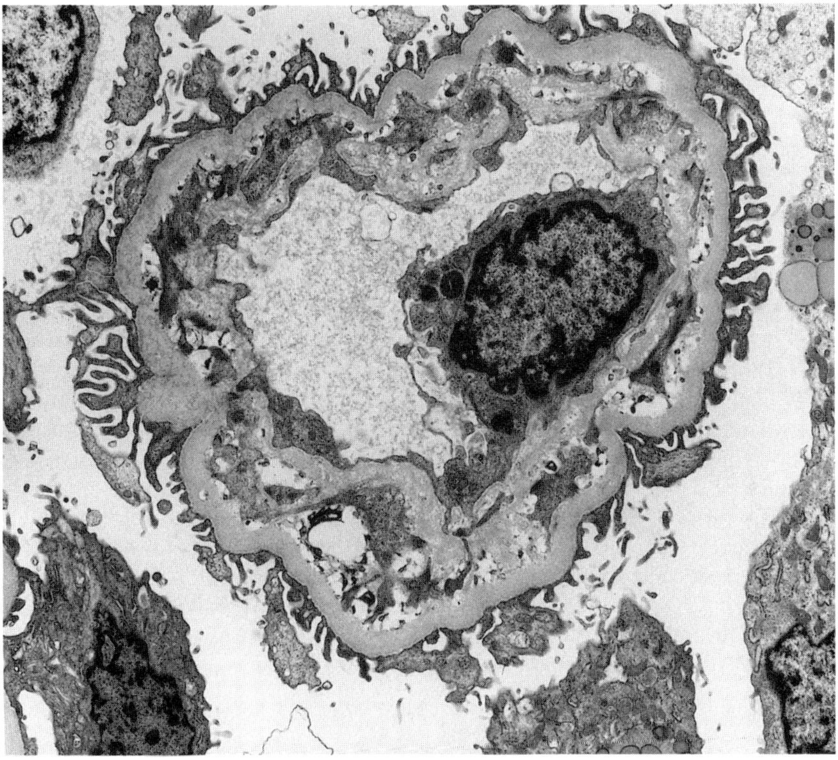

Fig. 2 Hepatic glomerulosclerosis. Doubling of the glomerular basement membrane with subendothelial depositions of lucent zones with granular material (EM ×9000)

Glomerulonephritis in viral hepatitis

Glomerulonephritis in chronic hepatitis B and C virus infection

Case report: A 65-year-old Italian woman with biopsy confirmed chronic aggressive hepatitis, positive for HBsAg and HBeAg in serum developed microscopic haematuria, proteinuria and hypertension (170/80 mmHg). Serum creatinine was 0.9 mg/dl, serum uric acid 6.3 mg/dl, C3 and C4 were low. Microscopy of the urinary sediment showed 20 red blood cells/high-power field with hyaline and granular casts. Quantitative urinary protein was 2.5 g/24 h. The tentative clinical diagnosis was hepatitis B-associated membranous glomerulonephritis.

A *renal biopsy* showed increased mesangial matrix and thickening of the glomerular capillary walls. By electron microscopy subepithelial osmiophilic deposits (Fig. 3) were identified, together with a few osmiophilic deposits along the mesangial basement membrane. Immunofluorescence showed IgG along the capillary walls and mesangial IgA deposits.

The *biopsy diagnosis* was: mixed-type glomerulonephritis; membranous glomerulonephritis and mesangial proliferative glomerulonephritis (IgA nephropathy).

Comment: the membranous pattern fits well with hepatitis B virus-associated glomerulonephritis, and the presence of IgA is consistent with chronic liver disease of any aetiology.

Membranous (=epimembranous) glomerulonephritis (MGN) remains the best-recognized glomerulopathy associated with hepatitis B virus (HBV) infection (Fig. 3). The condition has been known since 1971 when a chronic HBsAg carrier developed nephrotic syndrome and MGN[14]. As the prevalence of HBsAg carrier state varies widely, HBV-MGN is most frequently reported from Southeast Asia, where the virus is endemic[15,16]. In Taiwan about 95% of non-lupus MGN in children is related to HBV infection[16]. The natural course indicates that 30–60% of the patients have spontaneous remission. They usually remain symptomatic for more than 12 months with proteinuria, often within the nephrotic range, and microscopic haematuria. Renal insufficiency is very infrequent. Children with HBV-MGN seldom have any evidence of liver disease, whereas in adults there is often a history of acute hepatitis months to years before the onset of kidney disease. Glomerular subepithelial immune complexes containing HBsAg, HBeAg and HBcAg have been identified by immunohistochemistry in the capillary walls[16].

Membranoproliferative glomerulonephritis is also associated with HBV, and is found in children and adults with nephrotic syndrome accompanied by

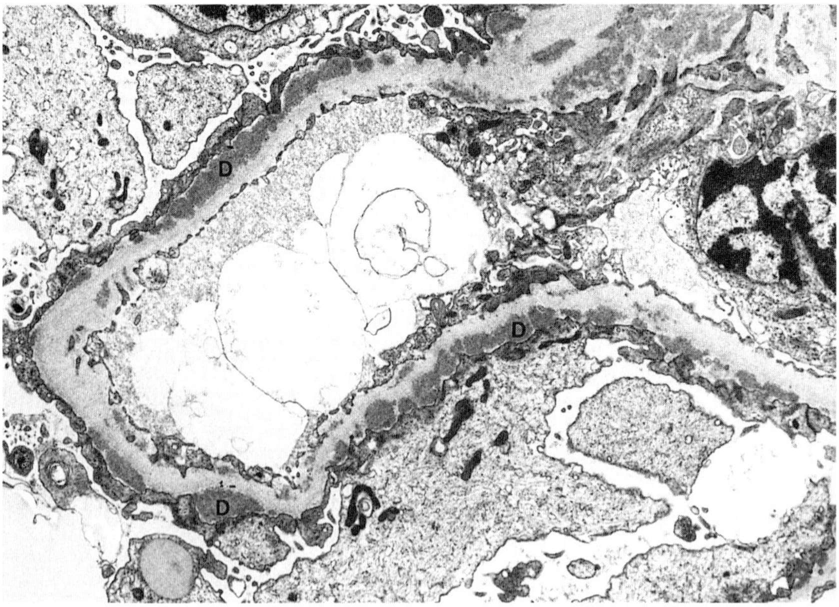

Fig. 3 Membranous glomerulonephritis. Thickening of glomerular capillary walls with subepithelial deposits (D) (EM ×6485)

microscopic haematuria. Hypertension and renal failure are found more often than in patients with MGN. Morphologically glomerular hypercellularity with subendothelial deposits and mesangial interposition are noted (Fig. 4). Most likely circulating immune complexes which contain HB antigens deposit subendothelially.

Finally, *mesangial proliferative glomerulonephritis*, with non-IgA deposits, as seen in post-infectious nephritis of other aetiology, has been observed in HBsAg carriers. Aspects of IgA nephritis in hepatitis are outlined below.

Several mechanisms by which virus may induce tissue damage are proposed. The demonstration in biopsy material of viral antigens, immunoglobulins and complement factors or dense deposits is in favour of an immune complex-mediated disease[15]. A possibility for direct infection of the mesangial cell has also been suggested[17].

Co-infection with hepatitis delta virus does not seem to influence the renal manifestations of hepatitis B virus infection.

A proven effective treatment of HBV-GN is not available[15]. As cell-mediated immunity is important in eliminating the HB virus, administration of steroids in treatment of the renal disease may be harmful and worsen the underlying hepatic disease. However, clinical assessment of antiviral therapy is indicated, as case studies describe improvement of both liver and kidney disease with interferon therapy[18].

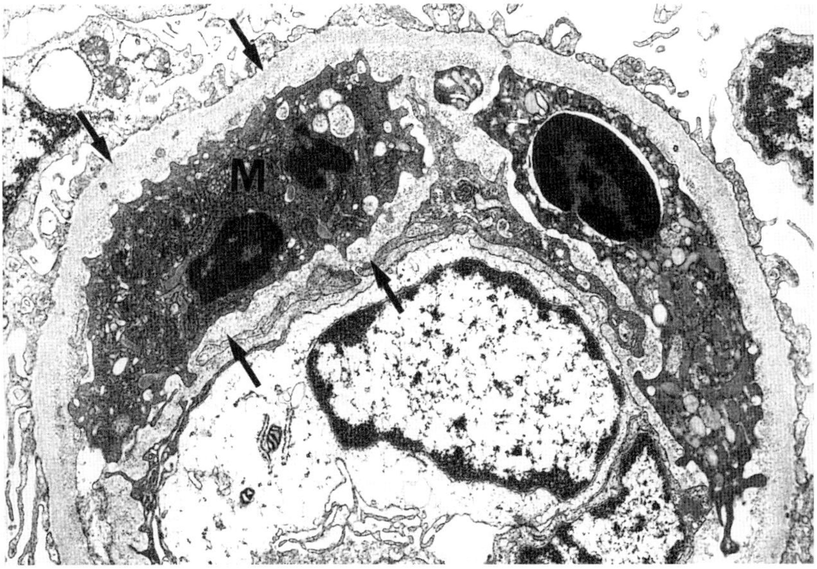

Fig. 4 Membranoproliferative glomerulonephritis. Interposition of mesangial cell (M) in the capillary wall between two layers of basement membrane material (arrows) (EM ×9400)

Serum sickness-like syndrome

A serum sickness-like syndrome with fever, arthritis and rash may affect 10–20% of patients with acute hepatitis B infection. Only a few of these patients have proteinuria and haematuria, and the symptoms are usually transient. Few patients undergo renal biopsy, so the morphology in acute serum sickness is better known from animal studies[19]. The glomeruli show diffuse hypercellularity, mainly due to influx of monocytes, with scattered subepithelial deposits. The lesions are completely reversible.

Systemic diseases in chronic HBV/HCV infection

Panarteritis nodosa (PAN)

PAN in the context of HBV infection is rather infrequent, although vasculitis with hepatitis B antigenaemia is probably the best-known example of viral infection-related vasculitis in humans. The presence of HBsAg in serum of patients with PAN has been reported to vary between 0% and 54%, being highest in cities in Europe and the USA where the virus mostly is transmitted by intravenous drug abuse or in homosexuals. PAN is very seldom reported from endemic areas, such as Southeast Asia or Africa (for references, see ref. 20). The condition often occurs weeks to months after a clinically mild acute hepatitis, but may appear years after a chronic active hepatitis has developed. PAN starts with fever, arthritis and skin exanthem and may later involve any organ. Eighty-five per cent have renal involvement, presenting clinically with hypertension, proteinuria, haematuria and even renal failure.

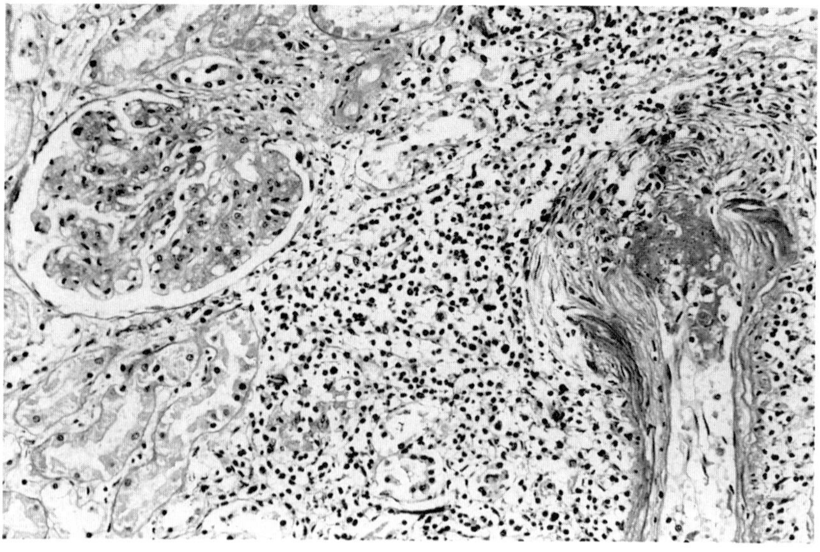

Fig. 5 Panarteritis nodosa. Focal inflammation and necrosis of interlobular artery (PAS ×157)

The renal pathology of classical vasculitis with focal inflammation of small arteries (Fig. 5) and ischaemic damage to glomeruli is typical, but various proliferative types of glomerulonephritis are also observed. HBV-PAN tends to resolve over several months, but acute life-threatening disease is also reported[21].

Mixed-type cryoglobulinaemia

Renal disease is a frequent manifestation in patients with cryoglobulinaemia. In renal disease cryoglobulins of IgG and IgM types are usually found, and are therefore called mixed cryoglobulins. Cryoglobulinaemia is not uncommon. It occurs in a *primary* form (essential cryoglobulinaemia) and *secondary* to infections, autoimmune diseases, lymphoproliferative disorders and liver diseases. Several viruses, such as hepatitis A and B virus, have been implicated as aetiological agents. Chronic active hepatitis due to HCV is an important newly recognized aetiological factor in mixed IgG–IgM cryoglobulinaemia[22].

The classical symptoms of mixed-type cryoglobulinaemia are purpura, arthralgia, liver disease and glomerulonephritis, mostly of the membrano-proliferative type. The glomerular lesion in the acute phase is characterized by hyaline 'thrombi' and macrophages in the capillary loops (Fig. 6). The 'thrombus' represents local precipitate of IgG–IgM complexes and has a characteristic crystalloid structure by electron microscopy (Fig. 7). A small-vessel vasculitis is commonly seen.

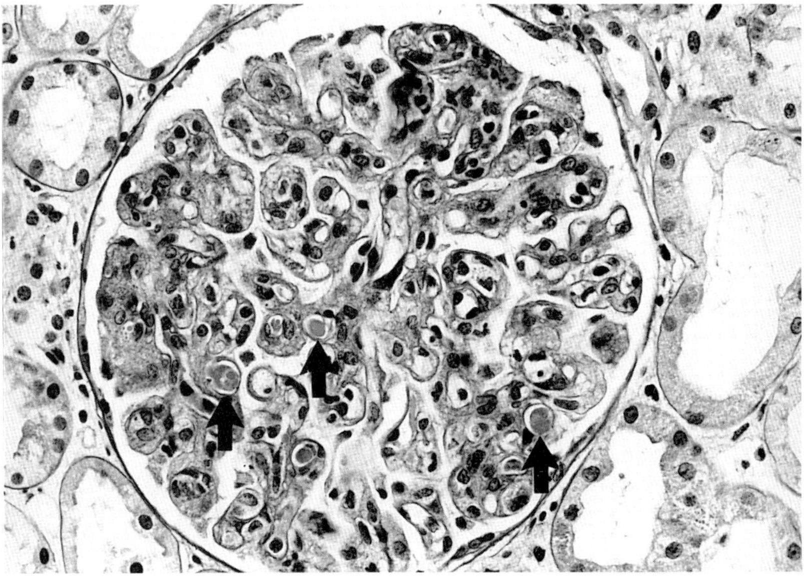

Fig. 6 Mixed-type cryoglobulinaemia. Hypercellular glomerulus with macrophages and protein 'thrombi' (arrows) in capillary loops (PAS ×315)

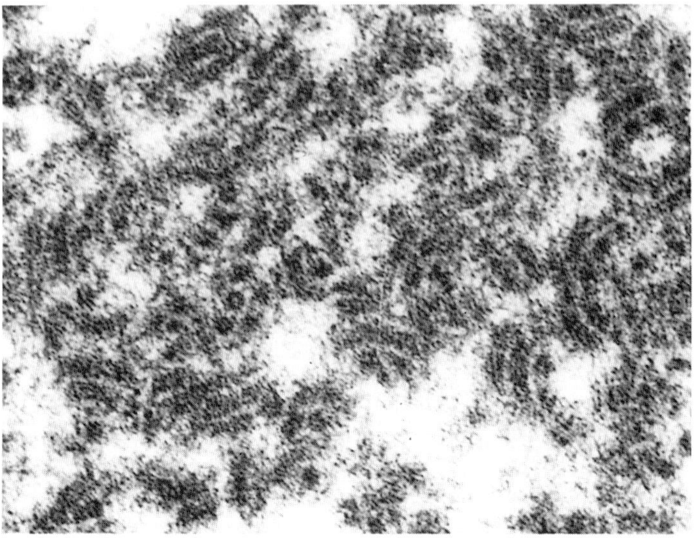

Fig. 7 Mixed-type cryoglobulinaemia. Characteristic crystalloid structure of protein precipitations (EM ×30 000)

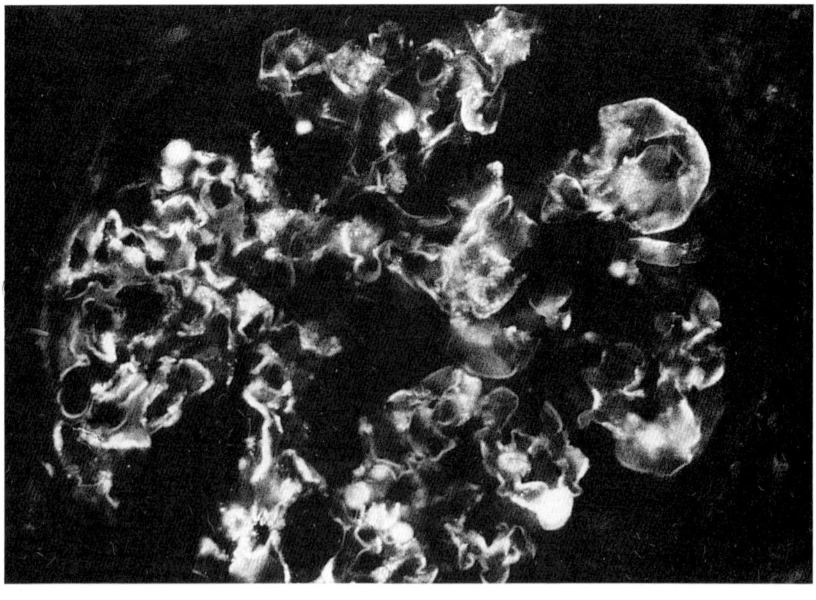

Fig. 8 IgA nephropathy. Mesangial and capillary deposition of IgA (IF ×315)

The clinical picture is variable with acute nephritic symptoms seen in 30% of patients. The majority have a more indolent and protracted renal course[5].

IgA nephropathy in liver disease

IgA nephropathy may occur in several clinical conditions, where the common feature is deposition of IgA in the glomerular mesangium (Fig. 8). The diagnosis cannot be made without a biopsy. *Idiopathic* IgA nephropathy (Berger's disease) is the most common type, and it is probably the most frequent cause of glomerular renal failure in several parts of the world. IgA nephropathy is also a manifestation of *Schönlein–Henoch disease*. IgA deposits in the kidney often accompany nephritis in *systemic lupus*, and finally, glomerular IgA deposition is a frequent finding in *chronic liver disease*.

Many cases previously considered as hepatic glomerulosclerosis (see above) are, with the help of immunohistochemistry, now classified as IgA nephropathy. Manigand *et al.*[23] described glomerular IgA and C3 deposits in biopsy specimens from 75% of patients with liver cirrhosis. Several studies on biopsy and autopsy material have confirmed the presence of glomerular morphological abnormalities in more than 50% of patients with liver cirrhosis[24].

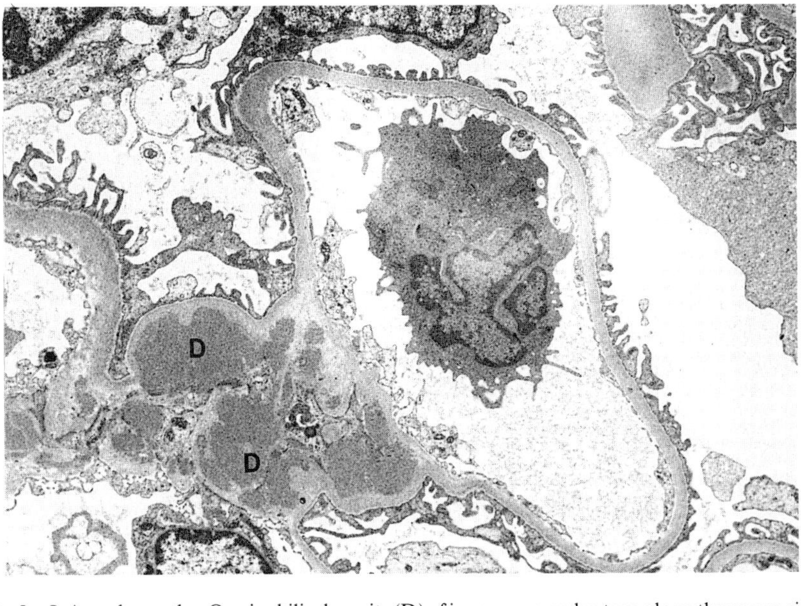

Fig. 9 IgA nephropathy. Osmiophilic deposits (D) of immune complex type along the mesangial basement membrane (EM ×4350)

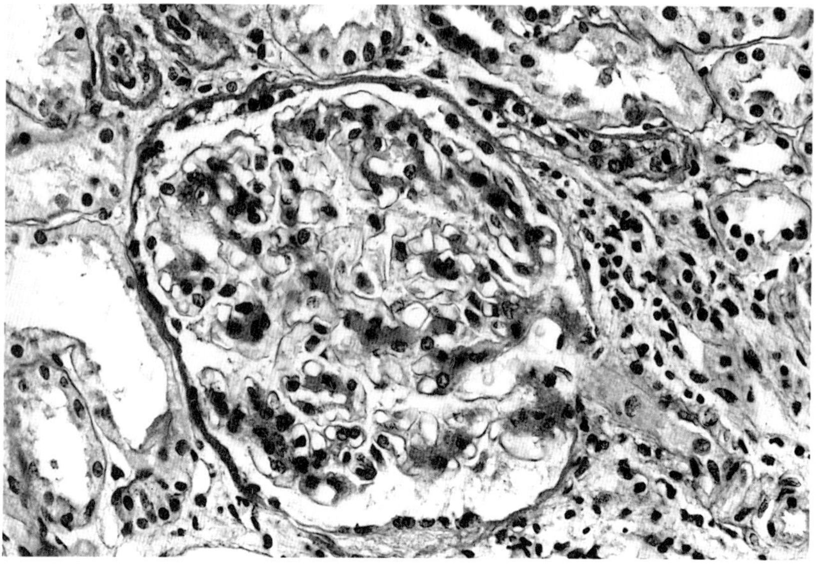

Fig. 10 IgA nephropathy. Mesangial matrix increase with only slight hypercellularity (=slight mesangial proliferative glomerulonephritis) (PAS ×315)

Comparison of light microscopic, electron microscopic and immunohistochemical features of idiopathic and liver-related IgA nephropathy

The renal pathological changes in hepatic IgA nephropathy are quite heterogeneous and are similar to the findings in idiopathic IgA nephropathy, but tend to be milder. The hallmark for the disease is the mesangial deposition of IgA (Fig. 8), and most often C3, where electron microscopy reveals electron-dense deposits in the mesangium (Fig. 9). Morphologically, an increase in mesangial matrix with slight hypercellularity is common (Fig. 10), although most types of glomerular lesions, from minimal change nephropathy to membranoproliferative glomerulonephritis, can be found. Membranous glomerulonephritis is not encountered. A few reports indicate that some features differ between idiopathic and hepatic IgA nephritis. Berger *et al.*[12] and Nakamoto *et al.*[25] noted a low frequency of focal lesions and segmental sclerosis. Cirrhotic IgA nephritis has more of a tendency to show mesangial interposition[25], and mesangial IgG and C1q may be present more frequently in cirrhosis-related glomerulonephritis[26].

IgA nephropathy in different types of liver disease

Several studies confirm the presence of IgA nephropathy in more than 50% of patients with liver cirrhosis. Nakamoto *et al.*[25] found no relationship between glomerular IgA and the aetiology of the cirrhosis. Sinniah[27] found no difference in the frequency of IgA deposition between *alcoholic* and *hepatitis-related* cirrhosis. Renal IgA deposits were found in 40% of patients with *cystic fibrosis*, who had either focal or multilobular biliary cirrhosis[28]. In *alpha-1-antitrypsin deficiency* membranoproliferative and mesangial proliferative glomerulonephritis associated with IgA deposits were found to be frequent[29]. IgA deposition is also noted to occur in alcoholic liver disease in the absence of cirrhosis in patients with steatosis or fibrosis, with or without portal hypertension[30].

The role of *hepatitis B virus* infection in IgA nephropathy is still controversial. Lai *et al.*[17] found a strong association between IgA nephropathy and hepatitis B antigenaemia in patients from Hong Kong, where the virus is endemic. HBsAg carrier rate was found more often among patients with IgA nephropathy than in the general population. HBV DNA was detected by *in-situ* hybridization in tubular cells and glomerular mesangium. However, no association between IgA nephropathy and HBV infection was found in a study from Japan, suggesting that hepatitis B virus plays no pathogenetic role in IgA nephropathy where the virus is not endemic[31].

Clinical features of hepatic IgA nephropathy

Most cases of IgA nephropathy in chronic liver disease lack clinical symptoms. Nakamoto *et al.*[25] found nephritic urinary changes in 9% of 752 consecutive patients with cirrhosis. In a study of 202 patients with IgA nephropathy and cirrhosis, 89 had signs of glomerular disease with microscopic haematuria and moderate proteinuria[30]. Gencrally, patients with non-proliferative glomerular changes have an unremarkable urinary sediment[12]. Nephritic urinary sediment correlates with the severity of glomerular lesions, mesangial cell proliferation and the presence of mesangial interposition[24]. Gross haematuria is rare in contrast to what is seen in idiopathic IgA nephropathy. Renal insufficiency in cirrhotic IgA nephropathy is exceptional, but is more likely to occur with membranoproliferative glomerulonephritis. The presentation of IgA nephritis with gross haematuria, oliguria and acute reduction of glomerular filtration rate, known to be associated with crescent formation in renal biopsies, is rarely observed in liver-related IgA nephropathy.

Very little is known about the prognosis of cirrhotic glomerulonephritis. The patient's overall prognosis is more likely dependent on the underlying hepatic disease. In support of this is the report by Ghabra *et al.*[32]. They recorded resolution of cirrhotic glomerulonephritis following liver transplantation, and conclude that liver transplantation may provide a means of treatment of severe and progressive hepatic glomerular disease.

In HBV-associated IgA nephropathy microscopic haematuria and asymptomatic proteinuria were often present[33]. In contrast to the relatively benign course in children with HBV-associated membranous glomerulonephritis, there are indications that HBV-associated IgA nephropathy is a slowly progressive disease that leads to renal insufficiency as in idiopathic IgA nephropathy[17].

Pathogenetic factors in hepatic IgA nephropathy

Experimental studies. Several immunological disturbances described in IgA nephropathy indicate that immunological mechanisms are involved in its pathogenesis: the occurrence of renal symptoms during infections, the presence of IgA in the mesangium and other organs, the elevation of serum IgA and IgM and the recurrence of IgA deposits in transplanted kidneys[34]. In idiopathic as well as in hepatic IgA nephropathy circulating IgA-containing immune complexes deposit in the glomeruli and cause the described immunohistological changes.

The pathogenesis of the renal deposition of IgA in liver disease may involve several mechanisms[35]:

1. *Impaired clearance* of IgA immune complexes from the circulation, being of less importance in idopathic IgA nephritis, may be very important in hepatic IgA nephropathy. Defective clearance by hepatic Kupffer cells is suggested by Gormly *et al.*[36]. They demonstrated IgA deposits in the glomeruli, circulatory immune complexes and elevated serum IgA levels in rodents rendered cirrhotic by inhalation of carbon tetrachloride. Rifai and Mannik[37] demonstrated the presence of a specific receptor on Kupffer cells that remove IgA containing immune complexes from the circulation. Likewise, extrahepatic mononuclear phagocyte function may be impaired secondary to accumulation of toxic substances induced by liver failure. Cryoglobulinaemia, being prevalent in liver cirrhosis[25,38], may reflect the impaired immune complex clearance.
2. Functional *portacaval shunts* in liver cirrhosis may allow immune complexes derived from the intestines to bypass hepatic degradation. Case reports illustrate the importance of a possible shunting of immune complexes in portal hypertension, even in the absence of liver pathology. A patient with a histologically normal liver and portal hypertension due to a splenic artery aneurysm developed IgA nephropathy and nephrotic syndrome. After removal of the aneurysm and restoration of the portal circulation, the renal symptoms disappeared[39].
3. The role of *biliary transport* of IgA has been demonstrated in experimental studies. Secretory IgA deposits were found in glomeruli of immunized mice with cholestasis induced by bile duct ligation[40]. The importance of biliary transport of IgA in humans has been controversial. However, studies in children with extrahepatic biliary atresia revealed IgA deposition in the glomeruli, and support the existence of an active hepatobiliary transport mechanism[41].
4. *Hypocomplementaemia* is frequently seen in liver failure and may be secondary to consumption of complement by the accumulating immune complexes. Since the liver synthesizes complement factors, liver failure *per se* may give rise to hypocomplementaemia. Complement is important in clearance of immune complexes by several mechanisms[42].
5. The role of *alcohol* was studied by Smith *et al.*[43]. In forensic autopsy material of alcoholic individuals from an American Indian population they found IgA nephropathy in 64%, with hepatic cirrhosis present in

only 9%. In an animal model they demonstrated that chronic alcohol ingestion was linked to renal disease even in the absence of liver cirrhosis[44]. Keeping ethnic variations in mind, these studies suggest a role for alcohol in the pathogenesis of IgA nephropathy, also in the absence of severe liver pathology. As a possible pathogenetic mechanism increased levels of circulating IgA and IgA-immune complexes secondary to an alcohol-induced defect in the hepatic immune complex clearance system has been suggested. Alternatively, alcohol abuse could imply excessive antigenic stimulation due to increased absorption of intestinal macromolecules induced by alcohol[45].

In alcoholic liver disease there is a polyclonal increase of serum immunoglobulins, where the increase in IgA levels exceeds that of IgG and IgM[46]. Most of serum IgA is polymeric, and in contrast to other conditions with elevated serum IgA, a shift towards the IgA_2 subclass seems to occur in alcoholic liver disease. Cirrhotic patients are also reported to develop anti-albumin antibodies, which may be part of the increased serum IgA levels[26].

6. The role of *Mallory bodies* as a potential antigen in the mesangial deposits in alcoholic patients has been extensively investigated by Lomax-Smith and Woodroffe[47]. From patients with alcoholic cirrhosis they eluted isolated glomeruli rich in IgA deposits and demonstrated antibody reactivity in these eluates to Mallory bodies by direct immunofluorescence on liver tissue from patients with alcoholic hepatitis. Mallory body-derived monoclonal antibodies have been found to react with glomeruli from alcoholic patients with liver and kidney disease[48]. However, we feel that these studies need further confirmation with specific and well-characterized antibodies.

Indeed, very little is known concerning the possible antigens involved in the formation of immune complexes in idiopathic as well as hepatic IgA nephropathy. Microbiological antigens, antigens in food and autoantigens have all been suggested.

Renal disease after liver transplantation

Lastly it should be mentioned that renal impairment occurs in more than 90% of patients after liver transplantation, and the majority develops chronic renal failure[49]. In a prospective study of non-alcoholic patients negative for HBsAg who underwent liver transplantation, all had abnormal renal biopsies. Glomerular minimal change and glomerular sclerosis were most frequently seen. These findings indicate that glomerular damage is universal in patients with end-stage liver failure[50].

SUMMARY AND OUTLOOK ON NEPHROPATHY IN LIVER DISEASE

Starting with the observation by Helwig[51], 60 years ago, of a 'liver kidney syndrome', the intimate relationship between renal and liver disease has been acknowledged. As mentioned in the introduction, primary liver disease often results in kidney disease, the opposite relationship being less common, and simultaneous involvement of both organs in disease processes is often recognized. Still today in many of the above-described conditions our knowledge of pathogenetic mechanisms is incomplete, especially in IgA nephritis. Other conditions, such as hepatic glomerulosclerosis, need to be redefined. Lastly, the role of hepatitis C virus infection in renal disease needs intensive study, and it is to be hoped that the ongoing liver studies may result in a better understanding of the renal diseases described here.

ADDENDUM

After submission of the manuscript we became aware of case reports linking HCV to glomerulonephritis (A. Gonzalo[a], R. Barcena[b], F. Mompaso[c], A. Zea[d], J. Artuno[a]. [Servicio de Nefrologia[a], Gastroenterologia[b], Anatomia Patologica[c], Reumatologia[d], Hospital Ramon y Cajal, Madrid, Espana] Membranoproliferative glomerulonephritis and hepatitis C virus infection. Nephron. 1993;63:475–6.)

References

1. Ehrich JHH, Brunkhorst R, Burdelski M, Ringe B, Kühn K. Klinische Syndrome mit Leber- und Nierenbeteiligung im Kindes- und Erwachsenenalter. Monatsschr Kinderheilkd. 1989;137:649–56.
2. Strøm EH, Westvik J, Pedersen SJ, Strømme P. Renal cysts in the carbohydrate deficient glycoprotein syndrome. Pediatr Nephrol. 1993; in press.
3. Galaske RG, Burdelski M, Brodehl J. Primär polyurisches Nierenversagen und akute gelbe Leberdystrophie nach Infusion von Zuckeraustauschstoffen im Kindesalter. Dtsch Med Wochenschr. 1986;111:978–83.
4. Glassock RJ, Cohen AH, Danovitch G, Parsa P. Human immunodeficiency virus (HIV) infection and the kidney. Ann Intern Med. 1990;112:35–49.
5. Striker LJ, Olson JL, Striker GE. The renal biopsy. Philadelphia: W.B. Saunders;1990.
6. Utz DC, Warren MM, Gregg JA, Ludwig A, Kelalis PP. Reversible hepatic dysfunction associated with hypernephroma. Mayo Clin Proc. 1970;45:161–9.
7. Lorenz R, Brauer M, Classen M, Tornieporth N, Becker K. Idiopathic portal hypertension in a renal transplant patient after long-term azathioprine therapy. Clin Invest. 1992;70:152–5.
8. Briggs JD. The recipient of a renal transplant. In: Morris PJ, editor. Kidney transplantation. Principles and practice. Philadelphia: W.B. Saunders; 1988:71–92.
9. Solez K. The pathology and pathogenesis of human 'acute tubular necrosis'. In: Solez K, Whelton A, editors. Acute renal failure. Correlations between morphology and function. New York and Basel: Marcel Dekker; 1984:17–42.
10. Iwatsuki S, Popovtzer MM, Corman JL, Ishikawa M, Pudnam CW, Katz FH, Starzl TH. Recovery from 'hepatorenal syndrome' after orthotopic liver transplantation. N Engl J Med. 1973;289:1155–9.
11. Koppel MH, Coburn JW, Mims MM, Goldstein H, Boyle JD, Rubini ME. Transplantation of cadaveric kidneys from patients with hepatorenal syndrome. N Engl J Med. 1969;280:1367–71.
12. Berger J, Yaneva H, Nabarra N. Glomerular changes in patients with cirrhosis of the liver. Adv Nephrol. 1978;7:3–14.
13. Magil A, Chase W, Frohlich J. Unusual renal biopsy findings in a patient with familial lecithin-cholesterol acyltransferase deficiency. Hum Pathol. 1982;13:283–5.
14. Combes B, Stastny P, Shorey J, Eigenbrodt EH, Barbera A, Hull AR, Carter NW. Glomerulonephritis with deposition of Australia antigen-antibody complexes in glomerular basement membrane. Lancet. 1971;2:234–7.

15. Lai KN, Lai FM-M. Clinical features and the natural course of hepatitis B virus-related glomerulopathy in adults. Kidney Int. 1991;40:Suppl 35:S40–5.
16. Lin C-Y. Clinical features and natural course of HBV-related glomerulopathy in children. Kidney Int. 1991;40:Suppl 35:S46–53.
17. Lai KN, Lai FM, Tam JS, Vallance-Owen J. Strong association between IgA nephropathy and hepatitis B surface antigenemia in endemic areas. Clin Nephrol. 1988;29:229–34.
18. Lisker-Melman M, Webb D, Di Bisceglie AM, Kassianides C, Martin P, Rustgi V, Waggoner JG, Park Y, Hoofnagle JH. Glomerulonephritis caused by chronic hepatitis B virus infection: treatment with recombinant human alpha-interferon. Ann Intern Med. 1989;111:479–83.
19. Fish AJ, Michael AF, Vernier RL, Good RA. Acute serum sickness nephritis in the rabbit (an immune deposit disease). Am J Pathol. 1966;49:997–1022.
20. Johnson RJ, Couser WG. Hepatitis B infection and renal disease: Clinical, immunopathogenetic and therapeutic considerations. Kidney Int. 1990;37:663–76.
21. McMahon BJ, Heyward WL, Templin DW, Clement D, Lanier AP. Hepatitis B-associated polyarteritis nodosa in Alaskan eskimos. Clinical and epidemiologic features and longterm follow-up. Hepatology. 1989;9:97–101.
22. Ferri C, Greco F, Longombardo G, Palla P, Moretti A, Marzo E, Mazzoni A, Pasero G, Bombardieri S, Highfield P. Association between hepatitis C virus and mixed cryoglobulinemia. Clin Exp Rheumatol. 1991;9:621–4.
23. Manigand G, Morel-Maroger L, Simon J *et al.* Lésiones glomérulaires et cirrhose du foie. Note préliminaire sur les lésions histologiques du rein au cours des cirrhose hépatiques, d'après 20 prélèvements biopsiques. Rev Eur Etud Biol. 1970;15:989–96.
24. Newell GC. Cirrhotic glomerulonephritis: incidence, morphology, clinical features, and pathogenesis. Am J Kidney Dis. 1987;9:183–90.
25. Nakamoto Y, Iida H, Kobayashi K, Dohi K, Kida H, Hattori N, Takeuchi J. Hepatic glomerulonephritis. Characteristics of hepatic IgA glomerulonephritis as the major part. Virch Arch (A). 1981;392:45–54.
26. Woodroffe AJ, Gormly AA, McKenzie PE, Wootton AM, Thompson AJ, Seymour AE, Clarkson AR. Immunologic studies in IgA nephropathy. Kidney Int. 1980;18:366–74.
27. Sinniah R. Heterogenous IgA glomerulonephropathy in liver cirrhosis. Histopathology. 1984;8:947–62.
28. Abramowsky CR, Dahms B, Swinehart G. IgA-associated glomerular deposits in liver disease. Hum Pathol. 1985;16:1243–6.
29. Davis ID, Burke B, Freese D, Sharp HL, Kim Y. The pathologic spectrum of the nephropathy associated with alpha-1-antitrypsin deficiency. Hum Pathol. 1992;23:57–62.
30. Nochy D, Druet P, Baran D, Bariety J. Chronic liver disease and IgA nephropathy. Plasma Ther Transfus Technol. 1985;6:725–31.
31. Iida H, Izumino K, Asaka M, Fujita M, Takata M, Sasayama S. IgA nephropathy and hepatitis B virus. IgA nephropathy unrelated to hepatitis B surface antigenemia. Nephron. 1990;54:18–20.
32. Ghabra N, Piraino B, Greenberg A, Banner B. Resolution of cirrhotic glomerulonephritis following successful liver transplantation. Clin Nephrol. 1991;35:6–9.
33. Lai KN, Lai FM-M, Chan KW, Chow CB, Tong KL, Vallance-Owen J. The clinico-pathologic features of hepatitis B virus-associated glomerulonephritis. Quart J Med. 1987;63:323–33.
34. Kincaid-Smith P, Nicholls K. Mesangial IgA nephropathy. Am J Kidney Dis. 1983;3:90–102.
35. Emancipator SN. Primary and secondary forms of IgA nephritis, Schönlein-Henoch syndrome. In: Heptinstall RH, editor. Pathology of the kidney, vol. 1, 4th edn. Boston/Toronto/London: Little, Brown; 1992:389–476.
36. Gormly AA, Smith PS, Seymour AE, Clarkson AR, Woodroffe AJ. IgA glomerular deposits in experimental cirrhosis. Am J Pathol. 1981;104:50–4.
37. Rifai A, Mannik M. Clearance of circulating IgA immune complexes mediated by specific receptor on Kupffer cells in mice. J Exp Med. 1984;160:125–37.
38. Nochy D, Callard P, Bellon B, Bariety J, Druet P. Association of overt glomerulonephritis and liver disease: a study of 34 patients. Clin Nephrol. 1976;6:422–7.
39. Babbs C, Warnes TW, Torrance HB, Ballardie FW. IgA nephropathy in non-cirrhotic portal hypertension. Gut. 1991;32:225–6.

40. Emancipator SN, Gallo GR, Razaboni R, Lamm ME. Experimental cholestasis promotes the deposition of glomerular IgA immune complexes. Am J Pathol. 1983;113:19–26.
41. Abramowsky CR, Christiansen DM. Secretory immunoglobulin deposits in renal glomeruli of children with extrahepatic biliary atresia: studies in a human counterpart of experimental ligation of the bile ducts. Hum Pathol. 1987;18:1126–31.
42. Emancipator SN, Lamm ME. IgA nephropathy: Overproduction or decreased clearance of immune complexes? Lab Invest. 1989;61:365–7.
43. Smith SM, Hoy WE. Frequent association of mesangial glomerulonephritis and alcohol abuse: a study of 3 ethnic groups. Mod Pathol. 1989;2:138–43.
44. Smith SM, Yu GSM, Tsukamoto H. IgA nephropathy in alcohol abuse: an animal model. Lab Invest. 1990;62:179–84.
45. Worthington BS, Meserole L, Syrotuck JA. Effect of daily ethanol ingestion on intestinal permeability to macromolecules. Am J Dig Dis. 1978;23:23–32.
46. Van Es LA, Valentijn RM. Circulating and mesangial IgA in IgA nephropathy. Henoch–Schönlein syndrome, and alcoholic liver disease. Plasma Ther Transfus Technol. 1985;6:669–76.
47. Lomax-Smith JD, Woodroffe AJ. Elution of antibodies to Mallory's hyaline from kidneys of patients with alcoholic liver disease and mesangial IgA deposits. J Clin Pathol. 1983;36:1416–17.
48. Burns J, D'Ardenne AJ, Morton JA, McGee JO'D. Immune complex nephritis in alcoholic cirrhosis: detection of Mallory body antigen in complexes by means of monoclonal antibodies to Mallory bodies. J Clin Pathol. 1983;36:751–5.
49. McCauley J, Van Thiel DH, Starzl TE, Puschett JB. Acute and chronic renal failure in liver transplantation. Nephron. 1990;55:121–8.
50. Crawford DHG, Endre ZH, Axelsen RA, Lynch SV, Balderson GA, Strong RW, Kerlin P, Powell LW, Fleming SJ. Universal occurrence of glomerular abnormalities in patients receiving liver transplants. Am J Kidney Dis. 1992;19:339–44.
51. Helwig FC, Scutz CB. A liver kidney syndrome. Clinical pathological and experimental studies. Surg Gynecol Obstet. 1932;55:570–80.

Section V
Liver and haematopoietic system

17

Haematopoiesis in liver diseases: haematological effects of alcohol

J. LINDENBAUM

INTRODUCTION

Rather than attempt to survey the myriad disorders of haematopoiesis associated with liver disease, I will focus in this brief review on alcoholic liver disease, and particularly on the haematological syndromes that have been shown to be induced by ethanol administration in human volunteers, or those in which effects of ethanol are strongly implicated in their pathogenesis. Our current understanding of the mechanisms of these haematological disorders will be summarized, and some common diagnostic problems faced by clinicians caring for alcoholic patients will also be highlighted. A more detailed review has been published elsewhere[1].

EFFECTS OF ETHANOL IN HUMAN SUBJECTS

Fortunately for them, but unfortunately for us, rats and baboons do not develop the haematological syndromes seen in alcoholic patients. This may be due to species differences or may reflect dosage effects. No baboon or rat would take ethanol as 75% or 100% of its total caloric intake, as do many of our patients. These animals have the good sense to prefer death by dehydration to the ingestion of such a high percentage of their caloric intake in the form of a dangerous toxin. Therefore, lacking an animal model, what we know of the mechanisms of the haematological effects of ethanol is based almost entirely on studies in human volunteers.

Table 1 lists the syndromes commonly encountered in alcoholic patients that have been shown to be experimentally induced by ethanol in human subjects. In the case of some of the haematological disorders, such as

Table 1 Haematological abnormalities induced by ethanol administration in human subjects

	Induced by ethanol with	
Abnormality	*Deficient diet*	*Nutritious diet*
Megaloblastic anaemia	+	0
Low serum folate	+	+
Ring sideroblasts	+	0
Vacuolization of pronormoblasts and promyelocytes	+	+
Thrombocytopenia	+	+
Granulocytopenia	+	0
Decreased granulocyte mobilization	n.s.	+

n.s. = Not studied under conditions of deficient diets
Reproduced with permission from ref. 1

megaloblastic and sideroblastic anaemia, a diet deficient in nutrients has had to be administered to the volunteers along with ethanol in order to produce the syndrome. In contrast, other effects such as thrombocytopenia, vacuolization of marrow red and white cell precursors, and decreased mobilization of neutrophils into sites of inflammation have been induced in subjects who were well nourished and in whom malnutrition presumably was not a contributing factor. In other words, some haematological actions of ethanol may result from 'conditioned' nutritional deficiency states, whereas others are apparently produced by alcohol via other mechanisms. All of these effects are completely reversible within a week or two of cessation of drinking.

RED CELLS

Megaloblastic anaemia

Our discussion of the haematological consequences of alcohol toxicity can well begin with the erythroid series, since anaemia is so common in those who imbibe heavily. In several large series of consecutively studied alcoholics, megaloblastic change was the most frequent abnormality in the bone marrow[2–4]. Megaloblastic anaemia in alcoholics is often difficult to diagnose. More than one-third of patients will not have an elevated MCV[4]. No test is perfect in identifying these patients. Serum and red cell folate levels are limited in both specificity and sensitivity[4]. The presence of neutrophil hypersegmentation on blood smears is a specific but not sensitive finding, and the reverse is true for the presence of macroovalocytes[4]. Megaloblastic anaemia in alcoholics is usually due to folate deficiency, but it is important to rule out cobalamin deficiency before potentially dangerous therapy with folic acid.

Sullivan and Herbert administered ethanol to patients with megaloblastic anaemia in a metabolic ward setting. The intake of wine, whisky or ethanol itself blocked the reticulocytosis that was occurring in response to small doses of folic acid, as long as alcohol was being administered[5]. These and subsequent studies[2,6-10] indicated that megaloblastic anaemia in alcoholics is due to the combination of a marginal dietary folate supply and an inhibitory effect of ethanol on metabolism of the vitamin.

The mechanism whereby ethanol interferes with folate metabolism is unclear. Eichner and Hillman infused ethanol intravenously to non-alcoholic human volunteers[6]. After 8 h of the infusion an abrupt fall in serum folate levels was noted. This effect of alcohol on serum levels of folate would therefore interrupt the supply of the vitamin to the bone marrow. Despite experiments in animals by many investigators, the cause of the decrease in circulating folate levels remains uncertain. A variety of widely differing animal models have been used (summarized in references 1 and 11) and the results have often been in conflict with each other[11] and of uncertain clinical relevance. Different workers have suggested that alcohol interferes with the enterohepatic circulation, the hepatic retention, the intestinal absorption or reabsorption or the renal retention of folate[1]. There are no conclusive data in humans, and it can only be said at this time that alcohol in some way compromises the folate status of alcoholics.

A few years ago we showed that when folic acid was added to the cheap wines commonly serving as the sole source of nutrients for many alcoholic persons living in New York City, it was soluble, stable for long periods of time and well absorbed along with intoxicating doses of the wines. We proposed that these wines be fortified with folic acid in order to prevent the morbidity and mortality associated with megaloblastic anaemia[12]. This idea was not acceptable, however. It was opposed out of a fear that such a fortification would encourage alcoholism; the same sort of thinking that perceives that the distribution of condoms in order to prevent AIDS will encourage licentious sex. Folate deficiency is common in imbibers of wine and whisky, which contain little or no folate, but is rare in beer drinkers. Many beers are already naturally very rich in folic acid in amounts sufficient to overcome the inhibitory effect of ethanol on folate metabolism.

Sideroblastic anaemia

Another established effect of alcohol is the induction of ringed sideroblasts in the bone marrow, which have been seen in about 30% of hospitalized alcoholics in some series[2,3]. The ringed sideroblasts, which are commonly identified by Prussian blue stains of bone marrow films, contain iron-laden mitochondria which are demonstrable ultrastructurally, arrayed in a ring or crown around the nucleus.

Ringed sideroblasts have been induced in human volunteers by alcohol administration[2,3,7,8], but the exact mechanism of this effect is again uncertain[1]. Most likely this is caused by a disturbance in haem synthesis, although it could be a non-specific effect of mitochondrial damage. There are conflicting data as to which enzyme in haem synthesis is blocked by ethanol[1]. This is almost never the only cause of anaemia in an alcoholic, and the clinical importance of this striking morphological finding has been difficult to unravel[4].

Vacuolization of marrow cells

Another alcohol-induced effect which may be no more than a morphological curiosity, or a marker that the patient is drinking, is vacuolization of red and white cell precursors in the bone marrow. Vacuoles in the cytoplasm of pronormoblasts and promyelocytes can be produced by giving alcohol to human volunteers, and are not prevented by the co-administration of folate or high-protein diets[13]. However, the vacuolization is not associated with evidence of marrow failure or impairment in haemoglobin production by the vacuolated red cells[13].

Macrocytosis

An increased erythrocyte mean cell volume, or MCV, is very frequently seen in alcoholics. Listed in Table 2 are the common causes of macrocytosis in alcoholics. Reticulocytosis may cause an elevated MCV because young red cells are larger than mature ones. Liver disease of any cause may be associated with increased deposition of cholesterol and phospholipid on red cell membranes[14], causing macrocytosis and often target cell formation as well. These changes have no adverse effect on cell survival. On the other hand, in some patients with extreme deposition of cholesterol on red cells, one finds spur cells on the blood smear, or acanthocytes. Typically, these patients have a brisk haemolytic anaemia in association with advanced liver disease that may or may not be caused by alcohol intake[14,15].

However, far and away the commonest cause of an elevated MCV in alcoholic patients is the more recently recognized condition called the macrocytosis of alcoholism[16,17]. This is an extremely common finding in chronic alcoholics[16,17]. The degree of macrocytosis is usually modest (MCVs characteristically in the 100–110 fl range) and associated with little in the way of anaemia. The cardinal findings of megaloblastic haematopoiesis on blood smears (hypersegmented neutrophils and macroovalocytes) are absent, and there is no evidence that the macrocytosis is due to folate deficiency[16–19]. No-one has produced the macrocytosis of alcoholism experimentally by giving ethanol to human volunteers, but there is good reason to suspect that this is an effect of alcohol by a currently obscure mechanism, distinct from the macrocytosis caused by liver disease.

Although this is also a benign phenomenon that has no apparent adverse consequences for the erythrocytes, it may serve to confuse the physician. An alcoholic with the anaemia of chronic disease may have an elevated MCV,

Table 2 Causes of macrocytosis in alcoholics

1. Folate deficiency
2. Reticulocytosis
3. Liver disease
4. Macrocytosis of alcoholism*

* Most common cause

therefore apparently having a 'macrocytic anaemia'. The macrocytosis is due to alcohol ingestion, but the anaemia is caused by the chronic disorder.

Iron deficiency anaemia

Iron deficiency is often seen in alcoholic patients, usually caused by blood loss. Diagnosis may be difficult, particularly because of the confounding effects of ethanol on red cell size. In a series of 48 patients with alcoholic liver disease and proven iron deficiency, 50% did not have a low MCV[4]. The most reliable test in the diagnosis of iron deficiency was the serum ferritin, which was either low or in the low end of the normal range in every patient. Summarized in Table 3 are the various possible results of serum tests of iron status. Many commonly obtained results are non-diagnostic. For example, the combination of a low serum iron and a low total iron binding capacity does not rule out iron deficiency in any way. It is often not appreciated by clinicians that a high normal or an elevated serum ferritin rules out iron deficiency even if the patient has active liver disease. In other words the hyperferritinaemia caused by liver disease, apparently the result of inflammation or of the release of ferritin from hepatocytes, is not seen in iron-deficient patients, regardless of the severity of hepatic dysfunction.

Other causes of anaemia

There may be other 'nutritional' causes of anaemia in alcoholics that we diagnose infrequently or fail to recognize. Severe hypophosphataemia may rarely cause a brisk haemolytic anaemia with spherocyte formation due to depletion of red cell ATP[20]. Severe protein malnutrition contributes to anaemia in children with kwashiorkor and in protein-starved monkeys. Whether it plays a role in alcoholics is not established. Whether vitamin E

Table 3 Use of serum tests to predict irons stores* in anaemic patients

Result	*Interpretation*
Definitive	
low ferritin	Deficient
high TIBC	Deficient
high normal or high ferritin	Not deficient†
Equivocal	
low normal ferritin	Uncertain
low serum iron	Uncertain
low or normal TIBC	Uncertain
low percentage transferrin saturation	Uncertain

* As documented by Prussian blue stain of bone marrow aspirates
† Even if inflammation, malignancy, liver disease or renal failure is present
TIBC = total iron-binding capacity

deficiency contributes to Zieve's syndrome[21,22] may be important only if there is such an entity as Zieve's syndrome, which is doubtful[1,14].

Anaemia in alcoholics presents a diagnostic challenge. In a recent study of 121 consecutive anaemic alcoholics admitted to hospital, more than 60% had several, at least two, underlying mechanisms for the anaemia[4]. The common causes of anaemia in alcoholics and their underlying mechanisms are listed in Table 4. A mild anaemia due to chronic disease is frequently seen in patients with various hepatic disorders. The clinician should also recognize that a mildly anaemic patient with liver disease may not be anaemic at all. When isotopic studies of the mass of circulating red cells in patients with cirrhosis have been performed, the number of circulating erythrocytes is often normal, and the apparent anaemia is purely due to an expansion of the plasma volume, particularly in patients with portal hypertension and splenomegaly, but not necessarily with ascites[23,24]. The haematocrit may be as low as 28% in patients with cirrhosis who have a normal red cell mass[23,24].

PLATELETS

Thrombocytopenia

Alcohol has been shown to have two separate damaging effects on platelets. Thrombocytopenia is very common in alcoholics[1,25], seen in perhaps 50% or more of alcoholic patients admitted to hospital. The experimental administration of ethanol to human volunteers causes thrombocytopenia[1,9,13] despite the concomitant intake of high levels of folate and protein[13]. The decreased number of circulating platelets induced by alcohol has been shown to be the combined result of ineffective thrombocytopoiesis by bone marrow cells (in other words, a failure to produce mature platelets despite normal to increased numbers of marrow megakaryocytes) and a shortened platelet life span[9].

However, this is not the only cause of thrombocytopenia that the clinician must consider in an alcoholic patient. Table 5 lists four other commonly seen mechanisms and some of the clinical clues to their detection. Alcohol-induced thrombocytopenia can be diagnosed only when these other aetiologies have been ruled out clinically. The diagnosis is clinched in retrospect after the rapid recovery that typically occurs after withdrawal of alcohol.

Table 4 Common causes of anaemia in alcoholics

Aetiology	*Mechanisms*
Megaloblastic	Decreased dietary folate Ethanol inhibition of folate metabolism
Acute blood loss	Gastrointestinal bleeding
Iron deficiency	Blood loss
Chronic disease	Hepatic inflammation
Haemodilution	Plasma volume expansion (portal hypertension, splenomegaly)

Impaired platelet function

In addition, ethanol interferes with platelet function, even in situations where the number of circulating platelets is maintained[26,27]. Alcohol in large doses can prolong the bleeding time[26]. In a study by Deykin and co-workers, an apparently trivial dose of ethanol (50 g) markedly potentiated the effect of 300 mg of aspirin on the bleeding time in four normal volunteers, even though this dose of ethanol taken by itself did not prolong the bleeding time[28]. This is a common clinical phenomenon in haemostasis: the interaction of multiple mild defects to cause clinical bleeding.

GRANULOCYTES

Granulocytopenia

There are two effects of ethanol on granulocytes that are worth highlighting. In perhaps 3% of patients, ethanol intoxication may be associated with granulocytopenia. This is at least in part due to depletion of the reserve of granulocytes in the bone marrow[29,30], where most of the mature neutrophils in the body normally reside. The marrow granulocyte reserve typically recovers rapidly after cessation of alcohol ingestion in such patients. Alcohol toxicity is implicated here but not proven experimentally. Other mechanisms may cause granulocytopenia in alcoholics, including folate deficiency, rapid mobilization of granulocytes into sites of infection and hypersplenism.

Impaired neutrophil adhesion

More important clinically, probably, is the profound suppression of the delivery of granulocytes into sites of inflammation, which has been shown by two groups[31,32] to be induced by small non-intoxicating doses of ethanol in human volunteers. The number of neutrophils accumulating in areas of slightly traumatized skin (so-called skin windows) over an 8 h period, was markedly reduced by single doses of ethanol. In fact, volunteers given cocktail doses of alcohol accumulated fewer neutrophils at sites of inflammation than

Table 5 Common causes of thrombocytopenia in alcoholics

Cause	*Helpful diagnostic findings*
Folate deficiency	MCV > 110 fl* neutrophil hypersegmentation, >3% macroovalocytes, LDH > 1000 U*
Hypersplenism	Enlarged spleen; other evidence of cirrhosis and portal hypertension
Septicaemia	Positive blood cultures
Disseminated intravascular coagulation	Decreased fibrinogen, other abnormal clotting tests, increased fibrin degradation products
Alcohol-induced thrombocytopenia	Absence of above findings; increase in platelet count within 5 days

* Present in only a minority of alcoholic patients with megaloblastic anaemia[4]
Reproduced with permission from ref. 1

did non-intoxicated patients in terminal shock[31]. This is almost certainly an effect of ethanol on the ability of granulocytes to adhere to the walls of capillaries[32], the adhesion step that occurs before they migrate into sites of inflammation. Whether the function of a particular adhesion molecule on the surface of granulocytes is disturbed by ethanol has not yet been demonstrated, but the impairment in cell migration may play an important role in the susceptibility of alcoholics to a variety of infections.

OTHER CELLS

The effects of ethanol on monocytes and macrophages have not been as extensively studied in humans, but it is likely that an impairment in cell adhesion similar to that seen with granulocytes is induced[1,33]. This may compromise host resistance to infections, such as tuberculosis, in which macrophages play a major role. Alcohol may also have subtle effects on lymphocyte function[1,30,32,34,35].

References

1. Lindenbaum J. Hematologic complications of alcohol abuse. Semin Liver Dis. 1987;7(3):169–81.
2. Eichner ER, Hillman RS. The evolution of anaemia in alcoholic patients. Am J Med. 1971;50:218–32.
3. Hines JD, Cowan DH. Anaemia in alcoholism. In: Dimitrov NV, Nodine JH, editors. Drugs and hematologic reactions. New York: Grune & Stratton; 1974:141–53.
4. Savage DS, Lindenbaum J. Anemia in alcoholics. Medicine. 1986;65:322–38.
5. Sullivan LW, Herbert V. Suppression of hematopoiesis by ethanol. J Clin Invest. 1964;43:2048–61.
6. Eichner ER, Hillman RS. Effect of alcohol on serum folate level. J Clin Invest. 1973;52:584–91.
7. Hines JD. Reversible megaloblastic and sideroblastic marrow abnormalities in alcoholic patients. Br J Haematol. 1969;16:87–101.
8. Hines JD, Cowan DH. Studies on the pathogenesis of alcohol-induced sideroblastic bone-marrow abnormalities. N Engl J Med. 1970;283:441–6.
9. Cowan DH. Thrombokinetic studies in alcohol-related thrombocytopenia. J Lab Clin Med. 1973;81:64–76.
10. Halsted CH, Robles EA, Mezey E. Intestinal malabsorption in folate-deficient alcoholics. Gastroenterology. 1973;64:526–32.
11. Weir DG, McGing PG, Scott JM. Folate metabolism, the enteropathic circulation and alcohol. Biochem Pharmacol. 1985;34:1–7.
12. Kaunitz JD, Lindenbaum J. The bioavailability of folic acid added to wine. Ann Intern Med. 1977;887:542–5.
13. Lindenbaum J, Lieber CS. Hematologic effects of alcohol in man in the absence of nutritional deficiency. N Engl J Med. 1969;281:333–8.
14. Cooper RA. Hemolytic syndromes and red cell membrane abnormalities in liver disease. Semin Hematol. 1980;17:103–12.
15. Powell LW, Halliday JW, Knowles BR. The relationship of red cell membrane lipid content to red cell morphology and survival in patients with liver disease. Aust NZ J Med. 1975;5:101–7.
16. Wu A, Chanarin I, Levi AJ. Macrocytosis of chronic alcoholism. Lancet. 1974;1:829–31.
17. Lindenbaum J. Folate and vitamin B_{12} deficiencies in alcoholism. Semin Hematol. 1980;17:119–29.
18. Wu A, Chanarin I, Slavin G, Levi AJ. Folate deficiency in the alcoholic – its relationship to clinical and haematological abnormalities, liver disease and folate stores. Br J Haematol. 1975;29:469–78.

19. Chalmers DM, Chanarin I, MacDermott S, Levi AJ. Sex-related differences in the haematological effects of excessive alcohol consumption. J Clin Pathol. 1980;33:3–7.
20. Jacob HS, Amsden T. Acute hemolytic anaemia with rigid red cells in hypophosphatemia. N Engl J Med. 1971;285:1446–50.
21. Zieve L. Jaundice, hyperlipemia and hemolytic anaemia: a heretofore unrecognized syndrome associated with alcoholic fatty liver and cirrhosis. Ann Intern Med. 1958;48:471–96.
22. Goebel KM, Goebel FD, Schubotz R, Schneider J. Red cell metabolic and membrane features in haemolytic anaemia of alcoholic liver disease (Zieve's syndrome). 1977;35:573–85.
23. Hyde GM, Berlin NI, Parsons RJ, Lawrence JH, Port S. The blood volume in portal cirrhosis as determined by P^{32} labeled red blood cells. J Lab Clin Med. 1952;39:347–53.
24. Hall CA. Erythrocyte dynamics in liver disease. Am J Med. 1960;28:541–9.
25. Lindenbaum J, Hargrove RL. Thrombocytopenia in alcoholics. Ann Intern Med. 1968;68:526–32.
26. Cowan DH. Effect of alcoholism on hemostasis. Semin Hematol. 1980;17:137–47.
27. Mikhailidis DP, Jenkins WJ, Barradas MA, Jeremy JY, Dandona P. Platelet function defects in chronic alcoholism. Br Med J. 1986;293:715–18.
28. Deykin D, Janson P, McMahon I. Ethanol potentiation of aspirin-induced prolongation of the bleeding time. N Engl J Med. 1982;306:852–4.
29. Liu YK. Leukopenia in alcoholics. Am J Med. 1973;54:605–10.
30. Liu YK. Effects of alcohol on granulocytes and lymphocytes. Semin Hematol. 1980;17:130–6.
31. Brayton RG, Stokes PE, Schwartz MS, Louria DB. Effect of alcohol and various diseases on leukocyte mobilization, phagocytosis, and intracellular bacterial killing. N Engl J Med. 1970;282:123–8.
32. MacGregor RR. Alcohol and immune defense. J Am Med Assoc. 1986;256:1474–9.
33. Rimland D. Mechanisms of ethanol-induced defects of alveolar macrophage function. Alcoholism. 1983;8:73–6.
34. Gluckman SJ, Dvorak VC, MacGregor RR. Host defenses during prolonged alcohol consumption in a controlled environment. Arch Intern Med. 1977;137:1539–43.
35. Drew PA, Clifton PM, LaBrooy JT, Shearman DJC. Polyclonal B cell activation in alcoholic patients with no evidence of liver dysfunction. Clin Exp Immunol. 1984;57:479–86.

18

Haemostasis in acute and chronic liver disease

J. A. SUMMERFIELD

INTRODUCTION

The liver has a central role in the control of coagulation, and this is reflected in the fact that about 75% of patients with liver disease will develop haemostatic problems at some time during their illness. The clinical problems include petechiae, ecchymoses, epistaxis and variceal haemorrhage. Furthermore liver patients may bleed abnormally following procedures such as venepuncture, liver biopsy and liver transplantation.

The liver is the site of synthesis of all the coagulation proteins except von Willebrand factor (vWF), which is synthesized by vascular endothelial cells. It is also the site of synthesis of the inhibitors of coagulation such as antithrombin III, protein C and protein S. Furthermore, the liver synthesizes most of the proteins involved in fibrinolysis. The other role of the liver in the control of haemostasis is the clearance of activated coagulation and fibrinolysis proteins.

The coagulation abnormalities that develop in liver disease depend on the balance between the hepatic synthesis and clearance of coagulation proteins, coagulation inhibitors and fibrinolysis proteins. Furthermore, coagulation abnormalities are dependent upon the presence of thrombocytopenia, dysfibrinogenaemia and disseminated intravascular coagulation. Although the coagulation disorders that develop are complex, and reflect the balance between a variety of factors, they can be broadly classified into three types. First, there are haemostatic disorders due to reduced concentrations of coagulation factors. Secondly, there are disorders due to hyperfibrinolysis. Thirdly, there is a hypercoagulable state that develops immediately after liver transplantation.

REDUCED LEVELS OF COAGULATION PROTEINS

The vitamin K-dependent proteins (prothrombin (II), Factor VII, Factor IX, and Factor X) are synthesized in hepatocytes in the rough endoplasmic reticulum. Vitamin K carboxylates the 10 terminal glutamic acid residues. This carboxylation enables the proteins to bind to phospholipids and function as coagulation proteins. In vitamin K deficiency states (such as cholestasis) non-functional precursor proteins are secreted into the serum[2]. Furthermore inactive precursor proteins can also be detected in patients with liver disease (who are not vitamin K deficient). This indicates that an acquired defect of carboxylation can develop in liver disease[3]. The other abnormalities that develop in liver disease are qualitative abnormalities of coagulation proteins. Two examples will be given. First, acquired dysfibrinogaenemia: this is due to increased sialylation of fibrinogen. Acquired dysfibrinogenaemia should be suspected in any patient with prolongation of the plasma thrombin time in the absence of low levels of fibrinogen or increased fibrinogen degradation products (FDPs). This abnormality is common and develops in more than 50% of patients with liver disease[4]. Another example of a qualitative abnormality of coagulation proteins is the accumulation of Factor VIIIC and vWF antigen in liver disease. However, the activities of these factors, as measured in functional assays, are within the normal range. This discrepancy is due to accumulation of non-functional antigens in the blood[5].

In addition to the reduction in the levels of coagulant proteins and the qualitative abnormalities in these proteins that develop in liver disease, the protease inhibitors of coagulation and fibrinolysis are also affected. Specifically, protein C and antithrombin III levels are decreased in advanced liver diseases such as cirrhosis. Futhermore, the major inhibitor of the fibrinolytic system, alpha$_2$-antiplasmin, is also decreased. These changes correlate with serum albumin concentrations, indicating that they reflect decreased hepatic synthesis of these protease inhibitors[6,7].

HYPERFIBRINOLYSIS

Fibrin has only a temporary function in blood clotting and the fibrinolysis system is responsible for removing it (Fig. 1). Fibrin is degraded to fibrin degradation products (FDPs) by plasmin. Plasmin is formed upon activation of plasminogen by a plasminogen activator such as tissue plasminogen activator (t-PA) and urokinase plasminogen activator (u-PA). Plasminogen activator inhibitor I (PAI-1) controls fibrinolysis by inhibition of t-PA and to a lesser extent of u-PA. Histidine-rich glycoprotein (HRG) regulates the amount of free plasminogen in the circulation by binding to plasminogen. Alpha$_2$-antiplasmin (alpha$_2$-AP) is the most important inhibitor of plasmin in the circulation. It acts by forming plasmin–alpha$_2$-AP complexes. Alpha$_2$-antiplasmin can also bind to plasminogen and crosslink to fibrin. The crosslinking of alpha$_2$-antiplasmin to fibrin is mediated by coagulation Factor

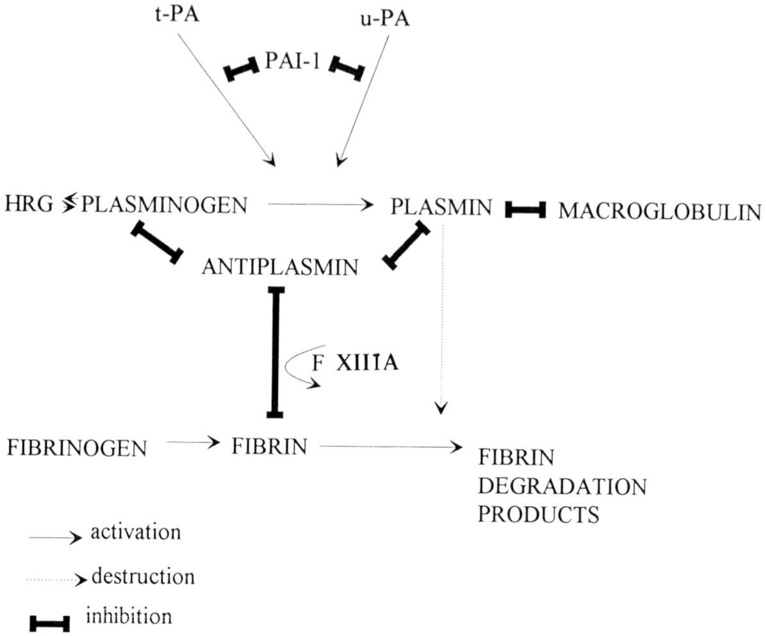

Fig. 1 The normal fibrinolysis system. Fibrin is degraded to fibrin degradation products (FDPs) by plasmin. The levels of plasmin are regulated by the profibrinolytic factors, plasminogen activators (t-PA and u-PA) and their inhibitor (plasminogen activator inhibitor 1 [PAI-1]) on the one hand and the antifibrinolytic factors which are alpha$_2$-antiplasmin and alpha$_2$-macroglobulin on the other (see text for details)

XIIIA. Alpha$_2$-macroglobulin is also a plasmin inhibitor but is much less efficient than alpha$_2$-antiplasmin.

Hyperfibrinolysis develops in advanced cirrhosis. This is due to an imbalance between fibinolytic proteins and inhibitors. The serum levels of t-PA are increased whereas the levels of PAI-1 are reduced. This leads to increased plasmin production. Furthermore alpha$_2$-antiplasmin activity is decreased. The reduction of alpha$_2$-antiplasmin results in more fibrin being available for degradation by plasmin to FDPs. This change in the balance of the fibrinolysis system in cirrhosis is summarized in Fig. 2. The end-result is that increased levels of tissue plasminogen activator in the presence of decreased levels of inhibitors lead to increased amounts of plasmin which act on fibrin to form increased amounts of fibrin degradation products[8,9].

There are two areas where the presence of hyperfibrinolysis in chronic liver disease has been shown to be clinically important. These are in variceal haemorrhage and liver transplantation. The study of Violi *et al.*[10] clearly showed the predictive value of hyperfibrinolysis for variceal haemorrhage. These authors followed 61 cirrhotic patients for 3 years. Hyperfibrinolysis, defined as FDPs greater than 10 mg/ml, were found in 28 patients. In these patients the t-PA levels were increased three times normal, and the PAI-1

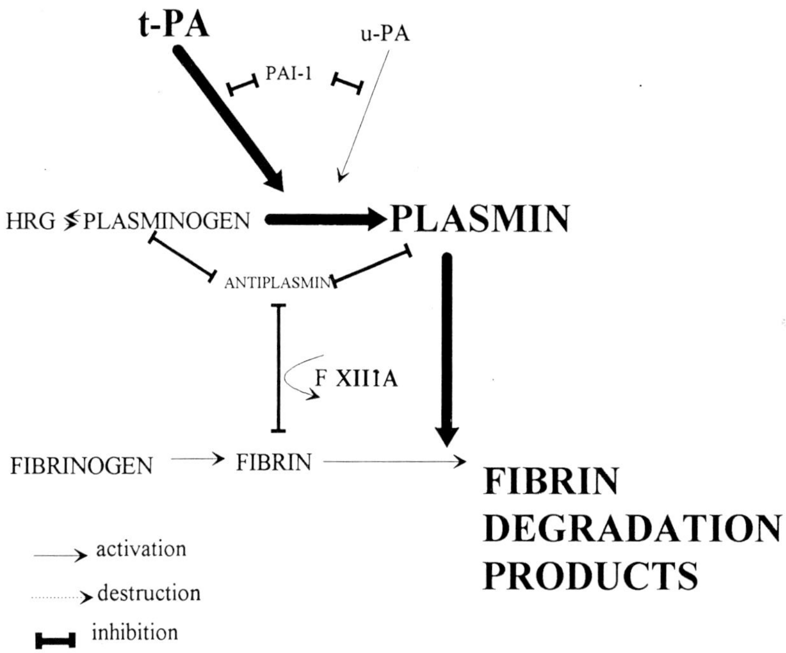

Fig. 2 Hyperfibrinolysis in cirrhosis. Serum levels of t-PA are increased whereas the levels of its inhibitor (PAI-1) are reduced. This leads to increased plasmin production. The parallel reduction in alpha$_2$-antiplasmin levels results in more fibrin being available for degradation by plasmin to fibrin degradation products. The consequence is hyperfibrinolysis

levels decreased three times normal. Of the 61 patients followed, 41 died in the course of follow-up. Twenty-two of these patients died of variceal bleeding. Analysis of the data showed that whereas nine of 33 patients with normal fibrinolysis bled, 21 of 28 patients with hyperfibrinolysis bled from varices. These authors found that hyperfibrinolysis in cirrhotic patients was the best predictor for variceal bleeding.

The other area where hyperfibrinolysis is clinically important is in liver transplantation. However, transplantation is complicated by the fact that after the operation a hypercoagulable state develops. I will deal with these two haemostatic complications in sequence.

During liver transplantation there is activation of the coagulation system, as judged by the presence of thrombin–antithrombin complexes. There is also evidence of hyperfibrinolysis as judged by increased levels of t-PA. It is unclear whether the increased t-PA levels are due to increased release of t-PA from the vascular endothelium or decreased clearance by the diseased liver. Hyperfibrinolysis starts during the anhepatic phase of liver transplantation (Fig. 3). However it continues and is often exacerbated during hepatic revascularization[11,12].

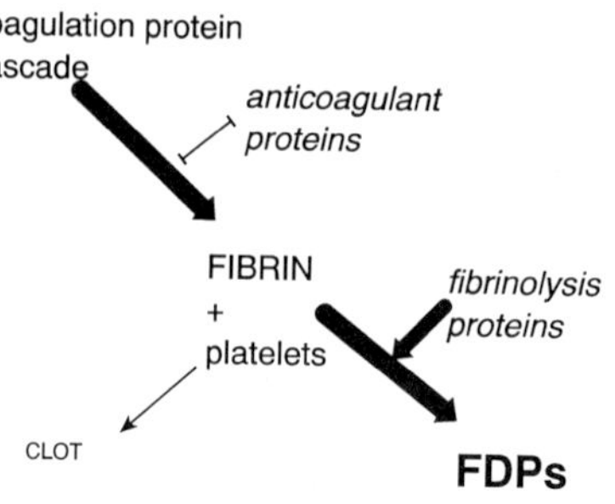

Fig. 3 Liver transplantation causes activation of both the coagulation cascade, as judged by the presence of thrombin–antithrombin complexes and hyperfibrinolysis as judged by increased levels of fibrin degradation products (FDPs). The coagulation cascade is increased because of lower levels of anticoagulant proteins (e.g. antithrombin III). Fibrinolysis is increased because of increased levels of fibrinolytic proteins (e.g. t-PA). Hyperfibrinolysis starts during the anhepatic phase of liver transplantation and is often exacerbated during hepatic revascularization

HYPERCOAGULABLE STATE FOLLOWING LIVER TRANSPLANTATION

In contrast, after liver transplantation a hypercoagulable state is common during the first 10 days. The cause of this appears to be an imbalance between procoagulant proteins and anticoagulant proteins. Most of the coagulant proteins have returned to normal levels by day 1 after transplantation. However Factor V and Factor VIII only recover by day 3. In contrast the recovery of anticoagulant protein levels is delayed. These include antithrombin III, protein C and protein S. Furthermore fibrinolysis is inhibited due to increased levels of PAI-1[13]. Data from Stahl *et al.*[14] showed the percentage of transplant patients with anticoagulant protein deficiency at day 3 and day 5 after liver transplantation. It is apparent that antithrombin III takes 5 days to return to normal in more than half the patients. Protein C and protein S levels are also depressed in a significant proportion of patients. Thus a hypercoagulable state commonly develops in the first 10 days after a transplant. It is noteworthy that this coincides with the incidence of hepatic artery thrombosis, and it seems probable that this major complication of transplantation may be due not to surgical problems like the anastomosis, but rather to the hypercoagulable state that develops.

EVALUATION OF THE RISK OF BLEEDING

The risk of bleeding in a patient depends on the balance between the synthesis and clearance of coagulation and fibrinolytic proteins. Clearly it is important to assess the risk of bleeding in patients undergoing liver biopsy or surgery. Unfortunately the risk of bleeding cannot easily be evaluated from routine haemostatic tests. For example, one cannot predict the risk of bleeding from a patient's platelet count, prothrombin time, fibrinogen level or thrombin time. The best indicator of the risk of bleeding appears to be the presence of hyperfibrinolysis. As pointed out earlier, hyperfibrinolysis is a good predictor of variceal haemorrhage and intraoperative bleeding during transplantation. However, in practice we need measures to evaluate the risk of bleeding for common procedures such as percutaneous liver biopsies. A good practical guide is to measure the prothrombin time (PT), the partial thromboplastin time (PTT) and the platelet count. If the PT or PTT are prolonged more than 3 s, vitamin K should be given for 3 days. If the platelet count is less than 60 000 platelet function tests should be performed and platelet infusions given prior to a biopsy. If the tests of coagulation do not return to normal, alternatives to percutaneous liver biopsy should be considered, such as transjugular liver biopsy.

PROGNOSTIC VALUE OF COAGULATION PROTEINS

Coagulation factors are sensitive indicators of liver function and in some situations have prognostic value. Two examples will suffice. Firstly, the study of Hillenbrand *et al.*[15], which showed that the Thrombotest result had useful prognostic value in patients with fulminant hepatitis. The second study is by Pereira *et al.*[16]. They also looked as fulminant hepatitis (in this case paracetamol poisoning) and examined the prognostic value of the coagulation factors in these patients. They showed the ratio of Factor VIII to Factor V gave good discrimination between survivors and non-survivors in this type of fulminant hepatitis.

THERAPY OF HAEMOSTATIC ABNORMALITIES

Fresh frozen plasma, vitamin K and platelet infusions remain the mainstay of treatment for bleeding in patients with liver disease. Several other treatments have been tried. These include desmopressin, antithrombin III concentrates, epsilon-aminocaproic acid, aprotonin and heparin. Here, I shall briefly describe the published experience of the value of these other agents.

Desmopressin

Desmopressin (D-amino-8-D-arginine vasopressin or DDAVP) causes a 2–3-fold increase in the level of Factor VIII and vWF. Agnelli *et al.*[17] showed that in cirrhotics DDAVP unexpectedly decreased the prothrombin time. Other studies have shown that both the PT and PPT are shortened by this agent. It has been claimed that DDAVP may be useful for patients with marginally deranged clotting tests who are undergoing liver biopsy. However, the use of DDAVP has not gained widespread acceptance.

Antithrombin III concentrates

Antithrombin III is an anticoagulant protein which inhibits the conversion of prothrombin to thrombin. It has been used to inhibit the coagulation cascade in patients with disseminated intravascular coagulation. There are anecdotal reports of success with antithrombin III concentrates in fulminant hepatitis and in acute fatty liver of pregnancy. However, in a recent randomized trial, antithrombin III concentrates were shown to have no effect on the transfusion requirements of patients undergoing liver transplantation, despite evidence of disseminated intravascular coagulation in these patients[18].

Epsilon-aminocaproic acid

There is a report of the use of epsilon-aminocaproic acid (EACA), a potent inhibitor of fibrinolysis, in liver transplantation[19]. In this study 1 g of EACA was given intravenously to 20 patients undergoing liver transplantation. The authors report that hyperfibrinolysis was reversed in all the patients. They further stated that there were no bleeding or thrombotic complications. However, this agent does not seem to have gained favour and is not in widespread use.

Aprotonin

Aprotonin is another story. It is being widely used during liver transplantation, because of its effect in reducing blood loss. There have been several reports of its use in transplantation and a consensus appears to be developing about the optimal dose and administration of aprotonin[20,21]. A loading dose of 2 million kallikrein international units is given at induction of anaesthesia. Throughout the operation an infusion of 0.5 million kallikrein international units per hour is maintained. One study has shown that a constant infusion is superior to just an initial bolus dose[22]. One of the problems of using aprotonin is cost. Using the above regime in the United Kingdom, the loading dose would cost £82 and the maintenance infusion would cost £21 per hour. However, when set against the saving in the use of blood products there is probably a net gain. In the trial reported by Grosse *et al.*[20], hyperfibrinolysis was largely reversed by aprotonin in transplant recipients. The consequence of this was a 50% saving in the use of packed red blood cells, fresh frozen plasma and platelet infusions.

Treatment of post-transplant hypercoagulable state

Finally there is a question of therapy for the hypercoagulable state that develops after liver transplantation. There is some evidence that this hypercoagulable state may be related to hepatic artery thrombosis. Stahl *et al.*[14] used the following protocol. Until the levels of anticoagulant proteins (ATIII, protein C and protein S) returned to normal they give regular infusions of fresh frozen plasma and low-dose heparin (300–400 units per hour). Although this protocol has not been submitted to a clinical trial they report that they have seen no hepatic artery thromboses in 65 consecutive patients with this regime. However, it must be said that another report using a similar protocol did not prevent hepatic artery thrombosis[13].

References

1. Friedman PA. Vitamin K. In: Arias I, Popper H, Schaffner D, Shafritz DA editors. The liver; biology and pathobiology. New York: Raven Press; 1982:359–65.
2. Stenflo J, Ganrot PO. Vitamin K and the biosynthesis of prothrombin: Identification and purification of a dicoumarol-induced prothrombin from bovine plasma. J Biol Chem. 1972;247:8186–92.
3. Blanchard RA, Furie CB, Jorgensen M *et al.* Acquired vitamin K dependent carboxylation deficiency in liver disease. N Engl J Med. 1981;305:242–8.
4. Francis JL, Armstrong DJ. Acquired dysfibrinogenaemia in liver disease. J Clin Pathol. 1982;35:667–72.
5. Kelly DA, O'Brian, Hutton RA *et al.* The effects of liver disease on factors V, VIII and protein C. Br J Haematol. 1985;61:541–8.
6. Sinclair TS, Booth NA, Penman SM *et al.* Protease inhibitors in liver disease. Scand J Gastroenterol. 1988;23:620–4.
7. Bell H, Odegaard OR, Andersson T, Raknerud N. Protein C in patients with alcoholic cirrhosis and other liver diseases. J Hepatol. 1992;14:163–7.
8. Leebeek FWG, Kluft C, Knot EAR *et al.* A shift in balance between profibrinolytic and antifibrinolytic factors causes enhanced fibrinolysis in cirrhosis. Gastroenterology. 1991;101:1382–90.
9. Huber K, Kirchheimer JC, Korninger C, Binder BR. Hepatic synthesis and clearance of components of the fibrinolytic system in healthy volunteers and in patients with different stages of liver cirrhosis. Thromb Res. 1991;62:491–500.
10. Violi F, Ferro D, Basili S *et al.* Hyperfibrinolysis increase the risk of gastrointestinal hemorrhage in patients with advanced cirrhosis. Hepatology. 1992;15:672–76.
11. Harper PL, Luddington RL, Jennings I *et al.* Coagulation changes following hepatic revascularisation during liver transplantation. Transplantation. 1989;48:603–7.
12. Dzik WH, Arkin CF, Jenkins RL, Stump DC. Fibrinolysis during liver transplantation in humans: role of tissue-type plasminogen activator. Blood. 1988;71:1090–5.
13. Harper PL, Edgar PF, Luddington RL *et al.* Protein C deficiency and portal thrombosis in liver transplantation in children. Lancet. 1988;ii:924–7.
14. Stahl RL, Duncan A, Hooks MA *et al.* A hypercoagulable state follows orthotopic liver transplantation. Hepatology. 1990;12:553–8.
15. Hillenbrand P, Parbhoo SP, Jedrychowski A, Sherlock S. Significance of intravascular coagulation and fibrinolysis in acute hepatic failure. Gut. 1974;15:83.
16. Pereira LMMB, Langley PJ, Hayllar KM *et al.* Coagulation factor V and VIII/V ratio as predictors of outcome in paracetamol induced fulminant hepatic failure: relation to other prognostic indicators. Gut. 1992;33:98–102.
17. Agnelli G, De Cunto M, Berretuni M *et al.* Desmopressin improvement of abnormal coagulation in chronic liver disease. Lancet. 1983;i:645.
18. Palareti G, Legnani C, Maccaferri M *et al.* Coagulation and fibrinolysis in orthotopic liver transplantation: role of recipient's disease and use of antithrombin III concentrates. Haemostasis. 1991;21:68–76.
19. Kang Y, Lewis JH, Navalgund A *et al.* Epsilon-aminocaproic acid for treatment of fibrinolysis during liver transplantation. Anesthesiology. 1987;66:766–73.
20. Grosse H, Lobbes W, Frambach M *et al.* The use of high dose aprotonin in liver transplantation: the influence on fibrinolysis and blood loss. Thromb Res. 1991;63:287–97.
21. Mallett SV, Cox D, Burroughs AK, Rolles K. The intra-operative use of trasylol (aprotonin) in liver transplantation. Transpl Int. 1991;4:227–30.
22. Himmelreich G, Kierzek B, Neuhaus P *et al.* Coagulation changes and the influence of the early perfusate in the course of orthotopic liver transplantation (OLT) when aprotonin is used intra-operatively. Blood Coagul Fibrinolysis. 1991;2:51–8.

Section VI

Liver and endocrine function

19

Liver and insulin

H. HARTMANN, A. MEYER-ALBER and J. SUBERG

The coincidence of liver disease and diabetes mellitus was described almost a century ago by Bernard Naunyn[1]. He coined the term 'liver diabetes' or 'hepatogenous diabetes'. About 30 years ago, after the development of radioimmunoassays for the measurement of insulin[2], it was recognized that patients with liver cirrhosis frequently not only show an impaired glucose tolerance but also hyperinsulinaemia, thus suggesting insulin resistance[3,4]. More directly, insulin resistance was demonstrated in these patients by a blunted decrease of blood glucose following intravenous injection of insulin[5,6] and of tolbutamide[7]. Epidemiological data for the association of liver disease and diabetes mellitus and the early pathophysiological studies were reviewed by Creutzfeldt *et al.* in 1970[8]. Since that time new techniques have successfully been applied to examine individual aspects of altered carbohydrate metabolism (i.e. oral and intravenous glucose tolerance coupled to isotopic measurement of glucose turnover) and to study insulin secretion and action (i.e. euglycaemic and hyperglycaemic clamping). Most of these latter studies have been performed in rather small groups of heterogeneous patients at a single time-point and although single aspects of hepatogenous diabetes (like the localization and mechanisms of insulin resistance) have been fairly well characterized, a coherent pathogenic concept is still lacking. In 1982 Creutzfeldt *et al.* proposed a vicious circle for the pathogenesis of hepatogenous diabetes that would be initiated by a decrease of *hepatic* glucose uptake, leading to hyperglycaemia which in turn would stimulate compensatory pancreatic insulin secretion, followed by insulin resistance of peripheral target tissues and the liver and ensuing further reduction of glucose tolerance[9] (Fig. 1). Since the formulation of this hypothesis additional data have been obtained from patients with liver disease as well as from laboratory animals with experimental cirrhosis, that will be discussed in this chapter.

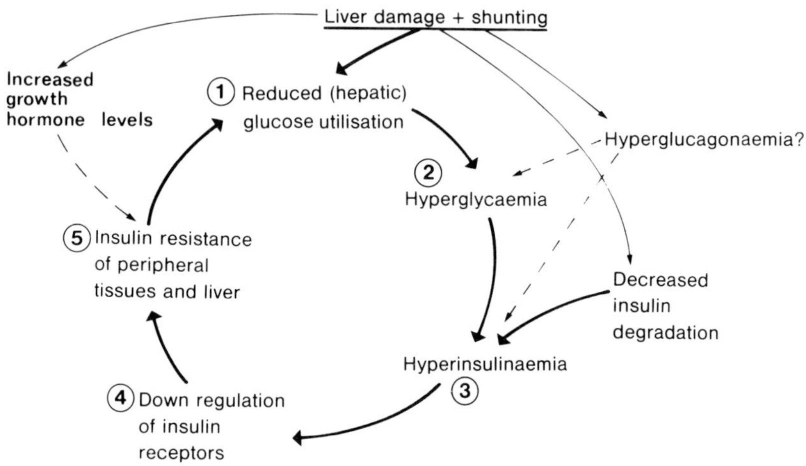

Fig. 1 Pathogenesis of hepatogenous diabetes. Reproduced from ref. 9

INSULIN RESISTANCE

Insulin action on the liver and on peripheral insulin-responsive tissues (of which skeletal muscle is quantitatively most important) has been studied employing the euglycaemic hyperinsulinaemic clamp technique in patients with cirrhosis of different aetiology and of various severity. These studies have unequivocally demonstrated a marked reduction of insulin-stimulated total body glucose disposal of up to 50% of maximal glucose utilization[9–19]. When dose–response curves for insulin (including physiological insulin concentrations) were obtained half-maximally effective plasma insulin concentrations were reported to be elevated in cirrhosis[10]. Similar data have been obtained in rats with CCl_4-induced cirrhosis of the liver[20]. Recently, we could demonstrate a 30% reduction of insulin-stimulated total-body glucose disposal during euglycaemic clamping in cirrhotic rats (Fig. 2). Since an unaltered insulin-mediated suppression of hepatic glucose production has been observed in cirrhotic patients[13,18,21], impaired peripheral tissue glucose utilization appeared to account for the reduction of total-body glucose disposal. Thus, insulin resistance has been localized to peripheral target tissues.

MECHANISM OF INSULIN RESISTANCE

Concerning affinity and number of cellular insulin receptors in patients with cirrhosis conflicting data have been reported. Since most binding studies were done on peripheral blood cells (e.g. erythrocytes and monocytes) the

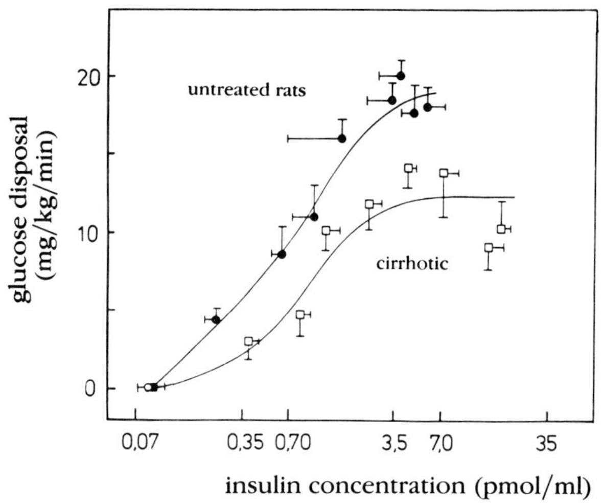

Fig. 2 Stimulation of total-body glucose disposal during euglycaemic hyperinsulinaemic clamping in rats with CCl_4-induced cirrhosis. Anaesthetized animals received continuous intravenous infusions of insulin. Exogenous glucose was infused to maintain euglycaemia. The amount of glucose infused at steady-state conditions was equivalent to whole-body glucose utilization. Arterial insulin concentrations were measured by radioimmunoassay. Values are means ± SD of at least five experiments each at individual doses. Reproduced from ref. 20

relevance of these data to insulin-responsive tissues remains questionable (for review see ref. 22). Among these latter tissues, only binding to adipocytes isolated from cirrhotic patients has been studied, again, yielding contradictory results[12,23]. Normal insulin binding has been reported for hepatocytes isolated from cirrhotic rats[24]. Therefore, reduced insulin receptor binding seems unlikely to explain insulin resistance in cirrhosis. Furthermore, several lines of evidence suggest that postreceptor events would be more important. Particularly when euglycaemic hyperinsulinaemic clamp studies were coupled to either isotopic measurements of glucose metabolism in rats[20] or to indirect calorimetry in humans[17–19], a marked decrease of non-oxidative glucose disposal (i.e. glycogen synthesis) was observed, while glucose transport and glucose oxidation appeared to be unaltered (Figs 3 and 4). In addition, insulin-stimulated skeletal muscle glycogen synthase activity was decreased in cirrhotic patients whereas pyruvate dehydrogenase activity was identical to control subjects[15]. The disparate effect of cirrhosis on individual intracellular pathways of glucose metabolism and on different intracellular enzymes strongly supports the view that insulin resistance in cirrhosis is associated with postreceptor events.

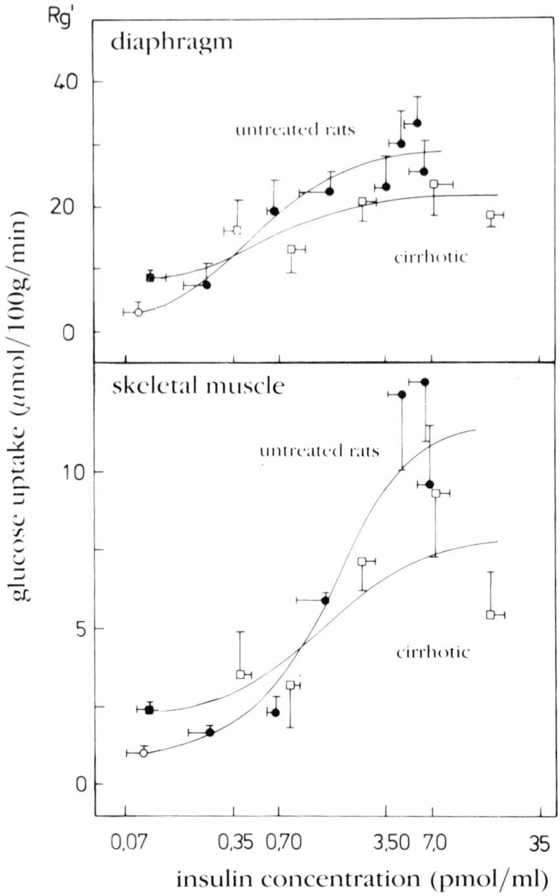

Fig. 3 Stimulation of 2-deoxyglucose uptake in diaphragm and red skeletal muscle during euglycaemic hyperinsulinaemic clamping in cirrhotic rats. Anaesthetized animals were treated as described in the legend for Fig. 2. After injection of labelled 2-deoxyglucose and subsequent tissue sampling, glucose metabolic index (Rg′) was calculated. Values are means ± SD of at least five experiments at each infusion rate. Reproduced from ref. 20

INSULIN SECRETION

Elevated plasma insulin concentrations in cirrhosis have been measured in fasted patients as well as following oral and intravenous glucose loads[25–28]. Since the normal liver degrades up to 50% of circulating insulin[29], the contribution of pancreatic secretion on the one hand and of decreased hepatic insulin clearance on the other hand, to the observed hyperinsuliaemia has been debated[30]. The recent availability of recombinant human c-peptide

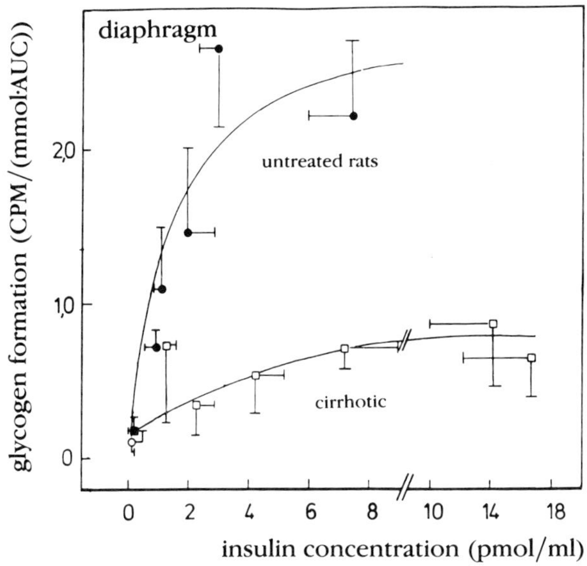

Fig. 4 Stimulation of glycogen formation in diaphragm during euglycaemic hyperinsulinemic clamping in cirrhotic rats. Anaesthetized animals were treated as described in the legend for Fig. 2. After injection of labelled glucose and subsequent tissue sampling glycogen synthesis was calculated. Values are means ± SD of at least four experiments at each insulin infusion rate. Reproduced from ref. 20

(which is not degraded by the liver) has permitted pharmacokinetic studies to measure c-peptide metabolic clearance rate (reported to be unaltered in cirrhosis), thereby allowing the calculation of pancreatic secretion rates from peripheral blood c-peptide concentrations[28]. Thus, while studying cirrhotic patients with normal tolerance to oral glucose, we were able to demonstrate increased insulin secretion in the fasted state as well as after oral glucose[26] (Fig. 5). Furthermore, pancreatic hypersecretion was described following intravenous glucose under hyperglycaemic clamp conditions[28]. Proinsulin, the single-chain biosynthetic precursor of insulin, apparently does not contribute to hyperinsulinaemia[26]. It should be noted, however, that in patients with abnormal tolerance to oral glucose, particularly in those with overt diabetes, relative hyposecretion of insulin has been documented[26,31]. Recently, a pronounced impairment of insulin secretion, i.e. a complete loss of first phase insulin response, has been observed in diabetic cirrhotic patients[32]. Studying glucose-stimulated insulin secretion in perfused pancreas from rats with experimental cirrhosis a reduction of about 40% was reported[33].

In conclusion, abnormalities of insulin secretion seem to depend on the stage of the disease. Hypersecretion may be an early feature when glucose tolerance is still normal, while in later stages (when insulin resistance is more pronounced) impaired glucose tolerance and relative hyposecretion ensues, eventually leading to frank diabetes.

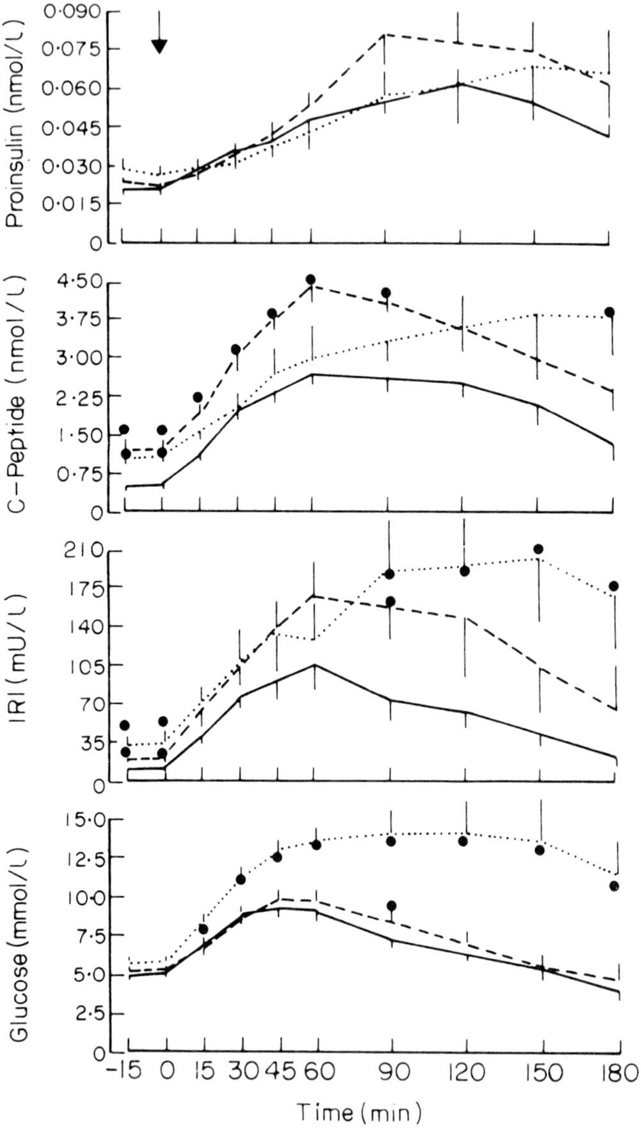

Fig. 5 Response of immunoreactive proinsulin, c-peptide, insulin and serum glucose to oral carbohydrate equivalent to 75 g glucose in healthy subjects (——) in patients with liver cirrhosis and normal glucose tolerance (– – – –) and in patients with liver cirrhosis and impaired glucose tolerance (···). Significant ($p < 0.05$) differences compared with healthy subjects are shown by (●). Reproduced from ref. 26

ROLE OF THE LIVER IN HANDLING ORAL GLUCOSE IN CIRRHOSIS

The question of a direct contribution of the diseased liver to impaired oral glucose tolerance has received little attention. It has been claimed that the normal liver takes up about 30% of an oral glucose load[34]. According to the hypothesis presented above (Fig. 1) a reduced hepatic glucose utilization secondary to liver damage could be the precipitating initial event. In fact, recent work employing a dual-isotope method (oral [^{14}C]glucose, intravenous [^{3}H]glucose) suggested an increase in the amount of ingested glucose appearing in the systemic circulation in cirrhotic patients, whereas suppression of hepatic glucose production by oral glucose was apparently unaltered[21]. It should be recognized, however, that this latter study was performed in patients with impaired oral glucose tolerance. Since insulin resistance has been documented in patients with normal tolerance to oral glucose[18,26], a decreased hepatic utilization of glucose can hardly explain the early presence of insulin resistance.

IS THERE A LIVER 'FACTOR' PROMOTING GLUCOSE METABOLISM OF PERIPHERAL TISSUES?

In 1954 Lang *et al.* studied glucose utilization of the hind limb in intact and in eviscerated dogs. They observed a decrease of glucose uptake (in the presence as well as in the absence of insulin) in eviscerated animals that could be restored by cross-circulation with an intact dog[35]. In addition, insulin resistance was demonstrated in acutely liver-damaged rabbits[36]. The existence of such a humoral liver factor capable of promoting glucose utilization of skeletal muscle has not been proved so far. Obviously, lack of such a factor due to diminished biosynthesis and/or secretion from the damaged liver and ensuing insulin resistance of peripheral tissues could contribute to the pathogenesis of hepatogenous diabetes. Interestingly, the liver has been shown to produce and secrete peptide hormones into the systemic circulation, which are known to affect carbohydrate metabolism. Particularly the insulin-like growth factors (IGF-I and IGF-II) are predominantly synthesized in adult liver[37,38]. Their serum concentrations are known to be decreased substantially in advanced liver disease[39,40] (Fig. 6). It should be noted, however, that IGF-I and IGF-II are bound to specific plasma binding proteins (predominantly synthesized in the liver too) that are equally diminished in liver disease[41], (Fig. 7) thus probably resulting in little change of free IGF plasma concentrations. Only this free form of IGF is believed to affect glucose metabolism[42]. However, as to the acute actions of IGFs in normal rats, we were recently able to demonstrate that IGF-I and IGF-II stimulated skeletal muscle glucose metabolism under euglycaemic clamp conditions with rather low potency, these effects probably being mediated through cross-activation of insulin receptors[43,44]. Since even a rather high insulin infusion rate could not restore the decreased hind limb glucose uptake in eviscerated dogs, mechanisms not involving skeletal muscle

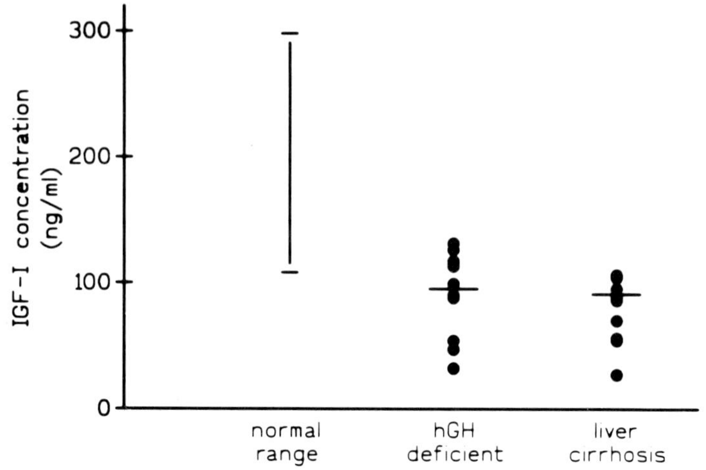

Fig. 6 Plasma insulin-like growth factor-I (IGF-I) concentrations in patients with cirrhosis of the liver and in patients with growth hormone (hGH) deficiency. Total plasma IGF-I was measured by radioimmunoassay after extraction by acid/ethanol precipitation

insulin receptors might be operative, thus arguing against a role of IGF-I. Clearly, the role of IGFs in extrahepatic manifestations of liver disease and in the pathogenesis of hepatogenous diabetes deserves closer attention.

RENAL INSENSITIVITY TO INSULIN-LIKE GROWTH FACTOR-I (IGF-I) IN CIRRHOSIS

IGF-I has been shown to contribute to the regulation of renal haemodynamics, e.g. it increases glomerular filtration rate and renal plasma flow in humans and laboratory animals[45,46]. Renal receptors for IGF-I have been demonstrated on cultured glomerular cells, proximal tubular epithelial cells, renal vascular endothelial and smooth muscle cells respectively[47]. In cirrhosis of the liver, renal disorders can represent a major clinical problem[48]. The pathogenesis of impaired renal function in advanced liver disease appears to involve hormonal and nerval responses to altered systemic and splanchnic haemodynamics, i.e. intense renal vasoconstriction secondary to peripheral and splanchnic vasodilation[49]. Using the rat model of CCl_4-induced cirrhosis of rats we have recently shown that the acute response of renal haemodynamics to IGF-I is blunted, suggesting renal resistance (Fig. 8). When renal IGF-I receptors were studied by quantitative autoradiography of kidneys from cirrhotic rats a 50% reduction of inner and outer cortical IGF-I receptors

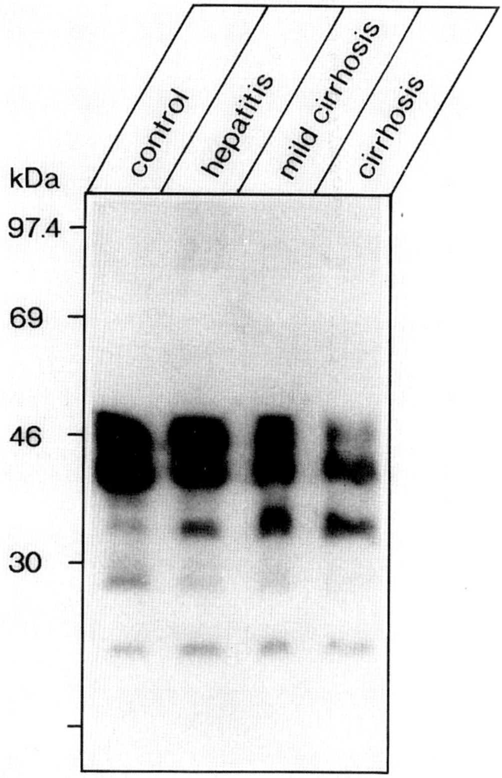

Fig. 7 Serum insulin-like growth factor binding proteins (IGFBP) in patients with liver disease. IGFBP were measured by Western ligand blotting using labelled IGF-I

was observed (unpublished data). Therefore, decreased plasma concentrations of IGF-I (due to reduced hepatic synthesis in cirrhosis), as well as resistance to IGF-I, might contribute to the pathogenesis of functional renal failure in advanced liver disease. Furthermore, it appears of interest to study the role of IGFs in the pathogenesis of skeletal muscle dystrophy, yet another extrahepatic manifestation of liver disease for which a clear pathophysiological concept is not available.

ACKNOWLEDGEMENT

We are grateful to Professor W. Creutzfeldt for reviewing this manuscript. The studies from our laboratory would not have been possible without his constant support and advice.

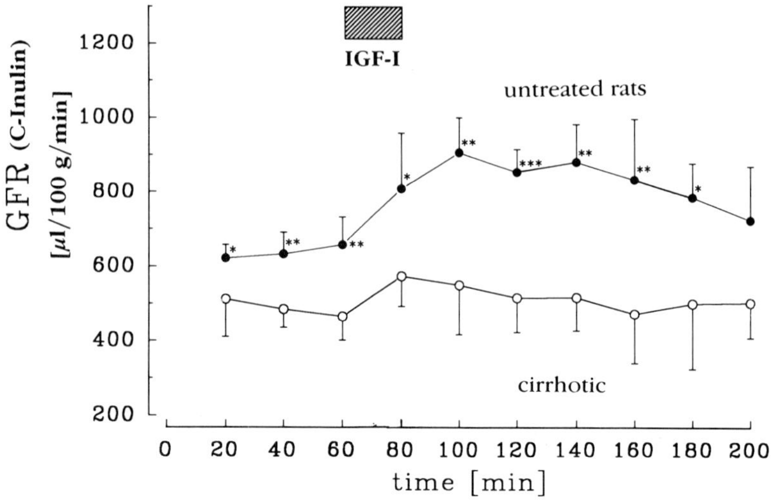

Fig. 8 Glomerular filtration rate (GFR) before, during and after infusion of IGF-I during euglycaemic clamping in cirrhotic rats. Anaesthetized animals received intravenous infusions of IGF-I from 60 to 80 min (hatched bar) at a dose of 3.2 pmol/100 g per minute. GFR was calculated from inulin clearance. Control animals received vehicle only. Data are means ± SD from seven experiments. *denotes $p < 0.05$, **$p < 0.01$, ***$p < 0.001$ by Student's *t*-test

References

1. Naunyn B. Der Diabetes mellitus. In: Nothagels Handbuch-Spez Path Ther Band VII, 1. Auflage, Wien; 1898.
2. Yalow RS, Berson SA. Immunoassay of endogenous plasma insulin in man. J Clin Invest. 1960;39:1157–75.
3. Iwasaki Y, Ohkubo A, Kajinuma H, Akanuma Y, Kosaka K. Degradation and secretion of insulin in hepatic cirrhosis. J Clin Endocrinol Metab. 1978;47:774–9.
4. Megyesi C, Samols E, Marks V. Glucose tolerance and diabetes in chronic liver disease. Lancet. 1967;2:1051–5.
5. Creutzfeldt W, editor. Beziehungen zwischen Leber und Zuckerkrankheit. 4. Congrès de la fédération internationale du diabète; 1961; Geneve. Fédération internationale du diabète; 1961.
6. West TET, Owens D, Sönksen PH. Metabolic responses to monocomponent human insulin infusions in normal subjects and patients with liver and endocrine disease. Clin Endocrinol. 1975;4:573–84.
7. Creutzfeldt W, Frerichs H, Kraft W. The intravenous tolbutamide test in liver disease. Acta Diab Latina. 1967;4:205.
8. Creutzfeldt W, Frerichs H, Sickinger K. Liver diseases and diabetes mellitus. In: Popper H, Schaffner F, editors. Progress in liver disease. New York: Grune & Stratton; 1970:371–407.
9. Creutzfeldt W, Hartmann H, Nauck M, Stöckmann F. Liver disease and glucose homeostasis. In: Bianchi L, Gerok W, Landmann L, Sickinger K, Stalder GA, editors. Liver in metabolic diseases. Lancaster: MTP Press; 1983:221–34.
10. Iversen J, Vilstrup H, Tygstrup N. Kinetics of glucose metabolism in relation to insulin concentration in patients with alcoholic cirrhosis and in healthy persons. Gastroenterology. 1984;87:1138–43.
11. Vannini P, Forlani G, Marchesini G, Ciavarella A, Zoli M, Pisi E. The euglycemic clamp technique in patients with liver cirrhosis. Horm Metab Res. 1984;16:341–3.
12. Taylor R, Heine RJ, Collins J, James OFW, Alberti KGMM. Insulin action in cirrhosis.

Hepatology. 15;5:64–71.
13. Cavallo-Perin P, Cassader M, Bozzo C, Bruno P, Nuccio M, Dall'Omo M, Marucci M, Pagno G. Mechanism of insulin resistance in liver cirrhosis. Evidence for a combined receptor and postreceptor defect. J Clin Invest. 1985;75:1659–65.
14. Marchesini G, Bianchi GP, Forlani G, Rusticali AG, Patrono D, Capelli M, Zoli M, Vannini P, Pisi E. Insulin resistance is the main determinant of impaired glucose tolerance in patients with liver cirrhosis. Dig Dis Sci. 1987;32:1118–24.
15. Kruszynska YT, Williams N, Perry M, Home PD. The relationship between insulin sensitivity and skeletal muscle enzyme activities in hepatic cirrhosis. Hepatology. 1988;8:1615–19.
16. Vetter D, Fratte S, Winiszewski P, Reville M, Hirsch E, Roze F, Blickle JF, Pinget M, Doffoel M, Bockel R. Conséquences de l'hyperglycémie sur le métabolisme glucidique et azote dans la cirrhose. Gastroenterol Clin Biol. 1990;14:483–91.
17. Müller MJ, Fenk A, Lautz HU, Selberg O, Canzler H, Balks HA, von zur Mühlen A, Schmidt E, Schmidt FW. Energy expenditure and substrate metabolism in ethanol-induced liver cirrhosis. Am J Physiol. 1991;260:E338–44.
18. Petrides AS, Groop LC, Riely CA, DeFronzo R. Effect of physiologic hyperinsulinemia on glucose and lipid metabolism in cirrhosis. J Clin Invest. 1991;88:651–70.
19. Müller MJ, Willmann O, Rieger A, Fenk A, Selberg O, Lautz HU, Bürger M, Balks HJ, von zur Mühlen A, Schmidt FW. Mechanism of insulin resistance associated with liver cirrhosis. Gastroenterology. 1992;102:2033–41.
20. Meyer-Alber A, Hartmann H, Stümpel F, Creutzfeldt W. Mechanism of insulin resistance in CCl_4-induced cirrhosis of rats. Gastroenterology. 1992;102:223–9.
21. Kruszynska YT, Meyer-Alber A, Darakhshan F, Home PD, McIntyre N. Metabolic handling of orally administered glucose in cirrhosis. J Clin Invest. 1993;91:1057–66.
22. Petrides AS, DeFronzo R. Glucose and insulin metabolism in cirrhosis. J Hepatol. 1989;8:107–14.
23. Harewood MS, Proietto J, Dudley F, Alford FP. Insulin action and cirrhosis: insulin binding and lipogenesis in isolated adipocytes. Metabolism. 1982;31:1241–6.
24. D'Arville CN, Le M, Kloppel TM, Simon FR. Alterations in the functional expression of receptors on cirrhotic rat hepatocytes. Hepatology. 1989;9:6–11.
25. Riggio O, Cangiano C, Capocaccia R, Cascino A, Lala A, Leonetti F, Mauceri M, Pepe M, Rossi Fanelli F, Savioli M, Tamburrano G, Capocaccia L. Glucose intolerance in liver cirrhosis. Metabolism. 1982;31:627–34.
26. Ballmann M, Hartmann H, Deacon CF, Schmidt WE, Conlon JM, Creutzfeldt W. Hypersecretion of proinsulin does not explain the hyperinsulinemia of patients with liver cirrhosis. Clin Endocrinol. 1986;25:351–61.
27. Marchesini G, Pacini G, Bianchi G, Patrono D, Cobelli C. Glucose disposal, β-cell secretion, and hepatic insulin extraction in cirrhosis: a minimal model assessment. Gastroenterology. 1990;99:1715–22.
28. Kruszynska YT, Home PD, McIntyre N. Relationship between insulin sensitivity, insulin secretion, and glucose tolerance in cirrhosis. Hepatology. 1991;14:103–11.
29. Field JB, Rodjimark S, Harding P, Ishida T, Chou MCY. Role of liver in insulin physiology. Diabetes Care. 1980;3:255–60.
30. Petrides AS, DeFronzo R. Glucose metabolism in cirrhosis: A review with some perspectives for the future. Diab Metab Rev. 1989;5:691–709.
31. Marchesini G, Melli A, Checchia GA, Mattioli L, Capelli M, Cassarani S, Pisi E. Pancreatic β-cell function in cirrhotic patients with and without overt diabetes. C-peptide response to glukagon and to a meal. Metabolism. 1985;34:695–701.
32. Kruszynska YT, Harry DS, Bergmann R, McIntyre N. Insulin sensitivity, insulin secretion and glucose effectiveness in diabetic and non-diabetic cirrhotic patients. Diabetologia. 1993;36:121–8.
33. Nakamura T, Otsuki M, Tani S, Okabayashi Y, Fujii M, Oka T, Fujisawa T, Baba S. Pancreatic endocrine function in cirrhotic rats. Metabolism. 1988;37:892–9.
34. Ferranini E, Bjorkmann O, Reichard GA, Pilo A, Olson M, Wahren J, DeFronzo RA. The disposal of an oral glucose load in healthy subjects. Diabetes. 1985;34:580–8.
35. Lang ST, Goldstein MS, Levine R. Influence of the liver on uptake of glucose by extrahepatic tissues. Am J Physiol. 1954;177:447–54.

36. Creutzfeldt W. Klinische Beziehungen zwischen Diabetes mellitus und Leber. Acta Hepatosplen. 1959;5:156–77.
37. Schimpff RM, Donnadieu M, Gasinovic JC, Warnet JM, Girad F. The liver as source of somatomedin (an *in vivo* study in dogs). Acta Endocrinol. 1976;83:365–72.
38. Schwander JC, Hauri C, Zapf J, Froesch ER. Synthesis and secretion of insulin-like growth factor and its binding protein by the perfused rat liver: dependence on growth hormone status. Endocrinology. 1983;113:297–304.
39. Wu A, Grant DB, Hambley J, Levi AJ. Reduced serum somatomedin activity in patients with chronic liver disease. Clin Sci. 1974;47:359–66.
40. Caufriez A, Reding P, Urbain D, Golstein, J. Copinschi G. Insulin-like growth factor I: a good indicator of functional hepatocellular capacity in alcoholic liver cirrhosis. J Endocrinol Invest. 1991;14:317–21.
41. Zapf J, Morell B, Walter H, Laron Z, Froesch ER. Serum levels of insulin-like growth factor (IGF) and its carrier protein in various metabolic disorders. Acta Endocrinol. 1980;95:505–17.
42. Zapf J, Hauri C, Waldvogel M, Froesch ER. Acute metabolic effects and half-lives of intravenously administered insulin-like growth factors I and II in normal and hypophysectomized rats. J Clin Invest. 1986;77:1768–75.
43. Schmitz F, Hartmann H, Stümpel F, Creutzfeldt W. In vivo metabolic action of insulin-like growth factor I in adult rats. Diabetologia. 1991;34:144–9.
44. Stümpel F, Hartmann H. Acute actions of insulin-like growth factor II on glucose metabolism in adult rats. Diabetologia. 1992;35:932–8.
45. Hirschberg R, Guler HP, Kopple JD. The effects of insulin-like growth factor I on renal hemodynamics. In: Spencer EM, editor. Modern concepts of insulin-like growth factors. New York: Elsevier; 1991:199–217.
46. Baumann U, Eisenhauer T, Hartmann H. Increase of glomerular filtration rate and renal plasma flow by insulin-like growth factor-I during euglycaemic clamping in anaesthetized rats. Eur J Clin Invest. 1992;22:204–9.
47. Hammermann MR. The growth hormone-insulin-like growth factor axis in the kidney. Am J Physiol. 1989;257:F503–14.
48. Ebstein M. The kidney in liver disease, 3rd edn. Baltimore: Williams & Wilkins; 1988.
49. Schrier RW, Arroyo V, Bernardi M, Epstein M, Henriksen JH, Rodes J. Peripheral arterial vasodilation hypothesis: a proposal for the initiation of renal sodium and water retention in cirrhosis. Hepatology. 1988;8:1151–7.

20

Hypothalamic–pituitary–gonadal function in liver disease

D. H. VAN THIEL and J. S. GAVALER

The liver, because of its central role in the biotransformation of endogenous as well as exogenous xenobiotics, has the potential to modify the functional status of many organ systems. One of these organ systems that is particularly susceptible to modulation by the functional state of the liver is the hypothalamic–pituitary–gonadal axis.

The hypothalamic–pituitary–gonadal axis consists of three organs; the function of each is interrelated and modulated by the performance of the other two components of the system. Within the hypothalamus, neurons within the medial lateral hypothalamus synthesize and secrete gonadotrophin-releasing hormone (GnRH) in a pulsatile manner determined by the net influence of cortical, other thalamic and hypothalamic influences and the levels of sex steroids present within the blood. GnRH exits the hypothalamus via the hypothalamic–pituitary portal circulation to reach the anterior pituitary, where it stimulates gonadotrophs to produce and secrete both follicle-stimulating hormone (FSH) and luteinizing hormone (LH) in a regular pulsatile manner that is dependent upon the net influence of GnRH, the sex hormone levels in blood and other factors that are capable of modulating gonadotrophin secretion. FSH and LH enter the systemic circulation and serve as trophic factors at the level of the gonads, the testes in the male and the ovary in the female.

The gonads are actually two organs in one. These two organs consist of a reproductive compartment (the seminiferous tubules in the testes and the follicles in the ovary) and an endocrine compartment (the Leydig cells in the testes and the granulosa as well as stroma cells of the ovary). In general, FSH is trophic for the reproductive compartment while LH is trophic for the endocrine compartment of the gonad.

The gonadal structure and function of the two sexes are quite different (Fig. 1). Males produce millions of new germ cells daily within the seminiferous tubules and essentially have lifelong Leydig cell function. In contrast, the reproductive compartment of the ovary is fixed prior to birth and steadily declines during the reproductive life of the individual until the time of menopause, at an age about 52 on average, when reproductive function ceases. The endocrine compartment of the ovary consists of the granulosa cells that exist about the ova, and form the follicles and produce oestrogens, and the stroma of the ovary that produces androgens. With the steady loss of reproductive potential during life, the number and function of the ova and the granulosa cells of the ovary decline steadily. In contrast, the ovarian stroma, although always important in determining the overall status of ovarian function, become increasingly important as the precursor source of endogenous oestrogens during the postmenopausal years.

The structural complexity of the ovary is reflected also in the functional complexity of ovarian function which varies cyclically as a result of the menstrual cycle in the non-pregnant state and declines in importance during pregnancy where the placenta becomes responsible for the bulk of sex steroid produced during pregnancy or after the menopause, when the cyclic pattern of sex steroid secretion ceases and is replaced by stable but diminished levels of oestrogen and sustained high levels of the two gonadotrophins.

Because of the complexity of hypothalamic–pituitary–gonadal function in females, most of the data available relating to the effects of liver disease upon this important neuroendocrine axis have been developed in males, where the consistency of function under normal circumstances can be disrupted and easily measured, particularly in men with hepatic disease. In contrast, only recently have any real data relating to the functional status of the hypothalamic–pituitary–gonadal axis of women with hepatic disease been reported in any meaningful way.

In general terms, gonadal failure, the end-result of disease or dysfunction of the hypothalamic–pituitary–gonadal axis, can be segrated into two main categories of disease: hypogonadotrophic and hypergonadotrophic forms of gonadal failure. The former, as the name implies, exists when gonadal failure exists in the presence of low or absent gonadotrophin levels and is either a consequence of pituitary (secondary) or hypothalamic (tertiary) dysfunction or organ failure. The latter, hypergonadotrophic form of hypogonadism, implies primary hypogonadism or gonadal failure with a failure of hypothalamic–pituitary compensation to correct or prevent the gonadal failure. The simplest form of primary gonadal failure to conceptualize is castration, where the organ of interest has been surgically excised. Other forms of primary gonadal failure exist, however, that can affect either one or both functional compartments of the testes. These include conditions such as mumps orchitis, varicocele, heat injury and other conditions.

The two principal disease processes that affect the liver and also affect the functioning of the hypothalamic–pituitary–gonadal axis are alcoholic liver disease and haemochromatosis. The first of these two is the more common, and represents a direct toxic injury to the testes and, to a lesser degree, to the hypothalamus and pituitary that results in a form of hypergonadotrophic

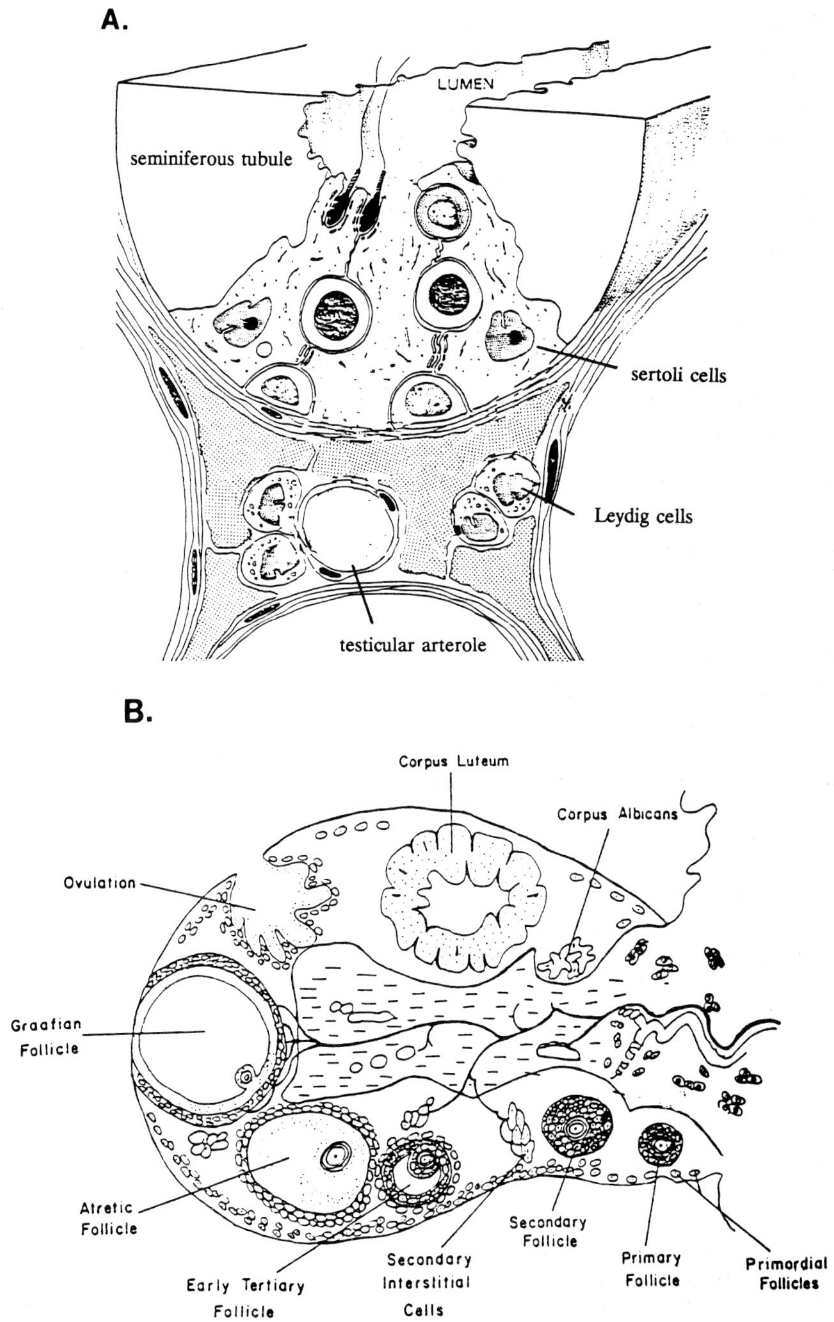

Fig. 1 Schematic representation of the anatomical structure of the testes (**A**) and the ovary (**B**). The testes has a continually renewing reproductive comportment while the ovary has a continuously declining reproductive comportment

hypogonadism or primary gonadal failure. The second of these two conditions, haemochromatosis, is also common, occurring at a rate of 3–8/1000 individuals, but is nonetheless less common than in alcoholism, which affects about 10% of the adult population. Haemochromatosis is due to excessive iron absorption and its subsequent deposition in tissues such as the liver, heart, hypothalamus and pituitary to name but a few of the overt sites of disease that occur as a consequence of the excess iron deposition in the tissues that causes clinical disease. In general, haemochromatosis produces a type of hypogonadotrophic hypogonadism as a result of hypothalamic or pituitary deposition of iron and a primary loss of gonadotrophic secretion[1]. As might be anticipated, as a result of these two different mechanisms responsible for the gonadal failure, the consequences of the gonadal failure in these two conditions also vary considerably.

The first definitive data relating to the mechanism responsible for the gonadal failure seen in chronic alcoholic men were reported in 1974[2]. In this study, testosterone levels in blood were shown to be low in chronic alcoholic men as expected, but the oestradiol levels were found to be normal, and not increased as had been expected, because of the many biochemical and clinical manifestations of 'hyperoestrogenization' or 'feminization' known to exist in chronic alcoholic men (Table 1)[3–7]. Moreover, the marked increase in sex steroid binding globulin reported in alcoholic men served only to simplify the hypogonadism by reducing further the plasma free testosterone level[2,3]. The first real insight into the mechanisms involved, however, was the observation that although increased in alcoholic men with liver disease, the plasma levels of the two gonadotrophins were lower than might otherwise reasonably be expected[2]. This finding suggested that a hypothalamic–pituitary defect might also exist in chronic alcoholic men, as well as a primary gonadal failure. This hypothesis has been borne out by the demonstration of inadequate gonadotrophin responses to clomiphene in these same alcoholic men[2].

The next steps in unravelling the mechanisms responsible for the hypogonadism seen in individuals with alcohol-associated liver disease were accomplished using a rat model of alcohol abuse[8,9]. In this model, either pre-pubertal or adult male rats fed alcohol could be shown to develop markedly reduced testosterone levels and overt testicular atrophy despite the fact that the experimental alcohol-induced liver disease failed to progress

Table 1 Manifestations of feminization in alcoholic cirrhotic men

Biochemical	*Clinical*
Increased levels of sex steroid binding globulin	Spider angiomata
Increased levels of prolactin	Palmar erythema
Increased levels of oestrone in blood and urine	Female escutcheon
Increased oestrogen receptor number	Female habitus
Increased levels of oestrogen responsive neurophysin	Gynaecomastia; loss of facial and body hair

beyond the stage of a fatty liver[8,9]. Coincident with this gonadal failure in the rat was the finding of reduced gonadotrophin levels not seen in alcohol-abusing men.

Because of this difference between what was seen in humans and the rat, the next step in unravelling the mechanism of gonadal failure induced by alcohol abuse was to examine the effect of alcohol upon Leydig cell function *in vitro*, first as isolated perfused testes and later as isolated Leydig cells in tissue culture[10–13]. In both systems, ethanol and, to an even greater degree, acetaldehyde were shown to be Leydig cell toxins that inhibited testosterone biosynthesis and secretion.

Subsequent studies in the rat demonstrated that the testes contain an alcohol dehydrogenase distinct from the alcohol dehydrogenase in the liver, and that this testicular alcohol dehydrogenase is responsible for the conversion of retinol to retinal within the testes. Retinal is essential for normal spermatogenesis[14,15]. The function of this enzyme can be inhibited competitively by ethanol, which is preferentially metabolized to acetaldehyde, a potent Leydig cell toxin[14,15]. Moreover, it has been shown that acetaldehyde production within the testes leads to testicular peroxidation injury manifested by the production of malonaldehyde and other markers of lipid peroxidation[16,17]. Interestingly, the lipid peroxidation observed in the testes is associated with, and followed sequentially by, a reduction or consumption of testicular glutathione levels[16,17]. Moreover, a direct linear relationship between the loss of testes mass and the glutathione content of the testes could be demonstrated, documenting that the germ cell injury and loss induced by ethanol abuse is, in large measure, due to a peroxidation injury.

The next step in the puzzle was resolved by returning to humans. Young adult males who ingested alcohol under metabolic ward conditions, and were receiving an adequate calorie intake rich in minerals and vitamins, could be shown to experience a reduction in serum testosterone levels followed by a compensatory increase in gonadotrophin levels. After about 2 weeks of steady alcohol ingestion the male volunteers developed a combined hypothalamic–pituitary as well as gonadal failure, manifested by low testosterone levels but without a compensatory increase in plasma gonadotrophin levels[18]. The gonadal injury induced in these normal men as a result of experimental alcohol ingestion was completely reversible. In contrast, the gonadal injury in chronic alcoholic men with variable degrees of histological liver disease often does not recover, even with long-term continued alcohol abstinence[19]. Moreover, attempts to drive recovery of gonadal function with the use of exogenous factors such as clomiphene, human chorionic gonadotrophin and even exogenous androgens have failed to correct the defect in gonadal function[19]. The latter finding was particularly interesting in that several times the usual replacement dose of an exogenous androgen failed to correct the signs and symptoms of androgen deficiency in these formerly chronic alcohol-abusing males. This suggested that these men might have reduced numbers of androgen receptors in their tissues, a finding that was subsequently confirmed in experimental animals[20]. Not only was a deficit in androgen receptors identified, but also an increase in oestrogen receptor number was noted in the tissues of chronic alcohol-abusing rats. This finding, coupled with the observations that ethanol ingestion induces aromatase activity, thereby enhancing the conversion of proandrogens to oestrogens, explains the apparent paradox of gonadal failure, low testosterone levels but normal oestradiol levels in chronic alcoholic men, particularly those with cirrhosis[6,7]. The presence of portal hypertension and portal systemic shunting in cirrhotics amplifies these effects by enhancing the delivery of proandrogens to sex steroid-responsive tissues such as peripheral fat stores, the skin and breast as a result of the disruption of the normal enterohepatic circulation[21].

The situation in men with haemochromatosis is characterized by hypogonadism but not a coexistent feminization. This is because in haemochromatosis there is no increase of aromatase activity, no disruption of the enterohepatic circulation of proandrogens and no up-regulation of oestrogen receptors as occurs in chronic alcoholic men with cirrhosis. Thus men with haemochromatosis do not often have gynaecomastia, a female habitus, a female escutcheon, spider angiomata or palmar erythema unless alcohol abuse coexists with their haemochromatosis[1]. Unfortunately, it appears anecdotally as if an increased rate of alcohol abuse may in fact exist in at least some men with haemochromatosis.

As noted earlier, the situation with women as to the relationships of liver disease and alcohol abuse with gonadal function has been much less investigated because of the complexity of the menstrual cycle. In contrast, postmenopausal women comprise an ideal study population. In one of the better studies examining this issue, the oestradiol levels in postmenopausal women with alcoholic liver disease or primary biliary cirrhosis were compared to those in normal postmenopausal women[22]. As the liver disease progressed from Child's Class A to Child's Class C, oestradiol levels in the alcoholic postmenopausal women increased. In contrast, as the liver disease progressed from Child's Class A to Child's Class B in PBC, the oestradiol levels fell. Nonetheless, in both groups of cirrhotic women the oestradiol levels were at least twice those in normal postmenopausal women. In contrast, when the serum testosterone levels of these three groups of women were compared in both cirrhotic groups, the serum testosterone level was nearly half that seen in normal postmenopausal women. As a result of the increased oestradiol levels, and the reduced testosterone levels, the calculated E/T ratio in the cirrhotic women, being an indirect measure of aromatase activity and peripheral aromatization of androgens to oestrogens, was increased significantly. Moreover, as was evident with the oestradiol levels, as the liver disease progressed (as manifested by the Child's score), the E/T ratio increased in the alcoholic women and declined in the women with PBC. Nonetheless, even in the group with the lowered E/T ratio, the cirrhotic women had E/T ratios at least twice those found in normal postmenopausal women.

The reduction in testosterone levels noted in the cirrhotic postmenopausal women as compared to the normal postmenopausal women was reflected probably, in large measure, as a consequence of the reduced serum LH concentration present in the cirrhotic women, with the reduction in LH levels increasing progressively with disease severity in both groups, but being more severe in the alcoholic women as compared to those with PBC. Similarly, the FSH levels of the cirrhotic postmenopausal women declined with increasing liver disease severity, and were considerably more reduced in those with alcoholic liver disease as compared to those with PBC.

Taken together, these data in postmenopausal women document that liver disease is associated with altered hormonal status in postmenopausal women, and that the pattern of hormonal changes observed differs between types of liver disease, as evidenced by the differences between postmenopausal women with alcoholic liver disease (predominantly hepatocellular disease) and those with PBC (predominantly cholestatic disease).

The best evidence that documents that the neuroendrocrine consequences of advanced hepatic disease differ in men and women is shown by an examination of the prolactin levels in men and women with advanced alcoholic liver disease[23–25]. The initial attention paid to prolactin in patients with advanced liver disease was a direct product of the false neurotransmitter hypothesis of hepatic encephalopathy, wherein a depletion of true neurotransmitters (norepinephrine and dopamine) was thought to occur and lead to a reduction in dopaminergic neurotransmission, while false neurotransmitters such as octopamine accumulate and produce abnormal rates and pathways of neurotransmission.

Dopamine is a powerful prolactin secretion inhibitor. Thus a reduction in dopaminergic transmission should result in an increase in the prolactin secretion, and the resultant prolactin measurements could be used as an indirect, albeit easily quantifiable, measure of assessing the degree of hepatic encephalopathy in a given individual. This has been shown to be the case in alcoholic men with cirrhosis having variable degrees of hepatic encephalopathy.

To determine if these findings could be replicated in alcoholic women, 36 postmenopausal women with alcohol-induced cirrhosis were studied[26]. These women could be divided into two groups based upon the presence ($n = 17$) or absence ($n = 19$) of any evidence for hepatic encephalopathy. The two groups were matched for age, body weight, body mass index and ovariectomy rates, as well as their age at menopause. As expected, the women with hepatic encephalopathy had more abnormal liver injury and function measures which were significant for the serum bilirubin level and the prothrombin time (both $p < 0.05$) (Table 2). Moreover, as might be expected, those with hepatic encephalopathy had a greater degree of hepatic decompensation as evidenced by the presence of ascites, oesophageal varices, a prior history of bleeding and spontaneous bacterial peritonitis, as well as higher Child's Class than did those without evidence of hepatic encephalopathy (Table 2).

Unexpectedly, the alcoholic postmenopausal women with hepatic encephalopathy did *not* have increased prolactin levels as compared to those without evidence of hepatic encephalopathy[26]. As noted, this finding differed markedly from the earlier reported findings in male alcoholics with cirrhosis of increased prolactin levels (Table 3). Moreover, the presence of an elevated prolactin level in alcoholic cirrhotic men was found to be associated with an increased risk of death during the same hospitalization[23–25]. This relationship could not be confirmed in alcoholic postmenopausal women[26] despite the fact that these studies were quite similar in size and characteristics of the patients being studied (Table 4).

Table 2 Liver disease status of 36 alcoholic menopausal women with alcohol-induced cirrhosis

	Encephalopathy	
	Present ($n = 17$)	*Absent* ($n = 19$)
Albumin (g/dl)	2.9 ± 0.2	3.1 ± 0.2
Total bilirubin (mg/dl)	7.9 ± 2.1*	3.3 ± 0.8
Prothrombin time (s)	15.9 ± 0.7*	14.2 ± 0.5
GGTP (mIU/ml)	115 ± 35	112 ± 25
ALT (mIU/ml)	55.1 ± 23.4	47.3 ± 18.2
AST (mIU/ml)	81.5 ± 27.4	76.8 ± 22.7
AST/ALT ratio	2.5 ± 0.3	3.5 ± 0.8
Ascites	100%*	36.8%
Varices	100%*	44.4%
H_x: variceal bleed	52.9%	26.3%
H_x: SBP	29.4%	5.2%
Child's Class		
A	0%*	47.4%
B	64.7%*	47.4%
C	35.3%*	5.2%

* $p < 0.05$

Table 3 Hormone* levels in 36 alcoholic menopausal women with alcohol-induced cirrhosis

	Encephalopathy		
	Present ($n = 17$)		*Absent* ($n = 19$)
Prolactin (ng/ml)	13.1 ± 2.3	nsd	14.3 ± 3.9
LH (mIU/ml)	1.3 ± 0.4	$p = 0.000$	8.9 ± 2.3
FSH (mIU/ml)	5.0 ± 1.8	$p = 0.005$	9.4 ± 2.2
Oestradiol (pg/ml)	80.0 ± 24.6	nsd	43.9 ± 7.7
Testosterone (ng/ml)	0.40 ± 0.06	nsd	0.53 ± 0.07
E_2:T ratio	245 ± 86	nsd	102 ± 18

* Logarithms used for statistical analysis
nsd = no significant difference

These findings of a difference in serum prolactin level patterns between alcoholic cirrhotic men and alcoholic postmenopausal women serve both to highlight the differences in neuroendocrine function in men and women with liver disease, and also add yet another obstacle to the universal acceptance of the false neurotransmitter hypothesis of hepatic encephalopathy.

ACKNOWLEDGEMENT

This work was supported by Grants NIAAA AA04425 and NIAAA AA06772.

Table 4 Prolactin* levels and portal systemic encephalopathy (PSE)

Reference	*PSE Absent*	*PSE Present*
McClain *et al.* (1981)[23]		
Prolactin (ng/ml)	18.7 ± 1.6	39.2 ± 4.6†
Number of men	21	21
Mortality	10%	62%
DeBesi *et al.* (1989)[24]		
Prolactin (ng/ml)	10.1 ± 2.6	22.9 ± 4.6†
Number of men	14	11
Mortality	n.a.	n.a.
Sharma *et al.* (1989)[25]		
Prolactin	2.16 ± 6.5	73.3 ± 28.8†
Number of men	24	20
Mortality	50%	90%†
Gavaler and Van Thiel (1992)[26]: study in postmenopausal women		
Prolactin	14.3 ± 3.9	13.1 ± 2.3
Number of women	19	17
Mortality		
Natural history group	4/14 = 29%	6/7 = 86%†
Transplanted group	2/3 = 67%	3/9 = 33%
Lost to follow-up	?/2	?/1

* Mean ± SEM
† Significantly different

References

1. McLaren GD, Muir WA, Kellermeyer RW. Iron overload disorders: natural history, pathogenesis, diagnosis and therapy. CRC Crit Rev Clin Lab Sci. 1984;19:205–40.
2. Van Thiel DH, Lester R, Sherins RJ. Hypogonadism in alcoholic liver disease: Evidence for a double defect. Gastroenterology. 1974;67:1188–99.
3. Van Thiel DH, Gavaler JS, Lester R, Loriaux DL, Braunstein GD. Plasma estrone, prolactin, neurophysin and sex steroid-bining globulin in chronic alcoholic men. Metabolism. 1975;24:1015–19.
4. Van Thiel DH, Lester R. Alcoholism: its effect on hypothalamic–pituitary–gonadal function. Gastroenterology. 1976;71:318–27.
5. Lester R, Van Thiel DH. The causes of feminization in chronically alcoholic men. In: Preisig R, Bircher J, Baumgartner G, editors. The liver: quantitative aspects of structure and function. Aulendorf: Editio. Cantor; 1976:205–11.
6. Van Thiel DH, Lester R. Sex and alcohol: a second peek (editorial). N Engl J Med. 1976;295:835–6.
7. Van Thiel DH. Feminization of chronic alcoholic men: a formulation. Yale J Biol Med. 1979;52:219–25.
8. Van Thiel DH, Gavaler JS, Lester R, Goodman MD. Alcohol-induced testicular atrophy: An experimental model for hypogonadism occurring in chronic alcoholic men. Gastroenterology. 1975;69:326–32.
9. Van Thiel DH, Gavaler JS, Cobb CF, Sherins RJ, Lester R. Alcohol-induced testicular atrophy in the adult male rat. Endocrinology. 1979;105:888–95.
10. Cobb CF, Ennis MF, Van Thiel DH, Gavaler JS, Lester R. Isolated testes perfusion: A method using a cell- and protein-free perfusate useful for the evaluation of potential drug and/or metabolic injury. Metabolism. 1980;29:71–9.

11. Van Thiel DH, Cobb CF, Herman GB, Perez HA, Estes L, Gavaler JS. An examination of various mechanisms for ethanol-induced testicular injury: studies utilizing the isolated perfused rat testes. Endocrinology. 1981;109:2009–15.
12. Chiao Y-B, Van Thiel DH. Biochemical mechanisms that contribute to alcohol-induced hypogonadism in the male. Alcoholism: Clin Exp Res. 1983;7:131–4.
13. Santucci L, Graham TJ, Van Thiel DH. Inhibition of testosterone production by rat Leydig cells with ethanol and acetaldehyde: prevention of ethanol toxicity with 4-methylpyrazole. Alcoholism: Clin Exp Res. 1983;7:135–9.
14. Van Thiel DH, Gavaler JS, Lester R. Ethanol inhibition of vitamin A metabolism in the testes: possible mechanism for sterility in alcoholics. Science. 1974;186:941–2.
15. Chiao YB, Van Thiel DH. Characterization of rat testicular alcohol dehydrogenase. Alcohol & Alcoholism. 1986;21:9–15.
16. Rosenblum ER, Gavaler JS, Van Thiel DH. Vitamin A at pharmacologic doses ameliorates the membrane lipid peroxidation injury and testicular atrophy that occurs with chronic alcohol feeding in rats. Alcohol & Alcoholism. 1987;3:241–9.
17. Rosenblum E, Gavaler JS, Van Thiel DH. Lipid peroxidation: a mechanism for ethanol associated testicular injury in rats. Endocrinology. 1985;116:311–18.
18. Van Thiel DH. Ethanol: its adverse effects upon the hypothalamic–pituitary–gonadal axis. J Lab Clin Med. 1983;101:21–33.
19. Gavaler JS, Van Thiel DH. Gonadal dysfunction and inadequate sexual performance in alcoholic cirrhotic men. Gastroenterology. 1988;95:1680–2.
20. Kahn D, Zeng Q, Kajani M, Eagon PK, Lai H, Makowka L, Starzl TE, Van Thiel DH. The effect of different types of hepatic injury on the estrogen and androgen receptor activity of liver. J Invest Surg. 1989;2:125–33.
21. Van Thiel DH, Gavaler JS, Slone FL, Cobb CF, Smith WI Jr, Bron KM, Lester R. Is feminization in alcoholic men due in part to portal hypertension? A rat model. Gastroenterology. 1980;78:81–91.
22. Gavaler JS, Van Thiel DH. The hormonal status of postmenopausal women with alcohol-induced cirrhosis: further findings and a review of the literature. Hepatology. 1992;2:312–19.
23. McClain CJ, Kromhout JP, Elson MK, Van Thiel DH. Hyperprolactinemia in portal systemic encephalopathy. Dig Dis Sci. 1981;26:353–7.
24. De Besi L, Zucchetta P, Zotti S, Mastrogiacomo I. Sex hormones and sex hormone binding globulin in males with compensated and decompensated cirrhosis of the liver. Acta Endocrinol. 1989;120:271–6.
25. Sharma MP, Acharya SK, Kamark AR. Significance of prolactin levels in portosystemic encephalopathy. J Assoc Physicians India. 1988;36:207–9.
26. Gavaler JS, Van Thiel DH. Pituitary hormone patterns in 36 alcoholic cirrhotic postmenopausal women with and without encephalopathy. Alcoholism: Clin Exp Res. 1992;16:357.

21
Liver and pregnancy

K. P. MAIER

Severe liver disease is rare in pregnancy, occurring in less than 0.1% of pregnancies[1,2]; therefore, most women are cared for primarily by their obstetricians. Thus, the pregnant woman suffering from a severe liver disorder poses a real challenge to the hepatologist. From a practical point of view it is useful to consider liver disease in pregnancy under three headings:

1. pregnancy in women with underlying liver disease,
2. liver disease not specific to pregnancy, and
3. liver disease unique to pregnancy.

PREGNANCY IN WOMEN WITH UNDERLYING LIVER DISEASE

Women with chronic liver disease, especially with cirrhosis, often exhibit severe gonadal failure; therefore, they rarely become pregnant. Since in most cases a pregnancy seems not to worsen a pre-existing liver disorder, the coincidence of the two is not usually regarded as an indication to terminate the pregnancy[3]. It is, however, very difficult to evaluate the individual risk of hepatic complications, since systematic studies are lacking.

Bleeding from oesophageal varices occurs in 18–32% of pregnant women with cirrhosis and in up to 50% in those with portal hypertension[4]; thus, maternal morbidity and mortality is markedly elevated (about 10%) in this high-risk group[5], as is the rate of fetal loss. The rates of premature birth and perinatal death are also increased; however, liveborn infants will generally be normal[5].

The course of pregnancies in women with autoimmune chronic active hepatitis has been followed[6]. There were no maternal deaths and no significant deterioration of chronic hepatitis during or after pregnancy. However, a high fetal loss and up to 30% prematurity have been reported[7]. Corticosteroid therapy must be continued in this group of women[7], in rare cases in increased doses.

There is only very limited experience with pregnancy in women with chronic hepatitis B and HBV-induced cirrhosis. Progressive liver failure has been the major cause of death.

Reports of pregnancy in primary biliary cirrhosis (PBC) are rare[8]. Moreover, pregnancies occurred mostly before the diagnosis has been established, i.e. in the (undiagnosed) asymptomatic stage of the illness.

Pregnancy has been reported in successfully treated Wilson's disease. D-Penicillamine therapy must be continued at relatively low doses (0.25–0.5 g/day), because withdrawal of the drug results in severe worsening of liver function. At least 65 normal infants have been born to women suffering from Wilson's disease, most of them on D-penicillamine therapy. Triethylene tetramine hydrochloride, an alternative drug for treating patients with Wilson's disease, also appears safe and effective, as has been demonstrated in seven women during 11 pregnancies[9]. It should be kept in mind that maternal caeruloplasmin concentration may increase during pregnancy[10]. This increase, however, does not indicate an improvement of the liver disorder!

Irrespective of the aetiology of the underlying liver disease, it seems advisable to monitor pregnancies in this group of patients very carefully. Management by an obstetrician in close co-operation with a hepatologist is recommended, particularly in patients with a previous bleeding episode.

LIVER DISEASE NOT SPECIFIC TO PREGNANCY

Hepatitis, probably virally induced, seems to account for most cases of clinical jaundice in pregnancy. Of 654 cases, 40% presumably were of viral origin[5]. However, the true incidence of hepatitis in pregnancy is unknown.

Pregnant women are not more susceptible to viral hepatitis as compared to non-pregnant women and to men. Women in all trimesters are equally affected. Except for hepatitis E (and herpes) infection, there is no difference in symptomatology, clinical course, complications and outcome of hepatitis in pregnant as compared to non-pregnant women.

The diagnosis of viral hepatitis is usually made with little difficulty, mostly by serologic testing.

Hepatitis A is not more severe in pregnancy and there seems to be no risk for the fetus, since the maternal antibody (anti-HAV) appears early during the illness and readily crosses the placenta. In an epidemic outbreak of hepatitis A in Shanghai in 1989 (292 301 cases reported) about 2% of patients were pregnant. HAV infection in pregnancy was not more severe and did not affect the fetus. The frequency of perinatal death associated with hepatitis A was similar to that without hepatitis (1.3% vs. 1.9%)[11].

The outcome of acute *hepatitis B* also does not differ between pregnant and non-pregnant women. However, nearly all infants born to HBeAg (HBV-DNA) positive mothers become infected. Long-lasting viral carriage will develop in more than 80% of these children.

Hepatitis C transmission from mother to the newborn is a rare event[12]. It has been speculated that vertical HCV infection may occur particularly in highly viraemic women[13]. A single family, in which HCV was transmitted from mother to child through two generations, has been described recently[14]. The baby's hepatitis was self-limited and transient. In many children, HCV positivity postpartum seems to reflect passive antibody transfer and not viral infection. However, true HCV infection has been documented especially in babies to HIV-positive mothers[15].

It is therefore advisable to look for HCV infection in all babies of anti-HCV positive mothers by specific tests, preferably by HCV-RNA (PCR). Pregnancies in chronic HCV infection were uncomplicated in 11 women, and all children did well during at least 1 year of follow-up[16]. Taken together, the available evidence suggests a remarkably low frequency of maternal–infant transmission. This may be referred to the low viral load in most patients with chronic HCV infection.

Hepatitis D infection is very uncommon in pregnancy. Unlike hepatitis B, HDV is rarely transmitted to the newborn[17].

Different from hepatitis A–D, *hepatitis E* infection exhibits a major threat to women in the third trimester of pregnancy. Endemics and epidemics of the disease have been observed in many countries, particularly in India, Nepal, Pakistan and the Middle East. The mortality rate in pregnant women in India is very high (17.3%) as compared to 2.1% in non-pregnant women and 2.8%, respectively, in men[18]. Therefore, HEV infection contributes significantly to the increased mortality in pregnant women from developing countries. HEV transmission to the fetus has not so far been described[19].

LIVER DISEASE UNIQUE TO PREGNANCY

Several liver diseases specifically occur in pregnancy, of which acute fatty liver may be life-threatening (Table 1). *Acute fatty liver of pregnancy* (AFLP) was first described as a catastrophic disease, typically complicating late pregnancy[20]. The condition is rare, but often fatal. It was previously said that if a woman survives, AFLP was not the correct diagnosis. Fortunately, this view has changed remarkably in recent years.

The disease belongs to the 'microvesicular fat disease group' (Table 2)[21], characterized histologically by swollen hepatocytes containing microvesicular fat droplets, metabolically by disturbed mitochondrial and ribosomal function.

AFLP is a disease of unknown aetiology and pathogenesis, affecting women usually in the third trimester of pregnancy. The presenting symptoms are very variable, ranging from signs of fulminant hepatic failure to nearly none.

Table 1 Liver diseases peculiar to pregnancy

Acute fatty liver of pregnancy (AFLP)
Intrahepatic cholestasis of pregnancy (ICP)
Pre-eclampsia–eclampsia
HELLP syndrome (*h*emolysis, *e*levated *l*iver enzymes, *l*ow *p*latelets)

Table 2 The microvesicular fat diseases

AFLP
Reye's syndrome
Jamaican vomiting disease (hypoglycin A toxicity)
Sodium valproate toxicity
Tetracycline toxicity
Congenital defects of the urea-cycle enzymes
Defect of fatty acid oxidation

Nausea, vomiting and right upper abdominal pain are common. Jaundice is variable, being present, however, in more than 90% of cases[19]. The physical examination at presentation is usually not very helpful[20]. It should be kept in mind that spider angiomas and palmar erythema are common in pregnancy!

The initial biochemical tests (see Table 3) are also variable. High serum uric acid levels, normally low in the third trimester, are a typical finding due to degradation of nucleic acids, released from necrotic hepatocytes. An increased uric acid concentration can be noticed very early during the course of the illness, in some patients preceding symptoms of AFLP[19]. Different from eclampsia, hyperbilirubinaemia is found without haemolysis[21]. Thrombocytopenia and neutrophilia are common. Leucocytosis may reach unusually high levels. Transaminases are moderately elevated[19], usually below 500 U/l.

Anaemia is not observed, unless bleeding or disseminated intravascular coagulation (DIC) is present. Clinically, AFLP should be suspected in every third trimester pregnant woman with hepatic dysfunction, and should be considered likely in patients with hepatic failure. Failure to recognize milder AFLP results from not considering the diagnosis in late pregnancy in a woman presenting with nausea and vomiting. In addition to the above-mentioned investigations, computed tomography has been described as mandatory to establish the diagnosis of fatty liver. Some investigators, however, strongly advocate ultrasound as the investigation of choice in this special situation, since it will demonstrate severe hepatic steatosis as accurately as computed tomography. Moreover, ultrasound seems able to identify mild and moderate changes of steatosis with greater sensitivity[22]. However, a normal sonogram does not exclude the diagnosis of AFLP and must not delay termination of pregnancy[23].

If clotting and bleeding times are normal, a liver biopsy can be performed. Given appropriate stains for fat on frozen sections, the hepatic histology is

Table 3 AFLP – laboratory findings

Elevated	
Alkaline phosphatase	100%
GPT/GOT	99%
Hyperbilirubinaemia	99%
Hyperuricaemia	84%
DIC	50%
Hypoglycaemia	34%

G. Freund *et al.*, Clin Chim Acta. 1990;191:125

characteristic, although not pathognomonic for AFLP.

The list of differential diagnoses of hepatic dysfunction in the third trimester is not long: only fulminant viral hepatitis or alcoholic hepatitis should pose any real problem. Acute cholecystitis and cholangitis may occur in pregnancy, but are not associated with hepatic failure or coagulopathy. Fulminant viral hepatitis may be difficult to distinguish, but severe leukocytosis, platelets below 100 000 and transaminases below 500 U/l are very uncommon in the early stage of virally induced liver disease.

Since there are no reports of spontaneous recovery from AFLP, prompt delivery of the baby is the treatment of choice. The termination of pregnancy correlates temporally with resolution of the disease.

There is only a single case of an AFLP-like syndrome following delivery[24]. In other forms of liver disease in pregnancy, e.g. in the case of hepatic failure due to viral hepatitis, delivery has no beneficial effect.

Generally, the clinical management of the mother is the same as in fulminant liver failure due to other causes. DIC is a common and often very severe complication of AFLP, resulting in excessive bleeding. Fresh frozen plasma, platelets and antithrombin III are given in this situation. Heparin therapy is not recommended[19]. If liver function continues to deteriorate despite immediate delivery, emergency liver transplantation remains an ultimate option[25].

There is no evidence that the fetal liver is subject to the same disease as the maternal organ, and liver failure seems not to be responsible for fetal deaths[26]. Indeed, liver function is usually normal in babies born to mothers with AFLP. However, fetal hypoglycaemia may occur and must be corrected appropriately[27]. The prognosis of AFLP in early series was very poor (Table 4). However, in recent series with earlier diagnosis, prompt supportive care and early delivery, the previously reported high mortality rate should improve. As in the case of fulminant hepatic failure due to viral infection, survivors of AFLP return to full health without signs of chronic sequelae. Following delivery, the clinical condition of most surviving mother–infant pairs improves within 2–3 days. A practical approach to the patients suspected of having AFLP is given in Table 5.

Does AFLP recur in subsequent pregnancies in a woman having survived the first episode? This question is particularly important, since about one-half of affected patients are in their first pregnancy. There are some reports of successful pregnancies without recurrence of AFLP[27,28]. Four women had two uneventful pregnancies[5]. Therefore, it has been generally accepted that subsequent pregnancies carry no additional maternal risk. However, apparent recurrence of AFLP in a 29-year-old woman, resulting in the loss of both

Table 4 AFLP – mortality rates

	Mother	*Child*
Early reports	80%	70%
Recent data	25%	25%
	(8–33%)	(14–66%)

Table 5 AFLP – approach to the patient

1. Consider AFLP in all women with liver dysfunction in late pregnancy
2. Exclude other causes of hepatobiliary disease:
   - good alcohol and drug history
   - hepatitis serology
   - ultrasound examination (biliary tree and liver)
3. Support the patient with:
   - i.v. fluids
   - antacids
   - (bowel catharsis)
4. Consider a liver biopsy if no other causes for liver disease are found (coagulation permitting)
5. Consider immediate termination of pregnancy (induced or operative delivery)
6. Treat acute liver failure appropriately

children at two successive pregnancies, has been recently described[29]. Both children suffered from a defect of fatty acid oxidation that proved fatal. In this situation we would recommend that the clinician should present parents with these facts. Many parents will avoid subsequent pregnancies because of the experience of a very severe illness and the fear of recurrence despite the above-mentioned data.

A variant of pre-eclampsia has been described under the acronym HELLP (*h*aemolysis, *e*levated *l*iver enzymes and *l*ow *p*latelet count). The disorder generally appears late in pregnancy. It is characterized by a microangiopathic haemolytic anaemia and low platelet count. Nearly all patients are hypertensive and many suffer from abdominal pain and vomiting. Therefore, the HELLP syndrome can be regarded as an extreme phase in the spectrum of pre-eclampsia/eclampsia. Maternal death and recurrence in subsequent pregnancies is rare[19]. However, fetal mortality reaches 20% and more[19]; therefore, prompt delivery is recommended to improve the chances of fetal survival. We are not aware of data showing a causal relationship between early delivery and decreased maternal mortality. Some characteristic aspects of the HELLP syndrome are summarized in Table 6.

Intrahepatic cholestasis of pregnancy (ICP) is the second most common cause of jaundice of pregnancy, following acute viral hepatitis[19]. The aetiology and pathogenesis of ICP is largely unclear. It has been hypothesized that ICP reflects a heritable sensitivity to the cholestatic effects of oestrogens[5]. Clinically, pruritus occurs first, followed by jaundice after 2–4 weeks. Serum bilirubin and transaminases are moderately elevated. Itching usually lasts for the duration of pregnancy. After delivery, pruritus quickly disappears, often within 1 or 2 days[5]. However, pruritus usually reoccurs with subsequent pregnancies. Itching has been treated with cholestyramine and with ursodesoxycholic acid[30]. Vitamin K administration seems advisable for women with prolonged cholestasis.

The prognosis of ICP for the mothers is good. There seems to be a trend towards increased fetal deaths; therefore, early delivery is recommended if signs of fetal distress occur. The main characteristics of this syndrome are summarized in Table 7.

Table 6 HELLP

Prevalence:	?
Symptoms	'Pre-eclampsia' Abdominal pain, headache, nausea Hypertension (diastolic BP >110 mmHg) Peripheral oedema
Biochemically	'Microangiopathic haemolysis' Haptoglobin ↓, LDH ↑, schistocytes Indirect bilirubin ↑, transaminases ↑
(Liver biopsy	Non-specific hepatitis)
Treatment	Prompt delivery Blood and blood products, AT III Steroids (maturity of fetal lung!) Plasma exchange
Prognosis	Maternal mortality approx. 3% (1.5–25%) Infant perinatal mortality approx. 35% (10–60%)

Table 7 ICP

Prevalence	1 in 1000–10 000 deliveries
Symptoms	Pruritus in the third trimester Dark urine Jaundice
Biochemically	Increased (less than 5 mg/dl) conjugated bilirubin Increased alkaline phosphatase, bile acids, cholesterol
Liver biopsy	Mild cholestasis
Therapy	Cholestyramine
Prognosis	Generally good

References

1. Krejs GJ. Jaundice during pregnancy. Sem Liv Dis. 1983;3:73–82.
2. Riely CA. Case studies in jaundice of pregnancy. Sem Liv Dis. 1988;8:191–9.
3. Schorr-Lesnick B, Lebovics E, Dworkin B, Rosenthal WS. Liver diseases unique to pregnancy. Am J Gastroenterol. 1991;86:659–70.
4. Britton RC. Pregnancy and oesophageal varices. Am J Surg. 1988;143:421–5.
5. Van Dyke RW. The liver in pregnancy. In: Zakim, G, Gojer TD, editors. Hepatology. Philadelphia: Saunders; 1990:1438–59.
6. Steven MM. Pregnancy in chronic active hepatitis. Q J Med. 1979;48:519–23.
7. Steven MM. Pregnancy and liver disease. Gut. 1981;22:592–614.
8. Whelton MJ, Sherlock S. Pregnancy in patients with hepatic cirrhosis. Management and outcome. Lancet. 1968;2:995–9.
9. Walshe JM. The management of pregnancy in Wilson's diseases treated with trientine. Q J Med. 1986;55:81–5.
10. Varma RR. Course and prognosis of pregnancy in women with liver disease. Sem Liv Dis. 1987;7:59–66.

11. Hu M, Kang L, Yao G. An outbreak of viral hepatitis A in Shanghai. In: Bianchi L, Gerok G, Deinhardt F, Maier KP, editors. Infectious Diseases of the Liver. Dordrecht: Kluwer;1990:361–6.
12. Alter HJ. The hepatitis C virus and its relationship to the clinical spectrum of NANB hepatitis. J Gastroenterol. Hepato!. 1990; Suppl. 1:78–94.
13. Rassam SW, Dusheiko GM. Epidemiology and transmission of hepatitis C infection. Eur J Gastroenterol Hepatol. 1991;3:585–91.
14. Inoue Y, Miyamura T, Unayama T, Takahashi K. Maternal transfer of HCV. Nature. 1991;353:609.
15. Weintrub J. Hepatitis C virus infection in infants whose mothers took street drugs intravenously. J Pediatr. 1991;119:869–74.
16. Wejstal R, Hermodsson S, Norkrans G. Mother to infant transmission of hepatitis C virus infection. J Med Virol. 1990;30:178–80.
17. Zenetti AR, Ferroni P, Magliano EM. Perinatal transmission of the hepatitis B virus and of the HBV-associated delta agent from mothers to offspring in northern Italy. J Med Virol. 1982;9:139–42.
18. Khuroo MS, Teli MR, Skidmore S. Incidence and severity of viral hepatitis in pregnancy. Am J Med. 1981;70:252–5.
19. Burroughs AK. Liver disease and pregnancy. In: McIntyre N, Benhamou IP, Bircher J, Rizzetto M, Rodes J, editors. Oxford Textbook of Clinical Hepatology. Oxford: Oxford Medical Publishers; 1991:1321–36.
20. Riely CA. Acute fatty liver of pregnancy. Sem Liv Dis. 1987;7:47–54.
21. Sherlock S. Acute fatty liver of pregnancy and the microvesicular fat diseases. Gut. 1983;24:265–9.
22. Kissin CM, Adam EJ, Joseph AEA. Acute fatty liver of pregnancy and diagnosis by computed tomography. Br Med J. 1988;292:622 (letter).
23. Campillo B, Bernuau J, Witz MO, Lorphelin JM, Degott C, Rueff B, Benhamou JP. Ultrasonography in acute fatty liver of pregnancy. Ann Intern Med. 1986;105:383–4.
24. Morrin PA, Handa SP, Walberg LS, Bencosome SA, Kiphie GF, Wyllie JC. Acute renal failure in association with fatty liver of pregnancy: recovery after fourteen days of complete anuria. Am J Med. 1967;42:844–51.
25. Ockner SA, Brunt EM, Cohn SM, Krul ES, Hanto DW, Peters MG. Fulminant hepatic failure caused by acute fatty liver of pregnancy treated by orthotopic liver transplantation. Hepatology. 1990;11:59–64.
26. Moise KJ, Shah DM. Acute fatty liver of pregnancy: etiology of fetal distress and fetal wastage. Obstet Gynecol. 1987;69:482–5.
27. Kaplan MM. Acute fatty liver of pregnancy. N Engl J Med. 1985;313:367–70.
28. Burroughs AK, Seong NH, Dojcinov DM, Scheuer PJ, Sherlock S. Idiopathic acute fatty liver of pregnancy in 12 patients. Q J Med. 1982;51:481–97.
29. Schoemann MN, Batey RG, Wilcken B. Recurrent acute fatty liver of pregnancy associated with a fatty-acid oxidation defect in the offspring. Gastroenterology. 1991;100:544–8.
30. Palma J, Reyes H, Ribalta J, Iglesias M, Gonzales MC, Hernandez I, Alvarez C, Molina C, Danitz M. Effects of ursodeoxycholic acid in patients with intrahepatic cholestasis of pregnancy. Hepatology. 1992;15:1043–1047.

Section VII

Liver and biotransformation

22
Drug metabolism in health and disease

U. A. MEYER

INTRODUCTION

This review will summarize present concepts of drug metabolism and the regulation of drug metabolism by genetic, environmental and disease-induced factors. More complete recent reviews of this topic are available[1-4].

BASIC PRINCIPLES OF DRUG METABOLISM

Most pharmacologically active molecules are lipophilic and remain un-ionized or only partially ionized at physiological pH. After glomerular filtration in the kidney they would be reabsorbed and remain in the organism. Biotransformation means that a lipid-soluble xenobiotic or endobiotic compound is enzymatically transformed by so-called functionalization reactions (phase I) and/or conjugation (phase II) reactions into polar, water-soluble and excretable metabolites (Table 1, Fig. 1). The major organ for drug biotransformation is the liver.

The metabolic products are often less active than the parent drug, or may even be inactive. However, some biotransformation products (metabolites) may have enhanced activity of toxic effects, including mutagenesis, teratogenesis and carcinogenesis. Thus biotransformation may include both 'detoxication' and 'toxication' processes.

Although every tissue has some ability to metabolize xenobiotics, the *liver* is the principal organ of biotransformation. At the subcellular level the major enzymes of biotransformation are either anchored in the membranes of the endoplasmic reticulum (P-450 monooxygenases, epoxide hydrolase, glucuronyl-transferases) or are cytosolic enzymes (acetyltransferases, sulphotransferases, xanthine oxidase).

Table 1 Drug-metabolizing enzyme reactions

Phase I
Conversion of functional groups
Dehydrogenation/hydrogenation
Oxidation
Hydrolysis (esterases)
Reduction
Monooxygenation
Phase II
Derivatization of functional groups
Glucuronidation
Sulphation
Acetylation
GSH conjugation
Methylation
Glycine/taurine conjugation

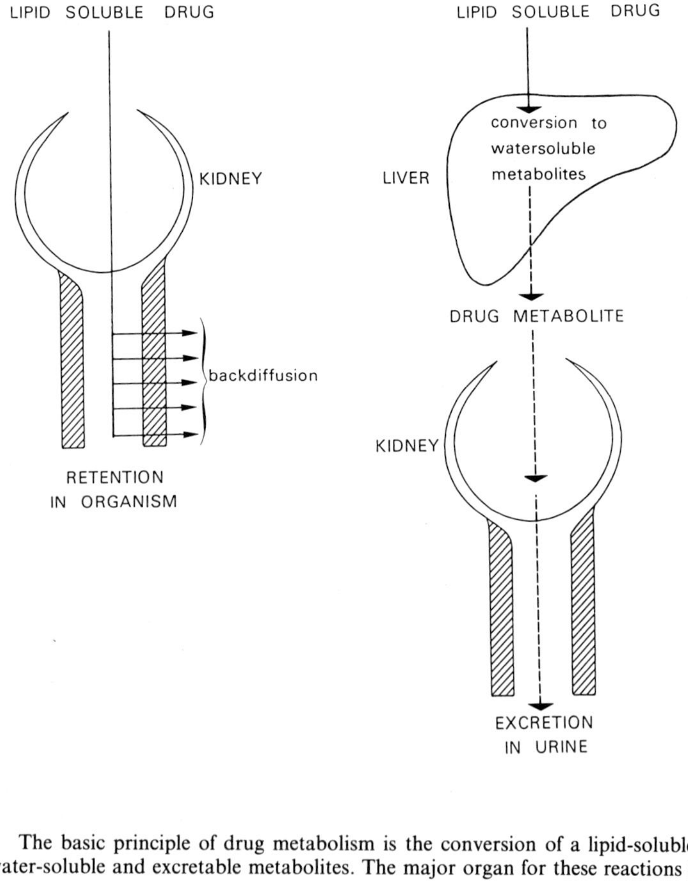

Fig. 1 The basic principle of drug metabolism is the conversion of a lipid-soluble substrate into water-soluble and excretable metabolites. The major organ for these reactions is the liver

When the lamellar membranes of the endoplasmic reticulum are isolated by homogenization and fractionation procedures, they are re-formed into vesicles called microsomes, which retain most of the morphological and functional characteristics of the intact membranes. The liver is particularly rich in endoplasmic reticulum and in enzymes responsible for oxidative drug metabolism, the most important class of drug biotransformation enzymes. Other tissues that display considerable activities of drug metabolizing enzymes are the intestinal tract, the lung, the skin, the kidneys and the olfactory mucosa. Recent studies also suggest that the brain has considerable capacities for drug metabolism.

CYTOCHROME P-450 MONOOXYGENASES

One of the major enzyme systems that determines the organism's capability of dealing with drugs and chemicals are the cytochrome P-450 monooxygenases. These enzymes are anchored in the endoplasmic reticulum and function as a multicomponent electron transport system. P-450 reactions have an absolute requirement for NADPH and molecular oxygen, and are also known as microsomal haemoprotein monooxygenases, or mixed-function oxidase. The enzyme system consists of two protein components: a haemoprotein called cytochrome P-450 of 45 000–55 000 molecular weight and a flavoprotein called NADPH-cytochrome P-450 reductase (Fp, Fig. 2). Cytochrome P-450 is the substrate- and oxygen-binding site of the enzyme system, while the reductase serves as an electron carrier, shuttling electrons from NADPH to the cytochrome P-450–substrate complex. One molecule of reductase is able to reduce 10–100 molecules of cytochrome P-450.

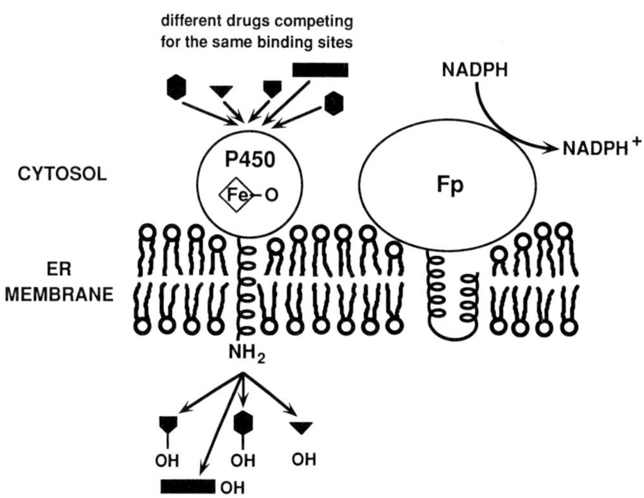

Fig. 2 Schematic view of the components of the microsomal cytochrome P-450 monooxygenase reaction. For details see text

Cytochrome P-450 has its designation from the fact that it is a red *p*igment that in the reduced form binds with carbon monoxide, yielding a complex with an absorbance maximum at *450* nm. Cytochrome P-450-dependent oxidations have been termed mixed-function oxidases because in reduced form the haemoprotein catalyses the consumption of a molecule of oxygen, with one atom of oxygen appearing in the oxidized form of the substrate and the other atom being reduced to form water.

MULTIPLICITY OF CYTOCHROME P-450 HAEMOPROTEINS

Studies in the past 15 years have provided evidence that cytochrome P-450 occurs in many different forms or 'isozymes', which differ in spectral, chemical and immunological properties and which have different but overlapping substrate affinities. These isozymes also differ in their regulation and tissue distribution. Recombinant DNA studies indicate that between 100 and 200 structural genes on different chromosomes may be coding for different cytochrome P-450 isozymes in a single organism. So far 28 human P-450 genes (designated CYP) have been characterized. The multiplicity of P-450 isozymes explains in part the literally thousands of substrates known to be metabolized by this system. Recent nomenclature proposals for this superfamily of genes are summarized in ref. 5.

GENETIC, ENVIRONMENTAL AND DISEASE FACTORS REGULATING DRUG METABOLISM

Numerous factors influence the concentration and activity of drug-metabolizing enzymes including age, nutrition, liver disease, environmental chemicals (e.g. cigarette smoking) and drugs themselves. A major source of interindividual differences in drug metabolism are common genetic polymorphisms, i.e. inherited deficiencies of single drug-metabolizing enzymes[6]. Recent studies also indicate that there are major interethnic differences in drug metabolism, particularly in the expression of cytochromes P-450 and glucuronosyltransferases, including different frequencies of genetic polymorphisms[7]. Most P-450 isozymes are regulated by multiple mechanisms, but transcriptional activation of P-450 genes is the predominant mechanism[3,4].

INDUCTION

A large number of P-450 enzymes (and also other drug metabolizing enzymes such as glucuronosyltransferases, epoxide hydrolase, etc.) are selectively induced by drugs such as phenobarbital, rifampicin, dexamethasone, etc., or by cigarette smoking and exposure to other chemicals[8,9] (Table 2). The induction response is dose-dependent and reversible. The exact mechanism of this induction response is still unknown, except for the induction of certain P-450s by polycyclic aromatic hydrocarbons such as TCDD (dioxin) via the

Table 2 Inducers of cytochromes P-450 and other drug-metabolizing enzymes in humans

Cigarette smoke	
Polychlorinated and polybrominated biphenyls	
Glutethimide	Phenobarbital
Rifampicin	Antipyrine
Phenacetin	Dexamethasone
Phenytoin	

Ah-receptor[10]. Induction leads to progressive drug tolerance and many clinically significant drug–drug interactions.

INHIBITION

Since one P-450 enzyme may bind many different substrates, competition at the site of drug binding by cosubstrates or other chemicals may cause inhibition. Known potent inhibitors of P-450 enzymes are quinidine (CYP2D6), cimetidine (numerous P-450s), furafylline (CYP1A2), gestodene (CYP3A subfamily).

DISEASE

Severe liver disease (hepatitis, cirrhosis, liver cancer), diabetes and starvation may affect drug metabolism by multiple mechanisms. Of particular importance are drugs whose metabolism is limited by liver blood flow (e.g. propropolol, lidocaine, nifedipine, verapamil, etc.). In cirrhosis with portal–systemic shunts these drugs can reach very high (toxic) plasma concentrations.

GENETIC POLYMORPHISM

Genetic variation in drug metabolizing enzymes can markedly affect drug kinetics[6,11]. Several of these genetic polymorphism are now well-studied at the epidemiological, protein and DNA level, and simple DNA tests to genotype individuals have been developed in this laboratory (Table 3).

The *debrisoquine/sparteine-type polymorphism* of drug oxidation affects the metabolism by cytochrome CYP2D6 of over 30 clinically used drugs including opioids, antidepressant, neuroleptic and antiarrhythmic drugs (Table 4). A cytochrome P-450 (CYP2D6) is deficient in poor metabolizers (PM) of debrisoquine[12]. In leucocyte DNA of PM subjects and their families mutant alleles *of CYP2D gene* associated with the PM phenotype were identified and sequenced (for review, see refs 13 and 14). Two point mutations and a deletion of the entire *CYP2D6 gene* account for most of the mutations causing deficient CYP2D6 function. DNA restriction fragment length analysis (RFLP) and a simple DNA test using PCR amplification can identify or predict $>90\%$ of poor metabolizers[13,14].

Table 3 Genetic polymorphisms of drug-metabolizing enzymes

Designation	*Archetypal examples*	*Other drug substrates*	*Incidence of 'poor metabolizers' in Caucasians*	*Enzyme involved*
Debrisoquine/sparteine polymorphism	Debrisoquine, sparteine, bufuralol	Antiidepressants, antiarrhythmics, beta-adrenergic receptor blocking drugs, codeine, dextrometorphan, neuroleptics	5–10% (Japanese, Chinese 0–2%)	Cytochrome P4502D6 (CYP2D6)
Mephenytoin polymorphism	Mephenytoin	Mephobarbital, hexobarbital, diazepam, omeprazol	3–5% (Japanese, Chinese 15–20%)	Cytochrome P4502C subfamily
Acetylation polymorphism	Isoniazid, sulphadiazine	Isoniazid, hydralazine, phenelzine, procainamide, dapsone, sulphamethazine, sulphapyridine	40–70% (Japanese, Chinese 10–20%)	*N*-acetyltransferase (NAT2)

Table 4 Examples of drugs whose metabolism is known to be under the same monogenic control as the debrisoquine/sparteine-type polymorphism

Antiarrhythmic agents	*Beta-adrenoceptor blocking drugs*
Encainide	Alprenolol
Flecainide	Bopindolol
Mexiletine	Bufuralol
Perhexiline	Metoprolol
Propafenone	Penbutolol
N-Propylajmaline	Propanolol
Sparteine	Timolol
Antidepressants	*Others*
(+)-Amiflamine	Codeine
Amitryptiline	Debrisoquine
Clomipramine	Dextromethorphan
Desipramine	Guanoxan
Imipramine	Indoramin
Nortriptyline	4-Methyoxyamphetamine
	Phenformin
	Tropisetron
Antipsychotics	
Perphenazine	
Thioridazine	
Clozapine	

The *mephenytoin-type polymorphism* affects the metabolism of mephenytoin and several other drugs. It is caused by a deficiency of a cytochrome P-450 of the CYP2C subfamily. However, which one of the multiple genes of this family is affected has not yet been conclusively determined[15].

The polymorphism of *N-acetyltransferase* (NAT) affects the metabolism of a wide variety of arylamine and hydrazine drugs, and several potential carcinogens. In livers of slow acetylators the enzyme NAT2 is reduced or absent[16]. We have identified three common mutant alleles of the *NAT2* gene which are responsible for slow acetylation in Caucasians. They now can be determined by a simple DNA test using PCR amplification[17].

NOVEL APPROACHES FOR THE STUDY OF HUMAN DRUG METABOLISM

One of the important questions in drug metabolism research is to what degree the metabolic pathways of a drug in humans can be predicted before application to animals or humans. For this purpose we have used a large human liver bank to study human drug-metabolizing enzymes *in vitro*. To identify the enzyme(s) responsible for a particular drug-metabolizing reaction, *reaction phenotyping* is performed with a panel of inhibitory antibodies or specific chemical inhibitors or by the correlation of an activity with the amount of enzyme–protein recognized on immunoblots. Final proof for the involvement of a particular enzyme is the demonstration of activity in cells *transfected with cDNA or gene* coding for the drug-metabolizing enzyme (see ref. 18 for an example). This is followed by the evaluation of the *in vivo* relevance of this particular step in the overall metabolism of the drug.

Once the enzymes are identified and specific assays developed, drug-metabolism interactions may be predicted from *in vitro* effects, e.g. inhibition of the enzyme reaction. For the assessment of the interindividual variation of a drug-metabolism reaction, a panel of livers from patients of different age, smoking history and drug history is used.

The described approach has been used to study the mechanisms of common genetic polymorphisms of drug metabolism. Moreover, these methods have been successful in the identification of the enzymes responsible for the metabolism of cyclosporin[18], midazolam, lidocain, and several other drugs.

OUTLOOK

Characterization of human drug-metabolizing enzymes has seen major progress in the past few years. An important aspect of this research are studies addressing the mechanisms causing interindividual or interpatient differences in the profiles and tissue distributions of these enzymes and the genetic and environmental factors that cause this heterogeneity, including interethnic differences. The evaluation of the clinical relevance of these variations will be an important area of research for the next few years.

ACKNOWLEDGEMENTS

The author's research is supported by the Swiss National Science Foundation.

References

1. Gibson GG, Skett P. Introduction to drug metabolism. New York: Chapman & Hall; 1986.
2. Watkins PB. Role of cytochromes P450 in drug metabolism and hepatotoxicity. Sem Liver Dis. 1990;10:235–50.
3. Porter TD, Coon MJ. Cytochrome P450, multiplicity of isoforms, substrates, and catalytic and regulatory mechanisms. J Biol Chem. (Minireview) 1991;226:13469–72.
4. Gonzalez FJ. Human cytochromes P450: problems and prospects. Trends Pharmacol Sci. 1992;13:346–52.
5. Nebert DW *et al.* The P450 superfamily: update on new sequences, gene mapping, and recommended nomenclature. DNA Cell Biol. 1991;10:1–14.
6. Meyer UA, Zanger UM, Grant D, Blum M. Genetic polymorphisms of drug metabolism, In: Testa B, editor. Advances in Drug Research, vol. 19. London: Academic Press; 1990:197–241.
7. Kalow W, Goedde HW, Agarwal DP. (eds) Ethnic differences in reactions to drugs and xenobiotics. New York: Alan R. Liss; 1986.
8. Okey AB. Enzyme induction in the cytochrome P450 system. Pharmacol Ther. 190;45:241–98.
9. Waxman DJ, Azaroff L. Phenobarbital induction of cytochrome P450 gene expression. Biochem J. 1992;281:577–92.
10. Whitlock JP. The control of cytochrome P450 expression by dioxin. Trends Pharmacol Sci. 1989;10:285–9.
11. Kalow W (ed.) Pharmacogenetics of drug metabolism international encyclopedia of pharmacology and therapeutics (executive editor A. C. Sartorelli), London, New York: Pergamon; 1992.

12. Zanger UM, Vilbois F, Hardwick JP, Meyer UA. Absence of hepatic cytochrome P450bufl causes genetically deficient debrisoquine oxidation in man. Biochemistry. 1988;27:5447–54.
13. Heim M, Meyer UA. Genotyping of poor metabolizers of debrisoquine by allele-specific PCR amplification. Lancet. 1990;336:529–32.
14. Broly F, Gaedigk A, Heim H, Eichelbaum M, Mörike K, Meyer UA. Debrisoquine/sparteine hydroxylation genotype and phenotype: Analysis of common mutations and alleles of *CYP2D6* in a European population. DNA Cell Biol. 1991;10:545–58.
15. Wilkinson GR, Guengerich FP, Branch RA. Genetic polymorphism of S-mephenytoin hydroxylation. In: Kalow W, editor. Pharmacogenetics of drug metabolism. New York: Pergamon Press; 1992:657–85.
16. Grant DM, Mörike K, Eichelbaum M, Meyer UA. Acetylation pharmacogenetics. The slow acetylator phenotype is caused by decreased or absent arylamine N-acetyltransferase in human liver. J Clin Invest. 1990;85:968–72.
17. Blum M, Demiere A, Grant DM, Heim M, Meyer UA. Molecular mechanism of slow acetylation of drugs and carcinogens in humans. Proc Natl Acad Sci USA. 1991;88:5237–41.
18. Kronbach T, Fischer V, Meyer UA. Cyclosporine metabolism in human liver: identification of a cytochrome P450 of the P450III gene family as the major cyclosporine-metabolizing enzyme explains interactions of cyclosporine with other drugs. Clin Pharmacol Ther. 1988;43:630–5.

23
Drug therapy in liver disease

M. H. DAVIES and E. ELIAS

INTRODUCTION

The liver is the principal organ of detoxification of a wide variety of drugs. In the presence of liver disease drug therapy frequently requires modification. This may be because of a change in the capacity to metabolize drugs, leading to higher than desired drug levels. Alternatively, there may be altered sensitivity to the intended effect, or to a particular side-effect. These, and other factors, frequently alter the balance of the risk/benefit equation, so that the dosage or choice of a particular therapeutic agent may have to be adjusted.

This chapter addresses some of the principal pharmacokinetic and pharmacodynamic alterations occurring in the presence of liver disease, and reviews recent literature in an attempt to recommend qualitative alterations in drug prescribing. The great heterogeneity of liver disease and the lack of precise means of predicting individual metabolic capacity, make it impossible to stipulate quantitative recommendations, other than in the broadest of terms.

PHARMACOKINETIC AND PHARMACODYNAMIC CONSIDERATIONS

Intestinal absorption of a drug may be altered in liver disease. This may result from changes associated with portal hypertension or diminished excretion of bile, which is important in the absorption of certain drugs, including cyclosporin. Concomitant medications, such as the bile acid binding resins, impede absorption of some drugs.

Protein binding may be altered, influencing the fraction of unbound drug. The change may directly reflect alterations in serum albumin level. More often protein binding shows wide fluctuations, which correlate imprecisely with hypoalbuminaemia alone, or with apparent level of hepatic dysfunction.

The precise mechanisms are likely to be multifactorial. Alterations in protein binding become more important for those drugs which are highly protein-bound. Hence a change from 98% bound to 96% represents a 100% increase in unbound concentration, compared to a change from 90% to 88%, an increase of 20%.

The influence of protein binding upon drug clearance may be modified by the ability of hepatocytes to metabolize both bound and unbound drug in some cases. Two types of extraction are described: restricted, in which extraction is limited to the free drug and non-restricted in which both bound and free drug may be metabolized. In general, the higher a drug's intrinsic free clearance, the less sensitive is its extraction to alteration in drug binding.

Table 1 Drugs exhibiting significant changes in binding in cirrhosis

Amylobarbitone	Frusemide
Azapropazone	Nifedipine
Cephazolin	Prednisolone
Clofibrate	Phenytoin
Diazepam	Valproic acid
Erythromycin	

The *volume of distribution* (V_d) is a mathematically defined relationship between the amount of drug in the intravascular and extravascular compartments of the body. Drugs which circulate highly bound to plasma proteins will have low apparent volumes of distribution, because they are predominantly confined to the intravascular compartment. The converse is true for drugs with low plasma protein binding. Alterations of drug binding and body composition in liver disease (e.g. ascites) will influence V_d. The volume of distribution does not necessarily have a physical equivalent and for lipid-bound drugs, such as propanolol, the V_d in liver disease may be several litres per kilogram body weight.

The half-life of a drug $T_{1/2}$ is related to its V_d:

$$T_{1/2} = \frac{(V_d)(0.693)}{\text{clearance}}$$

Thus prolongation of $T_{1/2}$ will occur when V_d increases, irrespective of the liver's ability to metabolize the drug. For a drug to reach its steady-state plasma concentration requires about 3–4 $T_{1/2}$ time-periods, and a similar interval is required for washout of the drug after cessation of treatment. Changes in $T_{1/2}$ do not necessarily represent changes in clearance.

The half-life is therefore a value which reflects a number of processes, which may be variably modified in patients with liver disease, sometimes in opposite directions. For this reason the study of drug metabolism should be considered in relation to hepatic clearance, rather than $T_{1/2}$.

Hepatic clearance is dependent on two processes, firstly the rate at which drug is delivered to the liver and secondly the efficiency of its removal:

$$\text{Hepatic clearance} = \text{liver blood flow} \times \text{extraction}$$

The rate of metabolism for a compound with a high extraction will depend closely upon blood flow, *flow limited*, whereas drugs which are of low extraction will be influenced proportionately less by blood flow, *capacity limited* (see Table 2). Several drugs are subject to a significant '*first-pass effect*'. Following oral administration, these undergo extensive metabolism when delivered by the portal venous system during their first pass through the liver.

Systemic availability is the ratio of plasma drug concentration after oral versus intravenous administration. For example the systemic availability of oral verapamil is about 22% of the dose administered[1]. Larger doses of a drug with a high first-pass effect have to be administered by the oral route compared with the intravenous route. The development of portal hypertension, whether due to parenchymal liver disease or portal vein thrombosis, will lead to major changes in the pharamacokinetics of such drugs. Systemic availability may be increased many-fold because of spontaneous portosystemic shunting, which allows a drug to avoid the first pass through the liver. Arteriovenous shunting occurs within the cirrhotic liver together with changes to sinusoidal fenestration, basement membrane thickening with collagenization of the space of Disse, which will diminish the extraction ratio of drugs as they traverse the liver. For drugs whose clearance is flow limited, the influence of liver disease is reasonably predictable. However, the complex outcome of changes in protein binding, hepatocyte uptake and enzyme metabolism may either increase or diminish the clearance of the various drugs by the liver.

The metabolic capacity of the liver is compromised as disease progresses. Whether this decline merely reflects a diminished mass of hepatocytes, which function to the same degree, but in reduced number, 'The intact hepatocyte theory', or reflects a qualitative loss of hepatocyte function, 'The sick

Table 2 Hepatic clearance of various drugs

Flow limited	*Capacity limited*
Acetylsalicylate	Aminopyrine
Alprenolol	Chlorpromazine
Chlormethiazole	Diazepam
Diltiazem	Digitoxin
Flumazenil	Nitrazepam
Fluorouracil	Phenobarbital
Indocyanine green	Phenytoin
Isosorbide dinitrate	Piroxicam
Labetalol	Tolbutamide
Lignocaine	Valproic acid
Metoprolol	Warfarin
Morphine	
Nifedipine	
Pentazoxin	
Verapamil	

Table 3 Effect of liver disease on the clearance of highly and poorly extracted drugs

Drug	*Percentage change in total systemic clearance in liver disease*
Highly extracted	
Lignocaine	−40
Metoprolol	−25
Morphine	−7
Pentazocine	−46
Pethidine	−50
Propanolol	−62
Verapamil	−50
Poorly extracted	
Ampicillin	−16
Atenolol	+23
Chloramphenicol	−65
Chlordiazepoxide	−54
Diazepam	−53
Frusemide	−15
Lorazepam	+8
Naproxen	+2
Oxazepam	+14
Prednisone	+9
Tolbutamide	+44
Warfarin	0

− = A reduction in clearance; + = an increase in clearance
This table is reproduced from Bass NM and Williams RL. Guide to drug dosage in hepatic disease. Clin Pharmacokinet. 1988;15:396–420.

hepatocyte theory' is subject to debate. Some metabolic processes are better preserved than others, for example glucuronidation is relatively well preserved[2,3], unless liver disease is advanced[4]. Particular liver diseases, such as primary biliary cirrhosis, may be associated with less decline in clearance capacity than others. Iqbal *et al.*[5] studied the activities of a variety of microsomal and cytosolic enzymes obtained from hepatectomy specimens removed at the time of liver transplantation. There was no significant difference in the activity of aminopyrine *N*-demethylase or ethoxycoumarin *O*-deethylase, in the group of PBC livers compared with a group of control livers, yet the activity of both groups of enzymes from a mixed group with other liver disease was significantly impaired.

Genetic polymorphisms create additional difficulties when trying to estimate individual capacity to metabolize specific drugs. Cytochrome P-450 IID6 has probably been the most extensively studied[6]. This is the target of the sparteine/debrisoquine polymorphism; 5–10% of Caucasians are poor metabolizers of these drugs, due to an absence of this enzyme. P-450 IID6 is an enzyme with wide substrate specificity. It is of prime importance in the metabolism of 15–20 different drugs. In addition, it may become saturated by some drugs at therapeutic levels, such as propafenone, and others will specifically inhibit it, e.g. quinidine. The study of genetic polymorphism is an important area for research, since marked metabolic dysfunction may be present in the absence of overt liver dysfunction (see Chapter 22).

SPECIFIC EXAMPLES

Sedation and analgesia

The requirement of sedation and/or analgesia in liver disease provides an example whereby the risk/benefit ratio of treatment is radically altered. (Chapter 24 discusses the use of narcotics in liver disease.) Psychotropic medication, including the phenothiazines, butyrophenones and benzodiazepines, is associated with the potential for increased cerebral sensitivity, in addition to impaired clearance. Use of these groups of drugs may precipitate or exacerbate encephalopathy. One compromise is to choose a benzodiazepine, since a specific antidote, flumazenil, is available. It is preferable to use a short-acting benzodiazepine, which is predominantly metabolized by glucuronidation (a relatively well-preserved phase II reaction). An example would be oxazepam.

Paracetamol is probably the safest analgesic agent when used in appropriate dosage. There are several anecdotal reports of hepatotoxicity resulting from standard doses in patients with alcoholic liver disease. Toxicity could theoretically arise in these cases, because of a combination of diminished glutathione reserves and cytochrome P-450 induction. These would compromise detoxification and increase production of the hepatotoxic P-450 metabolite. Hepatotoxicity is less likely to result from standard dosing in other circumstances. Several studies of paracetamol metabolism in liver disease have shown the drug to be well tolerated, despite a prolonged half-life, with no evidence of hepatotoxicity[7–10]. It is noted that, in advanced disease, impaired clearance may predispose to accumulation of parent compound, in which case dosage reduction is appropriate.

Non-steroidal anti-inflammatory drugs (NSAIDs) have a spectrum of side-effects in healthy individuals. Indomethacin or ibuprofen prescribed in standard doses in patients with liver disease reduced creatinine clearance[11]. This was ascribed to alterations in renal haemodynamics resulting from prostaglandin inhibition[12,13]. Renal prostaglandins play a major role in maintaining renal perfusion in patients with reduced renal blood flow. Administration of NSAID may precipitate overt renal decompensation. Patients at greatest risk are those with pre-existing renal disease or advanced hepatic dysfunction[14], with ascites and sodium retention. Indomethacin is the most potent prostaglandin inhibitor and is the most likely to cause nephrotoxicity and reduce glomerular filtration rate. Ibuprofen and naprosyn are intermediate in potency; aspirin and sulindac the least nephrotoxic, yet they are still capable of deleterious renal effects in susceptible patients. Impaired platelet function, damage to gastric mucosa and fluid retention are additional relative contraindications to the use of salicylates and NSAIDs in liver disease. In general, these agents are best avoided.

ANTIBIOTIC PRESCRIBING

Patients with cirrhosis are at increased risk of life-threatening Gram-negative infection. When a patient is considered septic, early antibiotic therapy is indicated, following appropriate bacteriological culture. Treatment is often commenced with a broad-spectrum agent on an empirical basis, whilst awaiting results of culture and sensitivity.

Aminoglycoside therapy may cause nephrotoxicity in paients with liver disease, even though these drugs are not metabolized by the liver, but are excreted unchanged in the urine. Toxicity may arise even when standard plasma levels are not exceeded. In one study, nephrotoxicity occurred in one-third of patients despite close monitoring of plasma levels, which remained in the appropriate range[15]. Aminoglycoside therapy should be avoided in advanced liver disease, unless results of bacteriological culture dictate their use. Close surveillance of renal function is then required.

Orally administered neomycin may be absorbed in small quantities in hepatic failure. Because of the increased susceptibility to the toxic effects of aminoglycoside therapy, it is best to avoid neomycin, other than for short-term use. In particular, long-term neomycin therapy of chronic hepatic encephalopathy is inappropriate.

Third-generation cephalosporins usually offer effective alternatives to aminoglycoside therapy. These have a high therapeutic index and, although clearance depends in part on hepatic metabolism, they appear safe in liver disease[16,17].

Penicillins and their derivatives are predominantly cleared by the kidneys. Dosage can remain unchanged in liver disease, if creatinine clearance is not impaired.

Therapy with metronidazole may be required. Although its clearance depends in part upon hepatic metabolism, it is appropriate to prescribe it in standard doses if renal function is normal[18], but in reduced dosage if creatinine clearance is reduced, since this was associated with a marked impairment of drug clearance[19].

BETA-BLOCKERS

When used in liver disease, all beta-blockers have the potential to impair renal function and can precipitate a marked decrease in creatinine clearance. Even atenolol, which has practically no hepatic extraction, can accumulate in liver disease, because of reduced renal clearance. Others, such as propanolol[20] and labetalol[21], have a marked first-pass effect with extensive hepatic extraction. Clearance of these will be impaired by liver disease. Propanolol may precipitate severe hepatic encephalopathy, even when used in small doses. It is unknown whether this relates to its lipid solubility and propensity to cross the blood–brain barrier.

If beta-blockers are used in liver disease, renal function and mental status must be monitored. Dose-related side-effects should also be monitored, because impaired clearance may lead to accumulation of the drug.

ANGIOTENSIN-CONVERTING ENZYME (ACE) INHIBITORS

Enalapril is a prodrug ester of the active compound enalaprilate. This bioactivation requires metabolism in the liver and may be impaired by liver disease. Captopril is not metabolized by the liver, so drug accumulation is not a problem.

ACE inhibitors were thought to have a potential therapeutic role in cirrhosis, because of the interplay between glomerular filtration rate, blood pressure, ascites and the renin angiotensin system. Some studies reported beneficial diuresis and natriuresis using ACE inhibitors alone or in combination with diuretics[22–24]. However, complications including severe hypotension[25] and increasing encephalopathy[26] were noted. It is suggested that the physiological conditions associated with resistant ascites resemble those in bilateral renal artery stenosis[25], in which case ACE inhibition has little therapeutic role. It appears, therefore, that in the presence of cirrhosis ACE inhibitors should be used with caution or avoided.

CALCIUM CHANNEL BLOCKERS

Verapamil[27,28], diltiazem and nifedipine are all extensively metabolized in the liver, with marked first-pass metabolism. Clearance of these drugs may be profoundly impaired, so that initial doses should be reduced and the patient monitored for dose-related side-effects. Verapamil is probably the most prone to cause constipation, which may create difficulties in those patients with chronic encephalopathy.

HISTAMINE ANTAGONISTS

The older H_1 blockers tend to cause drowsiness, which can be quite marked in the presence of impaired liver function. This is not the case with newer agents, which are generally well tolerated in patients with liver disease.

Peptic ulceration is a frequent complication of cirrhosis. The H_2 blockers have a high therapeutic index and are well tolerated. An agent with least oestrogenic side-effects is appropriate for male patients.

ANTIARRHYTHMICS

Treatment with antiarrhythmic drugs always requires close supervision, because of their frequent narrow therapeutic index, propensity to negative inotropism and pro-arrhythmicity.

Amiodarone has an extremely long terminal half-life and large volume of distribution. It is highly concentrated in the liver. Post-mortem studies have shown concentrations within the liver parenchyma of amiodarone to be as high as 1640 mg/kg wet weight and 8150 mg/kg of its active metabolite desethyl amiodarone[29]. This drug is of particular interest, since it is associated with several hepatic side-effects. Changes similar to alcoholic liver injury are commonly observed, with deposition of macro- and microvesicular fat, Mallory's hyaline and fibrosis. Electron microscopic study frequently reveals a phospholipidosis. The phospholipidosis may occur independently of the pseudo-alcoholic changes. Evidence of minor liver dysfunction is frequent and should not necessarily lead to withdrawal of the agent, since injury is minor in most cases and withdrawal of the drug might be associated with the resurgence of life-threatening arrhythmias. Some cases of hepatotoxicity will progress despite withdrawal of the drug.

The mechanism of amiodarone metabolism is not precisely known. There is no current recommendation for alteration of dosage in the presence of liver disease.

Although disopyramide is cleared predominantly extrahepatically, there is evidence of impaired clearance in liver disease[30]. There may also be quantitative and qualitative reduction of plasma protein binding[31,32]. Dosage reduction in the presence of impaired hepatic function is recommended.

Flecainide has extensive first-pass metabolism and high extraction. It is therefore prone to accumulation in the presence of liver disease or portosystemic shunting. Studies have shown that patients with cirrhosis have markedly reduced plasma clearance compared with controls[33,34]. Steady-state plasma levels will take longer to achieve in such patients, so dosage adjustments should be made cautiously, at intervals exceeding 4 days. Plasma level monitoring is strongly recommended.

The clearance of lignocaine relies to a large extent upon hepatic metabolism. Clearance is diminished as a result of liver disease[35] and half-life can be increased enormously[36]. Lignocaine clearance has been utilized as a sensitive marker of metabolic dysfunction in liver disease[37]. More recently its metabolism has been assessed in the field of liver transplantation. It may be used both as an indicator of disease progression, to assist in the appropriate timing of transplantation and as an indicator of donor liver function prior to transplantation.

Propafenone is another agent with high hepatic extraction and first-pass metabolism. Digoxin, on the other hand, undergoes minimal hepatic clearance and dosage is predicted according to creatinine clearance.

SUMMARY

Many factors contribute to the need for altered drug therapy in liver disease. Unfortunately, the degree of dysfunction in any particular case or disease group may differ greatly from another, who otherwise appear similar.

Hopes that hepatic drug clearance might be calculated by simple reproducible tests have been mostly fruitless. This is because of the great variety of drug-metabolizing enzymes and their partly overlapping substrate specificity.

It is therefore inappropriate and incorrect to provide dogmatic statements concerning specific dosage alterations which apply to all patients with liver disease. It is important to recognize that these patients are often more susceptible to adverse effects from therapeutic agents than others, which may alter the risk/benefit ratio.

It is essential to adopt a rational prescribing policy; to try to avoid those drugs with severe side-effects and to monitor closely the effects of all medication.

References

1. Somogyi A, Albrecht M, Kliems G, Schafer K, Eichelbaum M. Pharmacokinetics, bioavailability and ECG response of verapamil in patients with liver disease. Br J Clin Pharmacol. 1981;12:51–60.
2. Shull HJ, Wilkinson GR, Johnson RF, Johnson R, Schenker S. Normal disposition of oxazepam in acute viral hepatitis and cirrhosis. Ann Intern Med. 1976;84:420–5.
3. Kraus JW, Desmond PV, Marshall JP *et al.* The effects of aging and liver disease on the disposition of lorazepam in man. Clin Pharamacol Ther. 1978;24:411–19.
4. Hoyumpa AM, Schenker S. Is glucuronidation truly preserved in patients with liver disease? Hepatology. 1991;13:786–95.
5. Iqbal S, Vickers C, Elias E. Drug metabolism in end-stage liver disease. In vitro activities of some phase I and phase II enzymes. J Hepatol. 1990;11:37–42.
6. Brosen K. Recent developments in hepatic drug oxidation. Implications for clinical pharmacokinetics. Clin Pharmacokinet. 1990;18:220–39.
7. Forrest JAH, Finlayson NDC, Adjepon-Yamoah KK, Prescott LE. Antipyrine, paracetamol and lignocaine elimination in chronic liver disease. Br Med J. 1988;1:1384–7.
8. Arnman R, Olsson R. Elimination of paracetamol in chronic liver disease. Acta Hepatol Gastoenterol. 1978;25:283–6.
9. Forrest JAH, Adriaenssens P, Finlayson NDC, Prescott LF. Paracetamol metabolism in chronic liver disease. Eur J Clin Pharm. 1979;15:427–31.
10. Andreasen P, Hutters L. Paracetamol (Acetaminophen) clearance in patients with cirrhosis of the liver. Acta Med Scand. 1979; suppl 624:99–105.
11. Boyer TD, Zia P, Reynolds TB. Effect of indomethacin and prostaglandin A on renal function and plasma renin activity in alcoholic liver disease. Gastroenterology. 1979;77:215–22.
12. Zipser RD, Hoefs JC, Speckart PF *et al.* Modulators of renal function and pressor resistance in chronic liver disease. J Clin Endocrinol Metab. 1979;48:895–900.
13. Laffi G, Daskalopoulos G, Kronborg I *et al.* Effects of sulindac and ibuprofen in patients with cirrhosis and ascites. An explanation for the renal sparing effects of sulindac. Gastroenterology. 1986;90:182–7.
14. Kawasaki H, Nosaka Y, Yamada S *et al.* Effect of renal prostaglandins on survival in patients with liver cirrhosis. Am J Gastroenterol. 1989;84:285–9.
15. Cabrera J, Arroyo V, Ballesta AM *et al.* Aminoglycoside nephrotoxicity in cirrhosis. Value of urinary β2-microglobulin to discriminate functional renal failure from acute tubular damage. Gastroenterology. 1982;82:97–105.
16. Balant L, Dayer P, Auckenthaler R. Clinical pharmacokinetics of the third generation cephalosporins. Clin Pharmacokinet. 1985;10:101–43.
17. Felisart J, Rimola A, Arroyo V *et al.* Cefotaxime is more effective than is ampicillin-tobramycin in cirrhotics with severe infections. Hepatology. 1985;5:457–62.
18. Daneshmend TK, Homeida M, Kaye CM *et al.* Disposition of oral metronidazole in hepatic cirrhosis and in hepatosplenic schistosomiasis. Gut. 1982;23:807–13.
19. Farrell G, Baird-Lambert J, Cvejic M, Buchanan N. Disposition and metabolism of metronidazole in patients with liver failure. Hepatology. 1984;4:722–6.
20. Wood AJJ, Kornhauser DM, Wilkinson GR *et al.* The influence of cirrhosis on steady state blood concentrations of unbound propranolol after oral administration. Clin Pharmacokinet. 1978;3:478–87.
21. Williams RL, Mamelok RD. Hepatic disease and drug pharmacokinetics. Pharmacokinet. 1980;5:528–47.
22. Mantero F, Boscolo R, Zotti S *et al.* The renin–angiotensin–aldosterone system in liver disease. In: Langer M, Chiandussi L, Chopra IJ, Martini L, editors. The endocrines and

the liver. Proceedings Serono Symposia, vol. 51. Rome, June 1981. London: Academic Press; 1982:245–54.
23. Noto R, Bonanno G, Cantelmo R *et al.* Captopril and resistant ascites in cirrhotic patients with various stages of portal hypertension. Cur Ther Res. 1986;40:733–8.
24. Caramelo C, Berne JG, Salata H *et al.* Effect of captopril in sodium and water management in decompensated cirrhotic patients. Kidney Int. 1983;24:271–2.
25. Wood LJ, Goergen S, Stockigt JR *et al.* Adverse effects of captopril in treatment of resistant ascites. A state of functional bilateral renal artery stenosis. Lancet. 1985;2:1008–9.
26. Pariente EA, Bataille C, Bercoff E, Lebrec D. Acute effects of captopril on systemic and renal hemodynamics and on renal function in cirrhotic patients with ascites. Gastroenterology. 1985;88:1255–9.
27. Woodcock BG, Rietbrock I, Vohringer HF, Rietbrock N. Verapamil disposition in liver disease and intensive care patients: Kinetics, clearance and apparent blood flow relationships. Clin Pharmacol Ther. 1981;29:27–34.
28. Somogyi A, Albrecht M, Kleims G *et al.* Pharmacokinetics, bioavailability and ECG response of verapamil in patients with liver cirrhosis. Br J Clin Pharmacol. 1981;12:51–60.
29. Adams PC, Bennett MK, Holt DW. Hepatic effects of amiodarone. Br J Clin Pract. 1986;40(supp 44):81–95.
30. Bonde J, Graudal NA, Pedersen LE *et al.* Kinetics of disopyramide in decreased hepatic function. Eur J Clin Pharmacol. 1986;31:73–7.
31. Echizen H, Saima A, Umeda N, Ishizaki T. Protein binding of disopyramide in liver cirrhosis and in nephrotic syndrome. Clin Pharmacol Ther. 1986;40:274–80.
32. Pedersen LE, Bonde J, Graudal NA *et al.* Quantitative and qualitative binding characteristics of disopyramide in serum from patients with decreased renal and hepatic function. Br J Clin Pharmacol. 1987;23:41–6.
33. McQuinn RL, Pentikainen PJ, Chang SF, Conard GJ. Pharmacokinetics of flecainide in patients with cirrhosis of the liver. Clin Pharmacol Ther. 1988;44:566–72.
34. Pentikaeinen PJ. Pharacokinetics of flecainide in special situations: Effects of impaired liver function and enzyme induction on flecainide kinetics. Nordic Flecainide Symposium. 1986:53–59.
35. Benowitz NI, Meister W. Clinical pharmacokinetics of lignocaine. Clin Pharmacokinet. 1978;3:177–201.
36. Adjepon-Yamoah KK, Prescott LF. Gross impairment of hepatic drug metabolism in a patient with chronic liver disease. Br Med J. 1974;4:387–8.
37. Oellerich M, Burdelski M, Lautz HU *et al.* Lidocaine metabolite formation as a measure of liver function in patients with cirrhosis. Ther Drug Monit. 1990;12:219–26.

24

Use of narcotics in liver disease

R. K. OCKNER

Important functional interactions between brain and liver are well recognized. In health, for example, hepatic glycogenolysis and gluconeogenesis provide a level of plasma glucose sufficient to permit normal cerebral function, while in liver disease and portal hypertension the presence of encephalopathy is an indicator of insufficient hepatic processing of blood from the splanchnic circulation. In recent years a new dimension has been added to these liver–brain interactions which, while less well understood and still evolving, is clearly of major significance. This new element is the growing recognition of the relationships between the liver and the endorphin and γ-aminobutyric acid/benzodiazepine receptor systems, and their endogenous ligands. That the clinical use of *exogenous* ligands of these same receptor systems, i.e. the narcotics and the benzodiazepine drugs, should pose special challenges in the management of patients with liver diseases is not surprising. Although this chapter will refer briefly to the benzodiazepines to illustrate specific points, the major emphasis will be on the narcotic drugs and their interaction with the endorphin system in addressing three more or less related issues of potential concern in the care of patients with liver disease. These include: (1) pharmacokinetics, i.e. the determinants of drug clearance from plasma and thus the amount remaining available to exert a pharmacological effect (drug bioavailability); (2) pharmacodynamics, i.e. the determinants of the pharmacological effectiveness of the drug at its site of action; and (3) the effects of the drug on the liver itself, including intermediary metabolism and hepatotoxicity.

PHARMACOKINETIC AND PHARMACODYNAMIC CONSIDERATIONS

The general principles governing *pharmacokinetics*[1] were reviewed in Chapter 23, and will be considered here only briefly as they apply to narcotics and benzodiazepines. High-clearance drugs, e.g. meperidine[2], have high first-pass extraction by the liver, and are rapidly removed from plasma. For such agents a relatively small decrease in first-pass extraction, e.g. from 85% to 70%, would be reflected in an approximate doubling of their systemic bioavailability, e.g. from 15% to 30%, thus greatly increasing their clinical effects. In contrast, for low-clearance drugs, i.e. those with low first-pass extraction, the effect of liver disease on systemic bioavailability depends on the pathway of biotransformation. Thus, for those such as diazepam which undergo cytochrome P-450-mediated oxidation, a liver disease-related decrease in P-450 activity would result in increased systemic bioavailability. Conversely, oxazepam is mainly conjugated to glucuronic acid and excreted by the kidney; as these processes are relatively spared in liver disease, systemic bioavailability of this agent is generally normal. Morphine pharmacokinetics are unusual in that although it is a high-clearance drug, and therefore likely to be affected by liver disease, the studies of Patwardhan *et al.*[3] show that in cirrhosis it is apparently conjugated to glucuronic acid in extrahepatic sites, thus maintaining its relatively normal clearance and its systemic bioavailability despite severely impaired indocyanine green clearance. Changes in binding to plasma proteins may also affect clearance and bioavailability, especially for low-clearance agents.

Given these considerations it is evident that the influence of liver disease and portal-systemic shunting on the bioavailability of a given drug depend on its normal mechanisms of removal and biotransformation, and how these are modified by liver disease in the particular patient. It has become clear, however, that differences in narcotic drug effect do not depend on differences in rates of removal from plasma alone. Rather, there are additional factors, which modulate drug effect at the level of its interaction with its receptor.

For several reasons these *pharmacodynamic* considerations pose a more difficult challenge than the relatively simple matter of quantifying blood levels of a drug. First, there is the need to quantify drug effects, and this involves clinical assessment with its inherent inaccuracies, or more cumbersome but more quantitative approaches such as electroencephalography and psychometrics. Second, methods to quantify the effects of changes in receptor class, receptor number, ligand binding affinity, and the concentration of potentially competing endogenous ligands are methodologically difficult and for practical purposes are approachable only at the experimental level. Finally, it is likely that the biological consequences of the interaction of a drug with its receptor would be subject to influence by many factors, which are also difficult to quantify, affecting signal transduction and other cellular processes[4].

Morphine exemplifies the apparent dissociability of pharmacokinetic from pharmacodynamic factors. Recall that in cirrhosis the systemic bioavailability of morphine is relatively normal because of its extrahepatic glucuronidation. Despite this, Laidlaw *et al.*[5] demonstrated an increased sensitivity to morphine in cirrhotic patients, especially those who previously had encephalopathy. Although morphine clearance data were not provided in this study, other evidence indicates that profound changes in the endorphin system occur in clinical and experimental liver disease.

THE ENDORPHIN SYSTEM

The endorphin system encompases several classes of receptors, agonists, and antagonists, and an understanding of it is complicated by the large number and diversity of experimental approaches employed in studies of it. Necessarily, therefore, this can be only a brief overview of a very broad subject[6,7]. Endorphins were discovered as the result of a search for the natural, endogenous ligands of the receptors which had been shown previously to bind narcotic drugs and thus mediate their pharmacological effects. Endorphins, or endogenous morphine-like compounds, are products of one of three distinct genes, and are derived via cleavage of one of three corresponding large precursor or pro-proteins: (1) pro-opiomelanocortin is the precursor of β-endorphin, and also of β-lipotropin and ACTH; (2) pro-dynorphin is the precursor of dynorphin; and (3) pro-enkephalin the precursor of leucine-enkephalin (leu-enkephalin), methionine-enkephalin (met-enkephalin), and several other enkephalins. These precursor proteins are distributed widely throughout the body, each selectively enriched in certain areas: for example, pro-opiomelanocortin in the anterior pituitary (consistent with β-endorphin co-secretion with ACTH), pro-dynorphin in the posterior pituitary (consistent with dynorphin co-secretion with vasopressin), and pro-enkephalin in peripheral sympathetic ganglia nerves and (consistent with enkephalin co-secretion with catecholamines), the latter presumably including those in the liver itself.

The endorphins are characterized by a common amino-terminal tetrapeptide, and bind to four classes of opioid (i.e. endorphin and narcotic drug) receptors, all of which are coupled to K^+ or Ca^{2+} channels, and all of which bind all ligands, but with differing selectivity. Thus, the μ receptor preferentially binds β-endorphin and morphine, the κ receptor dynorphin, the δ receptor the enkephalins as well as β-endorphin, and the ε receptor β-endorphin. This multiplicity of ligand–receptor interactions participates in the regulation of a wide range of physiological functions, including: (1) water balance, temperature control, and the cardiovascular and respiratory systems; (2) responses to pain and stress, sensory-motor integration and gastrointestinal motility; and (3) appetite, eating behaviour, endocrine control, and intermediary metabolism.

ENDORPHINS IN LIVER DISEASE

The changes in the endorphin system that occur in liver disease not only provide a basis for understanding the pharmacodynamic changes affecting exogenous narcotics, but also contribute to the pathogenesis of the manifestations of the liver disease itself. Thus, Zeneroli *et al.*[8] showed that in dogs subjected to dimethylnitrosamine-induced liver damage and surgical portal-systemic shunt, there was an increase in specific, presumably receptor-mediated, naloxone binding to hypothalamic and cortical membranes, without a change in binding affinity, and that this was accompanied by a decrease in β-endorphin concentrations in both tissues. More recently, Swain *et al.*[9]

showed that plasma endorphin levels increase in rats after bile duct obstruction. Several clinical studies also clearly indicate that important changes in the endorphin system occur in liver disease. For example, plasma concentrations of leucine- and/or methionine-enkephalins are increased in liver diseases, including cirrhosis with ascites[10]. As plasma catecholamine levels are also increased in cirrhotic ascites, it is possible that these changes reflect, at least in part, enkephalin and catecholamine co-secretion from sympathetic nerve terminals. In addition, endorphin receptor antagonists have been shown to have beneficial effects in liver patients: naloxone infusion[11], but not a single dose[12], increases renal Na^+, K^+, creatinine, and osmolal clearance in cirrhotics with ascites, while naloxone[13,14] ameliorates pruritus in patients with primary biliary cirrhosis. There is also a loss of autonomic nerve fibres, presumably including those which secrete endorphins, in apposition to hepatocytes in the regenerating nodules of cirrhotic livers[15]. Thus, there is ample evidence that not only is the endorphin system deranged in liver disease, but also that this system may contribute to the pathophysiology of ascites, pruritus, and other manifestations of acute and chronic liver diseases, including encephalopathy. As a corollary, the deranged endorphin system can be expected to contribute significantly to aberrant responses which may follow the administration of its *exogenous* ligands, i.e. the narcotic drugs.

OPIOIDS, HEPATIC METABOLISM, AND HEPATOTOXICITY

The final issue to be considered is the effect of opioids on the liver itself, including intermediary metabolism and, related to it, hepatotoxicity. In regard to intermediary metabolism, the following paragraphs will focus specifically on the regulation of plasma glucose and free fatty acids (FFA).

Endorphins and intermediary metabolism

Although experimental results are varied and highly dependent on species, agent, dosage, and other parameters, administration of opioids typically causes an acute increase in plasma glucose, reflecting at least in part an increase in hepatic glycogenolysis and gluconeogenesis[16–18]. This response, associated with increased pancreatic glucagon secretion and a variable effect on insulin release, is mediated centrally via the μ class of receptors and by peripheral sympathetic nerves[19], associated with increased adrenal secretion of catecholamines. In addition, a possible paracrine effect of catecholamines and/or enkephalins released from sympathetic nerve terminals in the liver itself[20] is suggested both by the well-known hepatic effects of catecholamines, and by the finding that endorphins are abundant in liver[21] and stimulate glycogenolysis and gluconeogenesis in isolated hepatocytes[22]. Depending on experimental conditions, opioid administration may also cause hypoglycaemia, associated with depletion of hepatic glycogen.

Fatty acid metabolism is also influenced by endorphins. Thus, after opioid administration *in vivo*, plasma FFA, and therefore hepatic fatty acid uptake, are variably increased[19]. This reflects stimulation of adipocyte hormone-sensitive lipase and involves hormonal mechanisms similar to those contributing to glycogenolysis. Significantly, however, the central effect on FFA metabolism is mediated via different opioid receptors, namely μ–δ complexes, or ε[19].

Morphine hepatotoxicity *in vivo*

Just as the metabolic effects of endorphins on the liver are in part centrally mediated, so are important components of the hepatotoxic effects of morphine. Thus, in animal experiments, large doses of morphine cause aminotransferase elevations, sulphobromophthalein (BSP) retention, and diminished hepatic reduced glutathione (GSH)[23–27]. There is also hepatocellular accumulation of fat, in a microvesicular pattern similar to that associated with Reye's syndrome and valproate hepatotoxicity[24], and implying impaired mitochondrial fatty acid β-oxidation. While the mechanism of this effect in morphine hepatotoxicity is not known, stimulation of the hepatic sympathetic nerves has been shown to inhibit mitochondrial fatty acid oxidation and ketogenesis[28]; since this effect is only partially blocked by α-adrenergic antagonists, it is conceivable that it reflects in part a local endorphin effect. In any case, the increase in hepatic uptake of FFA which results from the rise in their plasma concentration, combined with impaired mitochondrial fatty acid β-oxidation, could readily contribute to both the microvesicular fatty liver and the accompanying functional impairment.

Morphine hepatotoxicity *in vivo* is more pronounced when the drug is administered into the cerebral ventricles[26,27,29], and is ameliorated by intracerebroventricular or peripheral administration of μ or δ opioid receptor antagonists within the first hour[24,29,30], implying early involvement of central opioid receptors in hepatotoxicity. Interference with the adrenergic transmission that results from central opioid stimulation is also protective. Thus, spinal cord transection prevents morphine-induced BSP retention[27]. In addition, morphine-induced GSH depletion *in vivo* is ameliorated by α-adrenergic antagonists via a mechanism that does not involve peripheral autonomic nerves or adrenal medullary release of catecholamines, implying that the participating α-adrenergic receptors are central rather than peripheral[26]. The findings in this study also suggest involvement of a hormonal component that includes a permissive effect of adrenal corticosteroids[26]. To what extent this apparently hormonal mediation of centrally induced morphine hepatotoxicity might involve the previously noted changes in fatty acid oxidation and other aspects of intermediary metabolism is unknown.

Morphine hepatotoxicity *in vitro*

Although morphine in the doses employed clinically is mainly conjugated to glucuronic acid, the much larger amounts used in *in vitro* toxicity studies overwhelm this pathway. As a result there is substantial biotransformation to morphinone via the 6-dehydrogenase pathway[31] and, to a lesser extent, to other intermediates via cytochrome P-450-mediated reactions[32,33].

Morphinone and other reactive intermediates form adducts with and thereby deplete cellular stores of reduced glutathione, associated with diminished cell viability[34]. Morphine may also inhibit cytochrome P-450 activity and accelerate turnover of its haem moiety[35]. Interestingly, the structural similarities to morphine that confer endorphin receptor antagonist activity on naloxone and naltrexone also render them inhibitors of morphine biotransformation[31]. As a result these agents ameliorate morphine hepatotoxicity *in vitro* by inhibiting its biotransformation and resulting glutathione consumption, whereas their protective effects *in vivo* primarily involve blockade of central nervous system endorphin receptors.

Thus, morphine hepatotoxicity may be viewed as having at least two components. The first, demonstrable *in vivo*, involves CNS endorphin receptors and adrenergic transmission, and is associated with diminished reduced glutathione as well as disturbed hepatic fatty acid metabolism and microvesicular fat accumulation. The second, demonstrable *in vitro*, reflects depletion of hepatocellular reduced glutathione by reactive intermediates of morphine biotransformation. Morphine antagonists ameliorate toxicity both *in vivo*, via endorphin receptor blockade in the central nervous system, and in the isolated hepatocyte via enzyme inhibition. Other possible effects of altered fatty acid metabolism, especially related to extramitochondrial oxidation, and of reactive drug intermediates are possible and remain to be defined. While overt clinical morphine hepatotoxicity is unusual, it could theoretically account for liver injury during periods of sustained high-dose administration, especially under conditions in which drug biotransformation is induced and glutathione stores are depleted.

SUMMARY AND CONCLUSIONS

In conclusion, both pharmacokinetics and pharmacodynamics of narcotic agents may be abnormal in patients with liver disease. Altered pharmacokinetics (impaired plasma clearance) reflects impaired hepatic extraction and/or biotransformation, may be minimized by use of low clearance agents which are primarily conjugated, and cannot be predicted reliably in individual patients. Altered pharmacodynamics (exaggerated CNS effects) may be present despite normal plasma levels, at least in part reflect liver disease-related changes in the endorphin system, are not predictable in individual patients, and require monitoring of their effects by means of clinical and/or psychometric assessment. Although clinical morphine hepatotoxicity is not common, the investigation of experimental morphine hepatotoxicity has provided new insights into mechanisms of chemically induced liver injury and the effects of opioids on hepatic metabolism. Finally, to the extent that endorphins, catecholamines, and other agents released from intrahepatic nerves modulate metabolism, toxicity, or other intrahepatic events, the impact of the denervation resulting from liver transplantation may be significant. Additional information is needed in this potentially important area.

ACKNOWLEDGEMENTS

This work was supported in part by grants from the National Institutes of Health: Liver Center (1 P30 DK 26743) and individual research grant (1 R37 DK 13328).

References

1. Bass NM, Williams RL. Hepatic function and pharmacokinetics. In: Zakim D, Boyer TD, editors. Hepatology: A Textbook of Liver Disease. Philadelphia: Saunders; 1990:235–54.
2. Pond SM, Tong T, Benowitz NL, Jacob P. Enhanced bioavailability of pethidine and pentazocine in patients with cirrhosis of the liver. Aust NZ J Med. 1980;10:515–19.
3. Patwardhan RV, Johnson RF, Hoyumpa A Jr, Sheehan JJ, Desmond PV, Wilkinson GR, Branch RA, Schenker S. Normal metabolism of morphine in cirrhosis. Gastroenterology. 1981;81:1006–11.
4. Kaiko RF. Relationships between opioid disposition and their pharmacological effects – an overview. Postgrad Med J. 1991;67:S44–9.
5. Laidlaw J, Read A, Sherlock S. Morphine tolerance in hepatic cirrhosis. Gastroenterology. 1961;40:389–96.
6. Akil H, Bronstein D, Mansour A. Overview of the endogenous opioid systems: anatomical, biochemical and functional issues. In: Rodgers RJ, Cooper SJ, editors. Endorphins, Opiates and Behavioural Processes. Chichester: John Wiley & Sons; 1988:1–23.
7. Watson SJ. The endorphin family of opioid peptides: biochemistry, anatomy, and physiology. In:Wyngaarden JB, Smith LH Jr, Bennett JC, editors. Cecil Textbook of Medicine. Philadelphia: Saunders; 1992:1204–6.
8. Zeneroli ML, Ventura E, Pinelli G, Casciarri I, Germini M, Cavalletti E, Tofanetti O, Baraldi M. Opiate receptors and β-endorphin levels in brain areas of dogs with portal-systemic encephalopathy. J Hepatol. 1985;1:619–27.
9. Swain MG, Rothman RB, Xu H, Vergalla J, Bergasa NV, Jones EA. Endogenous opioids accumulate in plasma in a rat model of acute cholestasis. Gastroenterology. 1992;103:630–5.
10. Thornton JR, Losowsky MS. Plasma leucine enkephalin is increased in liver disease. Gut. 1989;30:1392–5.
11. Leehey DJ, Gollapudi P, Deakin A, Reid RW. Naloxone increases water and electrolyte excretion after water loading in patients with cirrhosis and ascites. J Lab Clin Med. 1991;118:484–91.
12. Lee SS, Hadengue A, Moreau R, Girod C, Jiron MI, LeBrec D. Naloxone does not alter haemodynamics in cirrhosis: studies in humans and rats. J Hepatol. 1987;5:149–53.
13. Summerfield JA. Naloxone modulates the perception of itch in man. Br J Clin Pharmacol. 1980;10:180–92.
14. Bergasa NV, Talbot TL, Alling DW, Schmitt JM, Walker EC, Baker BL, Korenman JC, Park Y, Hoofnagle J, Jones EA. A controlled trial of naloxone infusions for the pruritus of chronic cholestasis. Gastroenterology. 1992;102:544–9.
15. Lee JA, Ahmed Q, Hines JE, Burt AD. Disappearance of hepatic parenchymal nerves in human liver cirrhosis. Gut. 1992;33:87–91.
16. Ipp E, Dhorajiwala J, Pugh W, Moossa AR, Rubenstein AH. Effects of an enkephalin analog on pancreatic endocrine function and glucose homeostasis in normal and diabetic dogs. Endocrinology. 1982;111:2110–16.
17. Matsumura M, Fukushima T, Saito H, Saito S. *In vivo* and *in vitro* effects of β-endorphin on glucose metabolism in the rat. Horm Metabol Res. 1984;16:27–31.
18. Ramabadran K, Bansinath M. Glucose homeostasis and endogenous opioid peptides. Int J Clin Pharmacol Ther Toxicol. 1990;28:89–98.
19. Gunion MW, Rosenthal MJ, Morley JE, Miller S, Zib B, Butler B, Moore RD. μ-Receptor mediates elevated glucose and corticosterone after third ventricle injection of opioid peptides. Am J Physiol. 1991;261:R70–81.
20. Bioulac-Sage P, Lafon ME, Saric J, Balabaud C. Nerves and perisinusoidal cells in human liver. J Hepatol. 1990;10:105–12.

21. Khawaja XZ, Green IC, Thorpe JR, Titheradge MA. The occurrence and receptor specificity of endogenous opioid peptides within the pancreas and liver of the rat. Biochem J. 1990;267:233–40.
22. Leach RP, Titheradge MA. The stimulation of glycogenolysis in isolated hepatocytes by opioid peptides. Biochem J. 1986;238:531–5.
23. Chang Y-YH, Ho IK. Effects of acute and continuous morphine administration on serum glutamate oxalacetate transaminase and glutamate pyruvate transaminase activities in the mouse. Biochem Pharmacol. 1979;28:1373–7.
24. Needham WP, Shuster L, Kanel GC, Thompson ML. Liver damage from narcotics in mice. Toxicol Appl Pharmacol. 1981;58:157–70.
25. James RC, Goodman DR, Harbison RD. Hepatic glutathione and hepatotoxicity: changes induced by selected narcotics. J Pharmacol Exp Ther. 1982;221:708–14.
26. Roberts SM, Skoulis NP, James RC. A centrally-mediated effect of morphine to diminish hepatocellular glutathione. Biochem Pharmacol. 1987;36:3001–5.
27. Hurwitz A, Looney G, Sullins M, Ben-Zvi Z. Hepatobiliary effects of morphine are mediated in the brain. Hepatology. 1990;12:1406–12.
28. Beuers U, Beckh K, Jungermann K. Control of ketogenesis in the perfused rat liver by the sympathetic innervation. Eur J Biochem. 1986;158:19–24.
29. James RC, Wessinger WD, Roberts SM, Millner GC, Paule MG. Centrally mediated opioid induced depression of hepatic glutathione: effects of intracerebroventricular administration of mu, kappa, sigma and delta agonists. Toxicology. 1988;51:267–79.
30. Hurwitz A, Fischer HR, Innis JD, Ronsse S, Ben-Zvi Z. Opioid effects on hepatic disposition of dyes in mice. J Pharmacol Exp Ther. 1985;232:617–23.
31. Nagamatsu K, Ohno Y, Ikebuchi H, Takahashi A, Terao T, Takanaka A. Morphine metabolism in isolated rat hepatocytes and its implications for hepatotoxicity. Biochem Pharmacol. 1986;35:3543–8.
32. Correia M, Wong J, Solivan E. Morphine metabolism revisited. I. Metabolic activation of morphine to a reactive species in rats. Chem Biol Interactions. 1984;49:255–68.
33. Ohno Y, Nagamatsu K, Kawanishi T, Ikebuchi H, Terao T, Takanaka A. Comparative evaluation of different pathways for the liver toxicity of morphine using freshly isolated hepatocytes. Biochem Pharmacol. 1988;37:2862–3.
34. Eklow-Lastbom L, Moldeus P, Orrenius S. On the mechanisms of glutathione depletion in hepatocytes exposed to morphine and ethylmorphine. Toxicology. 1986;42:13–21.
35. Gurantz D, Correia MA. Morphine-mediated effects on rat hepatic heme and cytochrome P-450 *in vivo*. Biochem Pharmacol. 1981;30:1529–36.

Section VIII

Extrahepatic manifestations of genetic liver diseases

25

Alpha-1-antitrypsin deficiency

F. CALLEA, G. FABBRETTI, M. BONETTI, M. BRISIGOTTI and V. J. DESMET

INTRODUCTION

Genetic alpha-1-antitrypsin deficiency (AATD) may result from impaired secretion, intracellular degradation or lack of synthesis of the molecule. Impaired secretion in turn results in intracellular accumulation and liver disease.

In this chapter we review the main experimental work carried out to unravel the molecular pathology of AAT storage and the mechanisms of liver cell damage in AATD.

AAT represents a unique model for analysing the polymorphism of protein secretion; the classical AAT deficiency variant has served as a prototype for clarifying intrahepatic protein retention and accumulation, contributing enormously to the development of the concept 'endoplasmic reticulum storage diseases'. The topic is reviewed under the following headings:

1. Biochemical and molecular properties of AAT.
2. Genetic variants of AAT.
3. Molecular pathology of AAT storage.
4. Morphology of AAT storage in hepatocytes.
5. The 'recruitment-secretory block' ('R-SB') phenomenon.
6. Endoplasmic reticulum storage diseases (ERSD).
7. Models for ERSD.
8. Mechanisms of liver damage in AATD.
9. AATD and hepatocellular carcinoma.
10. AAT in cells other than hepatocytes: the polymorphism of protein secretion.
11. The diagnosis of AATD.

BIOCHEMICAL AND MOLECULAR PROPERTIES OF AAT

AAT is a highly polymorphic secretory, acute-phase reactant protein with more than 75 electrophoretic variants. The AAT phenotype is determined by codominant expression of two parental alleles; the two alleles are expressed independently and each AAT molecule in the serum functions autonomously.

AAT is a 52 kD plasma glycoprotein with 394 amino acid residues and three oligosaccharide side-chains[1]. It is the major effector (90%) of the protease inhibitory capacity of serum. The AAT gene is expressed in several cell lines, the two major sites being hepatocytes and the mononuclear phagocyte cell family. The hepatocytes contain approximately 200-fold more AAT mRNA transcripts per cell than do mononuclear phagocytes (including blood monocytes and alveolar macrophages).

The biosynthesis pathway is typical of a secretory glycoprotein: AAT is synthesized in the liver from a 1.75 kb mRNA that is translated and the resulting polypeptide discharged into the rough endoplasmic reticulum (RER) as a 418 amino acid precursor protein containing a 24 residue signal peptide. N-linked carbohydrates are added to each of the three asparaginyl residues (Asn 46, Asn 83, Asn 247). The protein is translocated to the smooth endoplasmic reticulum (SER) where the high mannose carbohydrates are trimmed, and further to the Golgi apparatus where sialic acid is added. The fully glycosylated AAT is secreted as a mature protein of 394 amino acids.

The active site of the molecule is centred at residue Met 358, a part of a highly stressed, external loop protruding from the molecule.

AAT is capable of inhibiting a variety of proteases, including trypsin, chymotrypsin, thrombin, kallikrein, plasmin, acrosin and especially the neutrophil elastase.

GENETIC VARIANTS OF AAT

The AAT structural gene locus has been mapped to the q31–32.3 region of human chromosome 14[2] and is designated Pi (protease inhibitor). The AAT gene has three non-coding introns and four coding exons[3]. According to Brantly *et al.*[4] the AAT variants are grouped in:

1. normal alleles, with serum levels in the normal range (150–350 mg/dl);
2. deficient alleles, with serum levels lower than normal, which may or may not function normally;
3. null alleles in which no AAT in the serum can be attributed to the gene;
4. dysfunctional alleles, with normal amounts of non-functioning AAT.

The common normal variants are defined by an allelic frequence of over 10% and include M1 to M8[5]. Several normal and abnormal variants have been identified on the basis of isoelectric focusing (IF); each of them carries the name of the town where it was originally described. All sequenced variants and those with a partially known sequence have been recently reviewed[6]. Low plasma levels in AATD may result from hepatocytic storage, intracellular degradation or lack of synthesis.

Intracellular degradation occurs with the S variant; the substitution Glu–Val 264 probably causes a less stable protein which is more susceptible to intracisternal proteolysis. Lack of synthesis is characteristic for the Pi Null due either to a stop codon[8] or to large deletion[9].

Hepatocytic storage occurs with the common deficiency variant, the Z AAT, and with a few rare variants, i.e. M-like (among others Mmalton) and S-like[6] (among others Siiyama)[7].

MOLECULAR PATHOLOGY OF AAT STORAGE

The Z, Mmalton and Siiyama suffer from a molecular abnormality at the level of crucial points of the molecule. The Z mutation (glutamic acid at position 342 substituted by lysine) involves an amino acid at the base of the reactive centre loop of the molecule, resulting in the formation of insoluble polymers in the ER of hepatocytes, by interaction between the reactive centre loop of one molecule and the gap in the A-sheet of another[8]. Mmalton and Siiyama have gross mutation at position 52/53 (respectively deletion of Phe and Ser–Phe substitution) which cause polymerization and accumulation via a similar loop-sheet mechanism to that seen with the Z variant.

MORPHOLOGY OF AAT STORAGE IN HEPATOCYTES

Histological sections from PiZ, PiM-like, PiS-like livers show intracytoplasmic round eosinophilic inclusions, surrounded by a clear halo, eventually with a dark haematoxylinophilic dot at the centre. These inclusions are better visualized with PAS staining followed by diastase digestion, and are positively stained with a specific anti-AAT polyclonal antibody. Monoclonal antibodies specific to Z AAT do not stain M- or S-like variants[6,11]. The dark dots of AAT inclusions correspond to calcium precipitates[26].

Ultrastructurally, AAT appears as an amorphous material within dilated cisternae of the rough endoplasmic reticulum (RER). The amorphous material may be either fluffy, semi-electron-dense or more compact and dense. Very dark electron-dense, granular or crystalline precipitates can be found in some inclusions.

In a few PiZZ newborns and in about 25% of the heterozygous individuals (PiMZ), PAS diastase inclusions may be absent; however, appropriate immunohistochemistry invariably allows the recognition of AAT storage[9].

THE ‘RECRUITMENT-SECRETORY BLOCK’ (‘R-SB’) PHENOMENON

The heterozygous PiMZ phenotype is of particular interest from both a clinical and biological point of view. Individuals with this phenotype may have normal serum AAT levels under conditions of clinical stimulation, thus being virtually undetectable on the basis of the sole quantitative determination in serum. In contrast, under the same conditions they can be detected by immunohistochemical examination of liver tissue specimens because of the 'R-SB' phenomenon[10].

PiMM (normal homozygous) individuals synthesize two pools of M AAT which are regularly exported into plasma. PiZZ (abnormal homozygous) subjects synthesize two pools of Z AAT, which are retained within the cell resulting in hepatocytic storage and plasma deficiency. PiMZ individuals show partial AAT deficiency under basal conditions because the Z fraction of AAT is retained within the cell (Fig. 1a). When the liver is stimulated to synthesize acute-phase proteins including AAT, the M fraction is regularly exported, thus elevating the serum levels up to the normal range, while the Z fraction is retained in the hepatocytes (Fig. 1b).

Paradoxically, it follows that in PiMZ individuals the highest serum AAT levels may coincide with the maximal degree of storage. Under basal conditions AAT storage occurs in periportal (acinar zone 1) hepatocytes, which represent the 'routine' or 'professional' AAT synthesizing parenchymal cells, while under stimulation, AAT storage occurs in all hepatocytes, including the midlobular (zone 2) and centrilobular (zone 3) cells.

The staining pattern for AAT differs in the various acinar zones: in zone 1 it appears in the form of globules or granules in the entire cytoplasm (type I positivity); in zone 2 and 3 it appears in the form of granules marginated towards the cell periphery in crescent or rectilinear double rows along the sinusoids (type II positivity).

Whatever the type of positivity, ultrastructurally, AAT is always detected in the RER. As zone 2 and 3 hepatocytes represent newly recruited cells for AAT synthesis, the RER location of the newly synthesized AAT indicates that storage occurs at a very early stage of synthesis, and that translocation from the RER to the smooth endoplasmic reticulum (SER) does not take place (Fig. 2). The PAS diastase staining of AAT in the RER depicts the carbohydrate content, thus suggesting that the 'core' glycosylation is normally performed.

The immunostaining pattern of AAT correlates with the amount and the distribution of the RER in the normal human liver, according to lobular gradients[10] (Fig. 3). In newly recruited cells under conditions of clinical

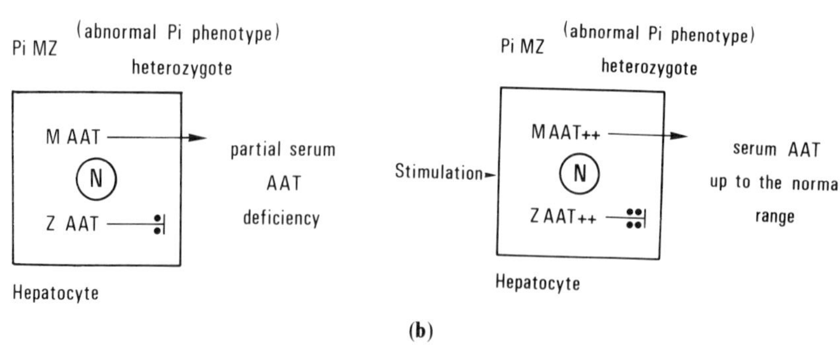

(a) (b)

Fig. 1 Under basal conditions PiMZ phenotype shows partial serum AAT deficiency (**a**); under stimulatory conditions there is simultaneous serum AAT elevation and increasing liver storage (**b**)

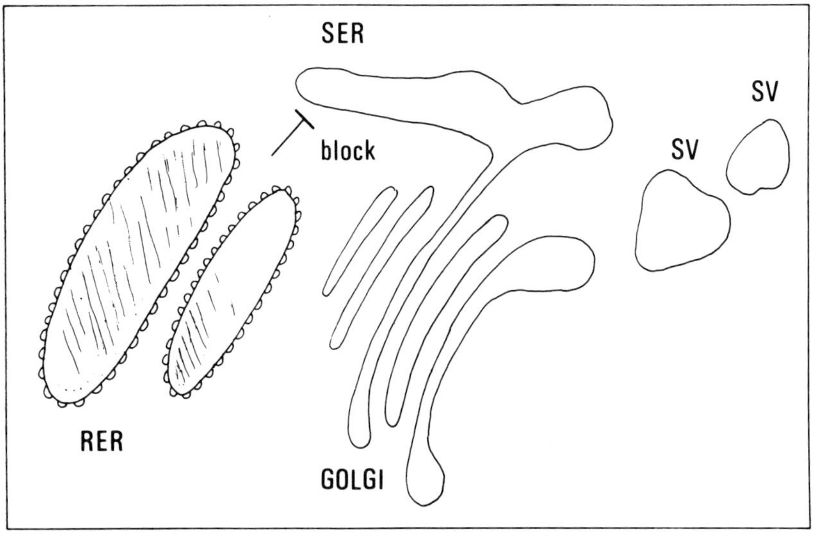

Hepatocyte

Fig. 2 Schematic representation of the concept ERSD: defective translocation of the mutant protein from the RER to the SER

stimulation, immunohistochemistry depicts the Z fraction of AAT which, due to the secretory block, is retained within the cell. For this reason the staining pattern illustrated in Fig. 3 is considered to be an expression of both recruitment of new hepatocytes and secretory block of the protein ('R-SB' phenomenon).

AAT inclusions remain negative on immunostaining for other secretory proteins. In PiMZ individuals, identical staining results are obtained with either a polyclonal anti-AAT or a monoclonal anti-Z AAT antibody. The latter observations prove definitely that the storage process selectively and exclusively affects the Z fraction of AAT.

The monoclonal anti-Z AAT antibody does not stain the retained M-like AAT[11], thus confirming that M-like mutations differ from that of PiZ[6].

To summarize, the 'R-SB' phenomenon allows a number of considerations:

1. All hepatocytes within the hepatic lobule are able to synthesize AAT, but they exert this function to different degrees, according to lobular gradients and the intensity of stimuli.
2. The recruitment of additional hepatocytes for the synthesis of AAT progresses through the lobule according to a portal–central gradient.
3. AAT storage occurs not only in periportal hepatocytes, as was previously thought, but in all hepatocytes throughout the entire lobule, with an immunohistochemical pattern that differs in the various acinar zones.
4. Staining patterns reveal the extent of engagement of the liver in the synthesis and the extent of derangement of the liver in the secretion of AAT.

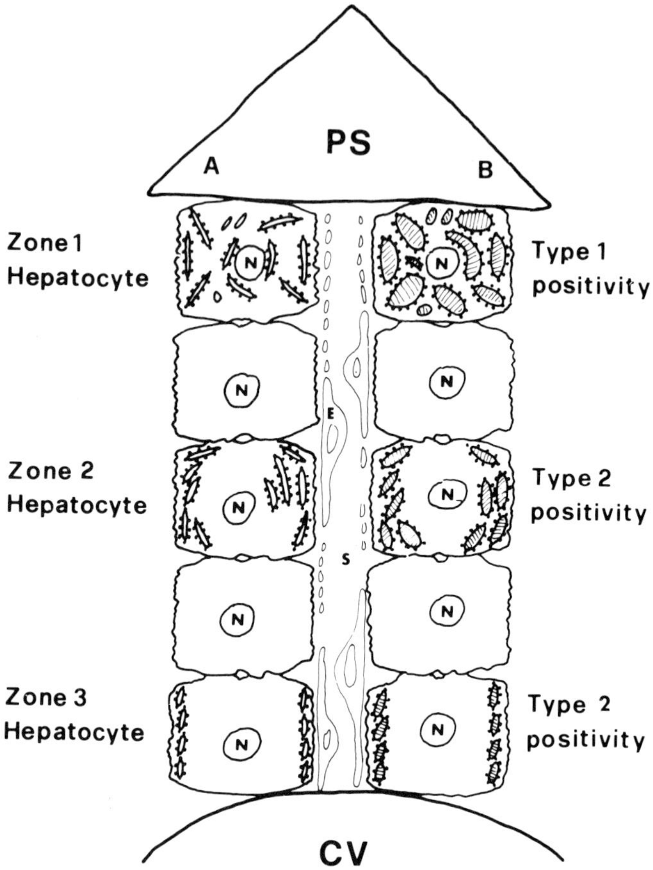

Fig. 3 Schematic representation of the amount and distribution of the RER (left liver cell muralium) and of the immunostaining pattern for AAT (right liver cell muralium), in the various acinar zones, according to a portal central gradient

5. Stimulation of the liver for AAT synthesis unavoidably results in increasing intracellular storage in PiZ individuals. This should discourage any attempt to induce an elevation of the serum levels of the Pi by drug (or any means) via an increased rate of synthesis without a parallel increase in the secretion rate of the Z protein.
6. The immunohistochemical staining patterns of the hepatocytes depend on the localization of the cells in the acinus, and reflect the amount and the distribution of the RER in the hepatic acinus.
7. In PiMZ individuals the storage phenomenon affects exclusively and selectively the Z fraction of AAT.
8. Immunohistochemistry is more sensitive than PAS diastase staining as the screening technique for AATD.
9. Translocation of the Z AAT from the RER to the SER is defective.

10. The Z AAT, retained in the RER, is glycosylated. In addition, the 'R-SB' is a basic biological phenomenon which presumably applies to other secretory proteins suffering from mutations which result in molecular abnormalities and insolubility in the cisternal milieu.

ENDOPLASMIC RETICULUM STORAGE DISEASES (ERSD)

The Z variant of AAT has served as a prototype for analysing intrahepatic protein retention and accumulation. The 'R-SB' phenomenon has contributed especially to the concept of endoplasmic reticulum storage diseases, and to its definition, i.e. 'inborn errors of metabolism affecting secretory proteins and resulting in hepatocytic storage and plasma deficiency. The storage phenomenon is due to a molecular abnormality that hinders the translocation from the RER to the SER. The storage is selective and exclusive for the mutant protein. The molecular abnormality is genetically determined, hence it is hereditary, congenital, familiar and permanent'[12].

A number of disorders analogous to AATD have now been identified[13]: fibrinogen storage in hereditary hypofibrinogenaemia[14,15], congenital deficiency of alpha-1-antichymotrypsin[16], alpha-2-antiplasmin deficiency[17] and the Lebanese low-density lipoprotein receptor defect[18].

MODELS FOR ERSD

A spontaneous disease in commercially grown turkeys characterized by pronounced cardiac dilation and, therefore, named round-heart disease, was first described in 1962[19]. Later it was observed that turkeys with spontaneous heart disease developed PAS-positive diastase-resistant globules in hepatocytes, and had either low plasma trypsin inhibitory capacity or hyperproteinaemia and serum alpha-globulin deficiency. These turkeys were proposed as a model for the study of AAT deficiency in humans[20].

Subsequent studies on furazolidine-induced round-heart disease in turkeys proved that the intrahepatocytic inclusions containing AAT were located not in the RER but in the lysosomes. Whatever the mechanisms for AAT storage in the turkey, the lysosomal localization points to a basically different defect than the human AATD.

Chronic galactosamine administration in rats depresses plasma trypsin inhibitory capacity and decreases plasma AAT concentration. In addition, galactosamine induces the formation of PAS-positive granules containing AAT, thus suggesting a similarity to the genetically determined AAT in humans[20]. It is not known whether, in the galactosamine model, AAT retention represents a selective and exclusive phenomenon, or whether AAT retention occurs in the RER.

Recently transgenic mice have been generated that bear a DNA construct containing the human structural gene for normal PiM AAT[22]. Immunohistochemical techniques combined with specific RNA analysis have shown that transgenic mice express AAT in multiple tissues[22] and analogous to the situation in humans[23]. Transgenic mice containing the human gene of Z AAT develop the ERSD as they accumulate the Z AAT in the RER[24]. The transgenic mice represent an extremely interesting model because they simultaneously express the endogenous normal AAT gene and the exogenous abnormal Z gene. One would expect from them a recapitulation of the experiment of nature[23] in humans, and further validation of the 'R-SB' phenomenon, originally described in human PiMZ phenotype individuals[10].

MECHANISMS OF LIVER DAMAGE IN AATD

The PiZZ condition is associated with neonatal cholestasis and hepatitis, childhood cirrhosis, juvenile pulmonary enphysema, and liver cirrhosis in adults. The heterozygous (PiMZ) condition also predisposes adults to the development of chronic hepatitis and cryptogenic cirrhosis. Both homozygotes and heterozygotes carry an increased risk for hepatocellular carcinoma (HCC)[24].

The mechanisms for liver damage in AATD are still unknown. There is no association with alcohol abuse or infectious agents. The insufficient neutralization of bacterial or intestinal proteases has been invoked as the main factor in severely deficient newborns[25]. A direct toxicity to the cell of the stored AAT is suggested ultrastructurally.

In addition to the classical electron microscopic appearance, i.e. fluffy, semi-electron-dense material (type a), AAT inclusions may acquire a very dense, compact and mummified appearance. The latter inclusions (type b) resemble intracellular stones and are associated with disruption of ER membranes (Fig. 4). Also apoptotic bodies (so-called Councilman bodies) stuffed with AAT, contain inclusions with a mummified appearance[23] (Fig. 5).

A variable number of inclusions, either fluffy or mummified, show a central core made up by dark, very electron-dense, granular or crystalline precipitates corresponding to calcium (Fig. 6)[26]. Disturbances in calcium homeostasis from whatever reason may trigger membrane alterations, organelle damage and cell death[26].

When examining successive biopsies from AATD patients one may observe fluctuating degrees of storage. Moreover, after portacaval shunt, cirrhotic PiZ livers may show a marked reduction in AAT storage[23,27], the vast majority of the retained protein corresponding to type b inclusions. These observations appear to indicate that AAT retained in the form of fluffy material can be progressively released, albeit more slowly than the normal AAT or, alternatively, that it can undergo intracisternal degradation. In contrast, the mummified 'stone-like' appearance reflects the impossibility of further translocation or degradation and consequently permanent segregation. Genetic engineering strategies should be addressed to suppressing the accumulation of the polymerized AAT or to allow the retained protein to be degraded.

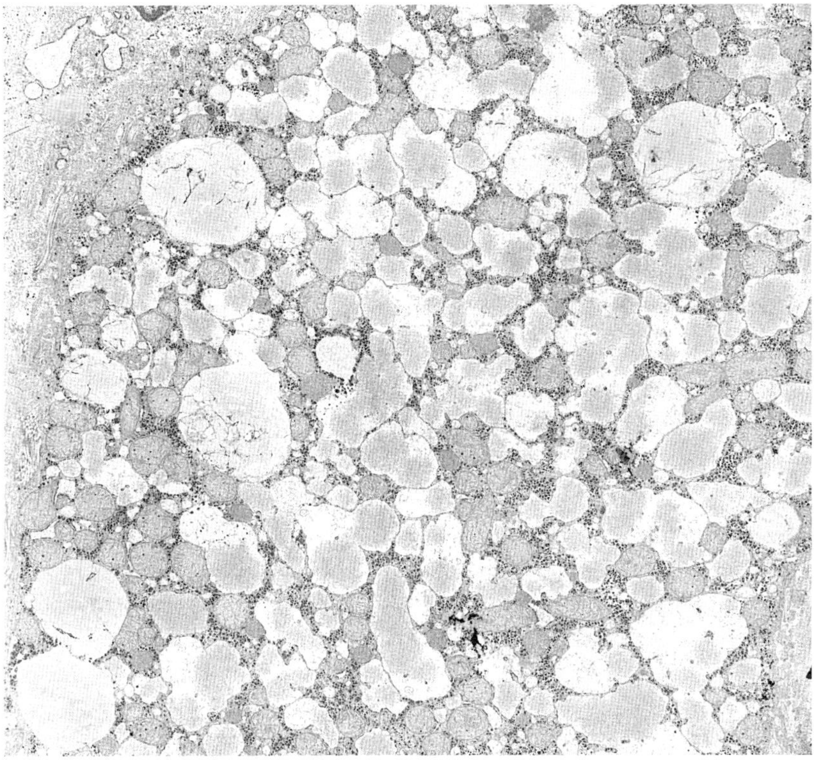

Fig. 4 The electron microphotograph shows type a and b AAT inclusions. Type b (dense, compact material) is associated with ER membrane disruption

AATD AND HEPATOCELLULAR CARCINOMA (HCC)

AATD patients are at high risk of developing HCC. Surprisingly, when PiZ individuals develop HCC, the tumour cells do not express (and consequently do not store) AAT, while non-tumorous hepatocytes continue to accumulate the Z AAT[28]. A similar phenomenon is known to occur in haemochromatosis with regard to iron storage. It is therefore speculated that during neoplastic transformation, in both metabolic disorders, hepatocytes may 'switch' their phenotype.

AAT IN CELLS OTHER THAN HEPATOCYTES: THE POLYMORPHISM OF PROTEIN SECRETION

It is common for histopathologists to obtain a negative hepatocytic staining for AAT in liver tissue specimens from normal PiM individuals. This happens because the normal M AAT is synthesized by hepatocytes and rapidly

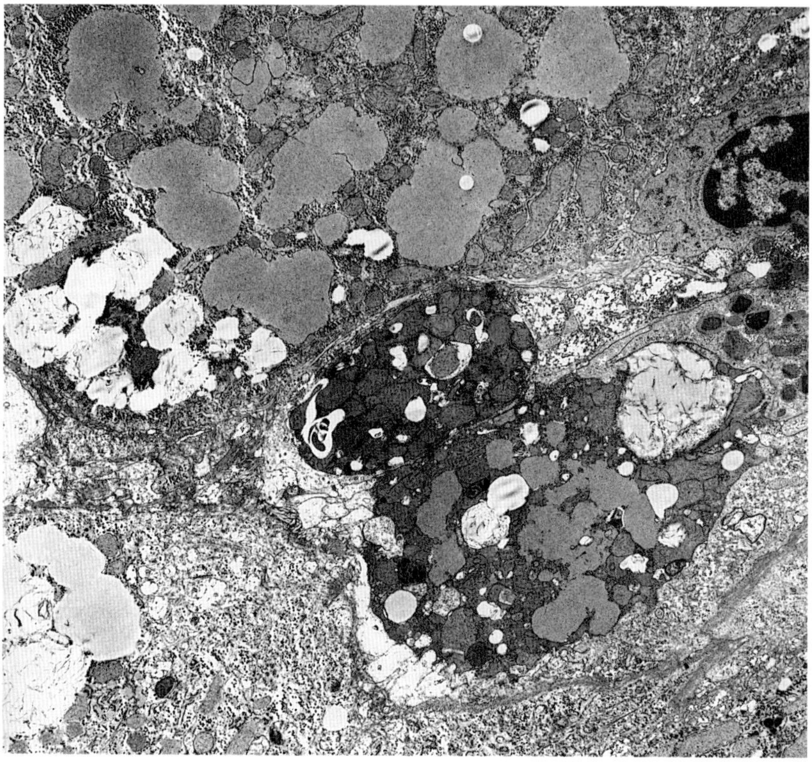

Fig. 5 An apoptotic parenchymal liver cell with dark appearance of the cytosol and condensed organelles, shows also mummified AAT within ER cisternae

exported, so that the intracellular concentration is usually very low and remains below the sensitivity of currently available detection techniques.

In the same tissue sections from PiM livers, immunohistochemistry for AAT gives a positive staining in Kupffer cells. Likewise, AAT can be demonstrated immunohistochemically in several tissues and cell lines from PiM individuals, including yolk sac, the monocyte–macrophage system, Paneth cells and mast cells, megakaryocytes, polymorphonuclear leucocytes, endocrine and paracrine cells in pancreas and gastrointestinal tract, sperm and renal proximal tubule cells[23].

Unequivocal signs of AAT storage in PiZ individuals have been found in cells of the intrahepatic biliary tree[29], in pancreatic islets[30] and in Kupffer cells[23]. However, in contrast to hepatocytes (all of which may undergo signs of AAT storage according to the intensity of the 'R-SB' phenomenon), only a limited number of biliary, pancreatic or Kupffer cells show storage of Z AAT. The latter observation would point to a different synthesis rate, fate and function of AAT in the various cells. Hepatocytes secrete AAT into the

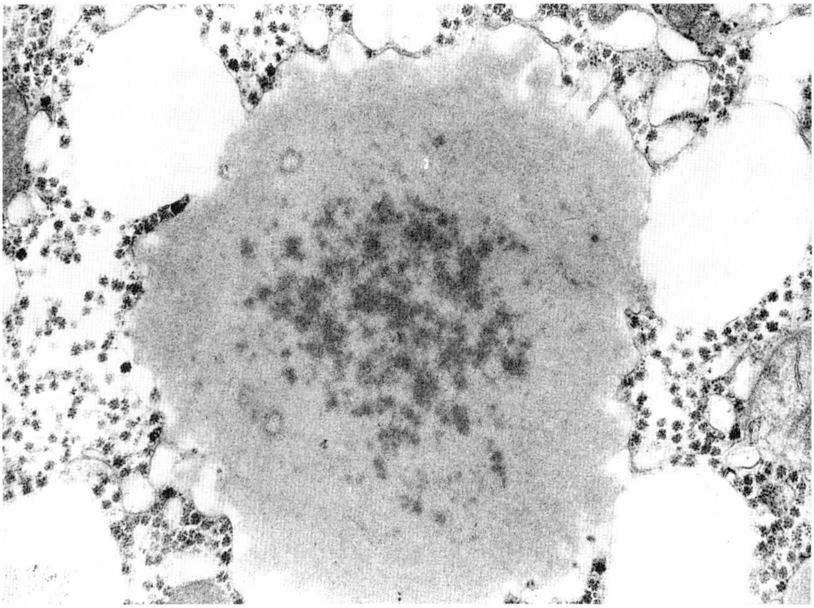

Fig. 6 AAT inclusion in the RER with a fluffy appearance and very dark electron-dense precipitates corresponding to calcium

blood; apparently they are the sole source for serum AAT. This is indirectly proven by the observation that PiZ individuals permanently acquire the donor's phenotype in serum after liver transplantation from a PiM graft[31]. Furthermore, the liver seems to be the exclusive target for acute-phase stimuli, as documented by the occurrence of the 'R-SB' phenomenon.

Biliary cells are likely to secrete AAT into bile via the conventional secretory pathway. AAT is indeed a normal component of human bile. Part of AAT, however, reaches the biliary lumen, moving as an AAT-dimeric IgA complex through the epithelium (Fig. 7).

Biliary cells do not respond to acute-phase stimuli and therefore are not predisposed to the 'R-SB' phenomenon. Macrophages (including Kupffer cells) dispose of secretory proteins in a way which differs from that of most epithelial cells, and as such are not responsive to acute-phase stimuli.

In Kupffer cells AAT may be coupled to proteases, similar to what happens in polymorphs, mast cells, and Paneth cells, thus probably protecting the cells from autodigestion by forming protease–antiprotease complexes (Fig. 8).

The presence of AAT in endocrine cells suggests a specific function. AAT in these cells may serve as an intraorganellar inhibitor of the proteolytic enzymes which activate prohormones into hormones by cleaving the secretory product, thus having a major regulatory role in hormone synthesis.

In sperm cells, AAT staining corresponds to the morphology of the acrosome[23]. In that location, AAT might inactivate the acrosomal proteolytic enzyme (acrosin), which allows sperm cells to penetrate the zona pellucida of the ovum, thus playing a role in capacitation and fertilization.

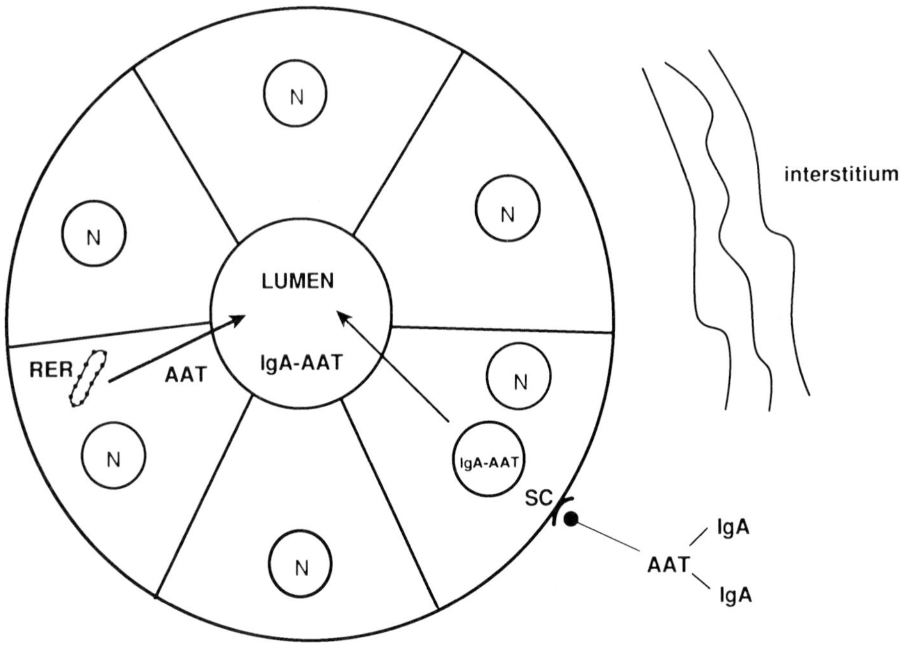

Fig. 7 Schematic representation of AAT secretion in bile and other excretory ducts. Primarily synthesized AAT is directly secreted into the lumen. Further amounts of AAT by-pass the epithelial cells bound to dimeric IgA

At present AAT is believed to have known biological functions in coagulation and fibrinolysis, immune response, cell proliferation, inflammation and tissue damage as extracellular Pi[32]. The presence of AAT in cells (other than hepatocytes) which synthesize but do not secrete the protein, raises the question of the significance of the intracellular AAT. AAT can be sent to organelles such as lysosomes by two alternative pathways: the pathway of cytoplasmic or the pathway of secretory proteins.

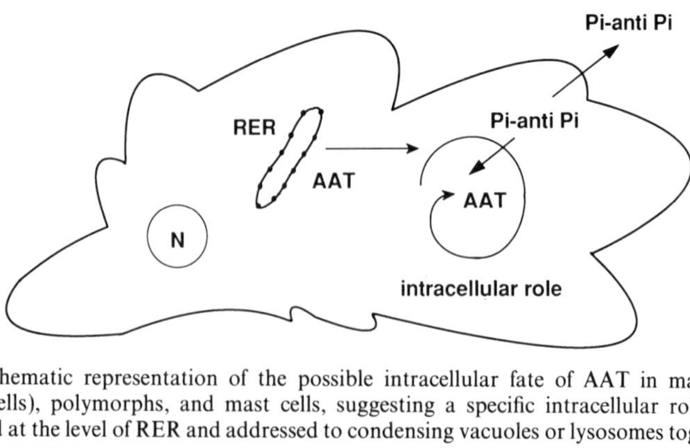

Fig. 8 Schematic representation of the possible intracellular fate of AAT in macrophages (Kupffer cells), polymorphs, and mast cells, suggesting a specific intracellular role. AAT is synthesized at the level of RER and addressed to condensing vacuoles or lysosomes together with proteolytic enzymes

The former are synthesized by free ribosomes and possess a 'primary organellar addressing signal' responsible for the post-translational transfer[33] through the cytosol to the organelles. The presence of a Pi in the cytosol of cells rich in proteolytic enzymes represents a potential protective mechanism against the possible intracellular action of these enzymes. Alternatively, AAT may reach the lysosomes via the intracisternal route as a secretory protein. At the GERL step the Pi would undergo a sorting-out process[33] and, instead of being exported, might be diverted towards the lysosomes to form complexes with proteases[34,35].

The control of proteolytic activity within cells and organelles opens new perspectives for the physiology of intracellular AAT. The protean behaviour of this polymorphic and multifunctional protein in various cells is summarized in the scheme (Fig. 9). For the sake of completeness the scheme also refers to the possibility that AAT is taken up from the circulation by specialized tissue and cells (e.g. kidney), for degradation.

THE DIAGNOSIS OF AATD

The Z gene of AAT can be identified with absolute certainty, irrespective of the serum level or the presence of hepatocytic inclusions, by serum ELISA[36] or in liver tisue by using the monoclonal anti-Z AAT[36] antibody immunohistochemically[11]. Besides being 100% specific, the ELISA system is far more sensitive than IF. In the same Swedish population 7.6% were found to carry the Z gene using ELISA, compared to 4.8% using IF[37]. Since results with polyclonal anti-AAT antibodies correlate fairly well with IF

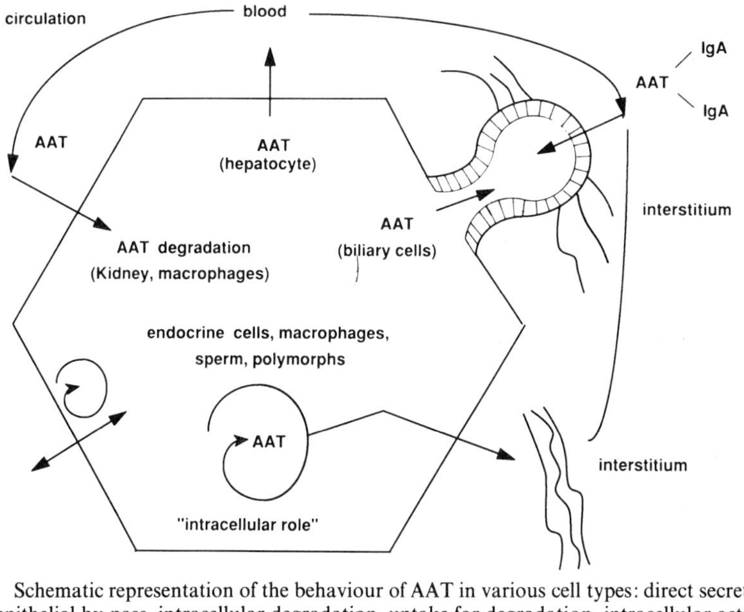

Fig. 9 Schematic representation of the behaviour of AAT in various cell types: direct secretion, trans-epithelial by-pass, intracellular degradation, uptake for degradation, intracellular activity

results[9,10], it is hoped that the monoclonal anti-Z AAT antibody will also increase the sensitivity of immunohistochemistry.

The monoclonal antibody can be extremely useful for identifying Z gene carriers in retrospective (both autopsy and biopsy) studies in patients for whom serum samples are not available. The monoclonal anti-Z AAT antibody is also crucial in suggesting M-like or S-like variants in the presence of hepatocytic AAT inclusions which do not react with the monoclonal anti-Z antibody.

Recently a variant of AAT has been described, characterized by a M2 M2 pattern on IF, severe plasma deficiency and massive liver storage of AAT (M-Cagliari)[11]. The monoclonal anti-ZAAT did not stain AAT inclusions in that patient, thus suggesting that the molecular abnormality in PiMcagliari differs from that of PiZ. By using immunohistochemical techniques and DNA analysis it has been possible to confirm that Mcagliari has antigenic and genetic properties other than the Z AAT[6]. A further M-like variant, the Mmalton, has now been characterized and its molecular abnormality[38] consists of a deletion at Phe 52. Recent progress in molecular biology and genetics has therefore made it possible to diagnose the Z gene as well as M-like and S-like variants by enzymatic amplification of human genomic DNA and direct sequencing of polymerase chain reaction products[39,40].

ACKNOWLEDGEMENTS

The authors thank Mrs L. Van Reykel, L. Salvi and F. Malaguti for technical assistance; Mr M. Rooseleers, R. Damiani and L. Camusso for preparing microphotographs, and Mrs M. Fereccio for editorial assistance. The work was supported by a grant from the Ministero della Sanità (Ricerca Finalizzata) and Istituto G. Gaslini (Ricerca Corrente).

References

1. Carrell RW, Jeppsson JO, Laurell LB *et al.* Structure and variation of human alpha-1-antitrypsin. Nature. 1982;298:329–34.
2. Rabin M, Watson M, Kidd V, Woo SLC, Breg WR, Ruddle FH. Regional location of alpha-1-antichymotrypsin and alpha-1-antitrypsin genes on human chromosome 14. Somatic Cell Mol Genet. 1986;12:209–14.
3. De Simone V, Ciliberto G, Hardon E, Paonessa G, Palla F, Lundberg L, Cortese R. *Cis* and *trans*-acting elements responsible for the cell specific expression of the human alpha-1-antitrypsin gene. EMBO J. 1987;6:2759–66.
4. Brantly M, Nukiwa T, Crystal RG. Molecular basis of alpha-1-antitrypsin deficiency. Am J Med. 1988;84:13–31.
5. Weidinger S. Reliable phenotyping of alpha-1-antitrypsin by hybrid isoelectric focusing in an ultranarrow immobilized pH gradient. Electrophoresis. 1992;13(4):234–9.
6. Fabbretti G, Sergi C, Consalez GG, Faa G, Brisigotti M, Romeo G, Callea F. Genetic variants of alpha-1-antitrypsin. Liver. 1992(special issue);12:296–301.
7. Seyama K, Nukiwa T, Takabe K, Takahashi M, Miyake K, Kira S. Siiyama (serine 53 (TCC) to phenylalanine 53 (TTC)). A new alpha-1-antitrypsin deficiency variant with mutation on a predicted conserved residue of the serpin backbone. J Biol Chem. 1991;266:12627–32.

8. Lomas DA, Evans DLI, Finch JT, Carrell RW. The mechanism of Z alpha-1-antitrypsin accumulation in the liver. Nature. 1992;357:605–7.
9. Callea F, Fevery J, De Groote J, Desmet VJ. Detection of PiZ phenotype individuals by alpha-1-antitrypsin (AAT) immunohistochemistry in paraffin embedded liver tissue specimens. J Hepatol. 1986;2:389–401.
10. Callea F, Fevery J, Massi G, Lievens C, De Groote J, Desmet VJ. Alpha-1-antitrypsin and its stimulation in the liver of PiMZ phenotype individuals. A 'recruitment-secretory block' (R-SB) phenomenon. Liver. 1984;4:325–37.
11. Callea F, Brisigotti M, Faa G, Lucini L, Eriksson S. Identification of PiZ gene products in liver tissue by a monoclonal antibody specific for the Z mutant of alpha-1-antitrypsin. J Hepatol. 1991;12:372–6.
12. Callea F, Desmet VJ. Endoplasmic reticulum storage diseases. In Fenoglio-Preiser *et al.*, editors. Progress in surgical pathology. Philadelphia PN: Field and Wood Med Publ 1993;13:in press.
13. Carlson J, Eriksson S. Alpha-1-antitrypsin and other acute phase reactants in liver disease. Acta Med Scand. 1980;207:79–83.
14. Pfeifer V, Ormans W, Klinge O. Hepatocellular fibrinogen storage in familiar hypofibrinogenemia. Virchows Arch (Cell Pathol.). 1981;36:247–55.
15. Callea F, De Vos R, Pinackat J, Fiaccavento S, Albertini A, Henschen A, Desmet VJ. Hereditary hypofibrinogenemia with hepatic storage of fibrinogen. A new endoplasmic reticulum storage disease. In: Lowe GDO *et al.*, editors. Fibrinogen 2: biochemistry, physiology and clinical relevance. Amsterdam: Elsevier; 1987:75–78.
16. Lindmark B, Millward-Sadler, Callea F, Eriksson S. Hepatocyte inclusions of alpha-1-antichymotrypsin in a patient with partial deficiency of alpha-1-antichymotrypsin and chronic liver disease. Histopathology. 1990;16:221–5.
17. Miura O, Hirosawa S, Kato A. Molecular basis of cogenital deficiency of alpha-2-plasma inhibitor. J Clin Invest. 1989;83:1598–604.
18. Lehrman MA, Schneider WJ, Brown MS. The Lebanese allele at the low density lipoprotein receptor locus: Nonsense mutation produces truncated receptor that is retained in endoplasmic reticulum. J Biol Chem. 1987;262:401–10.
19. Magwood SE, Bray DF. Disease condition of turkey faults characterized by enlarged and rounded hearts. Can J Comp Med. 1962;26:268–72.
20. Newmann FR, Meiron D, Rattner Z. Alpha-1-antitrypsin deficiency: animal model: round heart disease of turkey. Am J Pathol. 1976;84:427–30.
21. Balmer S, Kleinerman J. Isolation and characterization of alpha-1-antitrypsin in PAS-positive hepatic granules from rats with experimental alpha-1-antitrypsin deficiency. Am J Pathol. 1986;123:377–89.
22. Carlson J, Rogers BB, Sifers RN. Multiple tissues express alpha-1-antitrypsin in transgenic mice and man. J Clin Invest. 1988;82:26–36.
23. Callea F. Immunohistochemical study on alpha-1-antitrypsin. PhD thesis, Leuven, Acco. 1983;1–153.
24. Eriksson S, Carlson J, Valez R. Risk of cirrhosis and primary liver cancer in alpha-1-antitrypsin deficiency. N Engl J Med. 1986;314:736–9.
25. Udall JN, Black KJ, Walker WA. Transport of protease across neonatal intestine and development of liver disease in infants with alpha-1-antitrypsin deficiency. Lancet. 1982;1:1441–3.
26. Fabbretti G, Faa G, Riva A, Sergi C, Callea F. Mechanism of cell damage in AATD. A transmission, scanning electron microscopic and X-ray microanalysis study. It J Gastroenterol. 1992;24(5):274–5.
27. Starzl TE, Porter KA, Terblanche J. Interorgan communications with particular reference to hepatotrophic factors and intrinsic liver growth factors. In: Popper H *et al.*, editors. Communications of liver cells. Lancaster: MTP Press; 1980:93.
28. Callea F. The natural history of HCC as viewed by the pathologist. Appl Pathol. 1988;6:105–16.
29. Callea F, Fevery J, Massi G, De Groote J, Desmet VJ. Storage of AAT in intrahepatic bile duct cells in AAT deficiency (PiZ phenotype). Histopathology. 1985;9:99–108.
30. Callea F, Fevery J, Desmet VJ. Simultaneous accumulation of alpha-1-antitrypsin in liver and pancreas. Hum Pathol. 1984;15:293–5.
31. Hood JM, Koep LJ, Peters RL *et al.* Liver transplantation for advanced liver disease with

alpha-1-antitrypsin deficiency. N Engl J Med. 1980;302:272–5.

32. Fagerhol MK, Cox DW. The Pi polymorphism: genetic, biochemical and clinical aspects of human alpha-1-antitrypsin. In: Harris H, Hirschlon K, editors. Advances in Human Genetics, No. 11. New York: Plenum; 1981;1:1–62.
33. Sabatini DD, Kreibich G, Morimoto T. Mechanisms for incorporation of proteins in membranes and organelles. J Cell Biol. 1982;92:1–22.
34. Bainton DF, Farquhar MG. Segregation and packaging of granules enzymes in eosinophilic leukocytes. J Cell Biol. 1970;45:54–73.
35. Menson PM. The immunologic release of constituents from neutrophil leucocytes. J Immunol. 1971;107:1547.
36. Wallmark A, Eriksson S. Monoclonal antibody specific for the mutant PiZ alpha-1-antitrypsin and its application in a ELISA procedure for identification of PiZ gene carriers. Proc Natl Acad Sci. 1984;81:5690–3.
37. Carlson J. Alpha-1-antitrypsin and the liver. Clinical and biological studies. 1984 PhD thesis, Malmo.
38. Curiel DT, Holmes MD, Okayama H. Molecular basis of the liver and lung disease associated with the alpha-1-antitrypsin deficiency allele Mmalton. J Biol Chem. 1989;13938–45.
39. Newton CR, Kalsheker N, Graham A. Diagnosis of alpha-1-antitrypsin deficiency by enzymatic amplification of human genomic DNA and direct sequencing of polymerase chain reaction products. Nucleic Acids Res. 1988;16:8233–43.
40. Brind AM, McIntosh I, Brock DJH. Polymerase chain reaction for detection of the alpha-1-antitrypsin Z allele in chronic liver disease. J Hepatol. 1990;10:240–3.

26
Wilson's disease

I. STERNLIEB

Eighty years ago an English neurologist, Kinnier Wilson, described a syndrome characterized by involuntary movements, tremors, posturing of extremities, spasticity, abnormal gait, dysphagia, dysarthria, and mental symptoms, associated with an asymptomatic cirrhosis[1]. Wilson first considered the disorder to be familial. Within less than a decade its mode of inheritance was established as autosomal recessive. However, it took an additional 30 years before copper was identified as the toxin that Wilson had postulated[2], and even longer before a defect in the biliary route of excretion was recognized[3]. The resulting increased concentrations of copper are responsible for the ensuing toxicity and the pathological changes which affect the liver first and later the brain, kidneys, and corneas. As soon as the aetiology was established, rational therapy for the mobilization of the excess copper from the tissues followed[4]. Suddenly the natural history of the disease changed and the prognosis of patients lucky enough to have chelation therapy instituted in a timely fashion was strikingly improved[5].

GENETICS AND INCIDENCE

The genetic locus for Wilson's disease is found on the long arm of chromosome 13, specifically at 13q14–q21, at a single locus[6]. The Wilson's disease gene is present worldwide with a frequency of 1:180 and an incidence of affected homozygotes of 1:30 000 births. The disease occcurs in all continents and in virtually all populations[7].

BIOCHEMICAL ABNORMALITIES

There are several paradoxical observations that characterize Wilson's disease: first, the patients exhibit excess copper deposits in the tissues while the concentration of the major circulating copper-carrying protein of plasma, caeruloplasmin, is reduced or absent[8]. This deficiency, present in 95% of patients with Wilson's disease, is not an expression of the primary gene defect because caeruloplasmin synthesis is controlled by a gene localized to chromosome 3 and not to chromosome 13. Second, in contrast to other storage diseases in which the accumulation of the offending agent is progressive, in Wilson's disease the young, asymptomatic patients display higher concentrations of hepatic copper than the older, symptomatic individuals[7]. This astonishing finding indicates that the liver is the primary storage site for the excess copper. Third, the intracellular distribution of copper changes with the stage of the disease: early on the copper is diffuse in the cytoplasm, whereas at the stage of cirrhosis an important fraction of the hepatocellular copper is sequestered in lysosomes. Fourth, striking mitochondrial abnormalities are encountered during the early stages of the disease, which disappear from the hepatocytes by the time cirrhosis develops.

EXTRAHEPATIC MANIFESTATIONS

Central nervous system

After release from the liver into the circulation, copper is distributed to the brain and other organs. This sequence explains why the effects of copper toxicity on the central nervous system appear relatively late, and why patients manifesting neurological manifestations tend to be older than those with overt hepatic disease[7]. The neurological abnormalities (Table 1) can be classified into three syndromes: an akinetic-rigid syndrome, a dystonic syndrome, and a syndrome in which tremulousness predominates. Occasionally, these syndromes are accompanied by psychiatric abnormalities which differ from those exhibited by patients suffering from hepatic encephalopathy. Magnetic resonance imaging (MRI) can demonstrate abnormal signals in the lenticular, thalamic, caudate, and dentate nuclei, as well as in the brainstem, which generally correlate with symptoms. Although all the patients with neurological Wilson's disease display anatomical changes in their livers, routine biochemical liver tests may fail to show them.

Kidneys

Various alterations of renal functions are encountered in some patients with Wilson's disease (Table 2). Rarely, gross haematuria may be a first sign of the disease.

Table 1 Neurological signs of Wilson's disease

Tremors	Posturing of extremities
Rigidity	Retracted upper lip
Dystonia	Amimia
Dysarthria	Grimacing
Drooling	Abnormal gait
Athetosis	

Table 2 Renal defects in Wilson's disease

Proximal tubular dysfunction
Distal tubular dysfunction
Combined proximal and distal tubular dysfunction
Calculi
Nephrocalcinosis
Haematuria

Eyes

A striking, relatively late manifestation of Wilson's disease consists in the deposition of fine, opaque, golden-greenish, copper granules at the periphery of Descemet's membrane of the cornea. These circumferential or crescentic Kayser–Fleischer rings[9], are grossly visible in subjects with blue or green irises. Regardless whether they are or are not detectable on gross inspection, a slit-lamp examination is essential for their definitive identification. Occasionally, similar copper deposits are found on the anterior and posterior aspects of the lenses, where they appear as sunflower cataracts. Kayser–Fleischer rings are not necessarily pathognomonic for Wilson's disease because they are also seen in rare patients with long-standing cholestasis or primary biliary cirrhosis. The rings tend to fade and ultimately disappear in most patients treated with penicillamine or trientine, and following liver transplantation.

Skeleton

Several skeletal abnormalities have been observed in patients with Wilson's disease (Table 3).

Skin

Azure lunulae, bluish discolorations of the nailbeds, are present in some patients with Wilson's disease[10]. The pathogenesis of this pigmentation is unknown. These azure lunulae are pathognomonic for Wilson's disease in the absence of argyria.

A melanotic pigmentation of the shins occurs in some patients[7]. The nature of this pigmentation, resembling that caused by haemosiderin deposits, is unknown.

Table 3 Skeletal abnormalities in Wilson's disease

Osteoporosis	Osteochondritis dissecans
Osteomalacia	Chondromalacia
Spontaneous fractures	Chondrocalcinosis
Rickets	

Gonads

Primary or secondary amenorrhoea, miscarriages, and reduced fertility are encountered in some women, and delayed puberty and gynaecomastia occur in boys[7,11]. These seem to be the consequence of hormonal imbalance associated with hepatic dysfunction. They tend to disappear as liver function improves.

DIAGNOSIS

The diagnosis of Wilson's disease is certain when two congruent criteria are fulfilled: in the majority of patients an absence or deficiency of caeruloplasmin (less than 200 mg/l; normal 200–450 mg/l) and the presence of Kayser–Fleischer rings are sufficient for the diagnosis. In the absence of either of these abnormalities, a hepatic copper concentration of more than 4 μmol (250 μg) per gram of dry liver will clinch the diagnosis in the presence of compatible histological findings[7]. It should be noted that deficiency of serum caeruloplasmin alone is not a sufficient criterion for the diagnosis, because 20% of heterozygous carriers of one Wilson's disease gene also exhibit hypocaeruloplasminaemia without ever developing the disease. A urinary copper excretion in excess of 1.6 μmol (100 μg) over 24 h (normal, less than 0.8 μmol) is confirmatory for the diagnosis, provided strict precautions to avoid contamination of the collection with traces of copper are taken. Histological abnormalities, ranging from hepatocellular steatosis in young patients to fibrosis and cirrhosis in patients with more advanced disease, are almost always present in liver biopsy samples[12]. An elevated hepatic copper concentration, in the absence of other compatible findings, leaves the diagnosis of Wilson's disease in doubt because patients with long-standing cholestasis, primary or secondary biliary cirrhosis, and patients with Indian childhood cirrhosis may display values which are indistinguishable from those of patients with Wilson's disease.

TREATMENT

The past 40 years have seen tremendous advances in the therapy of Wilson's disease: from no therapy to a virtual plethora of choices: D-penicillamine, trientine, British anti-Lewisite (BAL), zinc, tetrathiomolybdate, and liver transplantation. Decoppering therapy can maintain or restore normal health and longevity to every patient with asymptomatic Wilson's disease, and in many of those who are ill, provided it is instituted in a timely fashion and is continued indefinitely. The drug of choice is D-penicillamine[7,13,14] at a dose of about 1 g. A beneficial response may require months or years of therapy and neurological symptoms may worsen initially before improvement occurs. When the response to therapy is suboptimal, particularly in a severely ill patient, a temporary increase to 2 g of D-penicillamine daily, and the addition of intramuscular injections of BAL, may achieve the desired improvement.

For patients who experience sensitivity reactions within the first few weeks of treatment, desensitization with slowly increasing doses of D-penicillamine, together with oral prednisone, is often successful[7].

In patients who develop more serious toxic manifestations (lupus, cytopenia, pemphigus, proteinuria) which mandate the discontinuance of penicillamine, trientine will maintain or produce further improvement[15]. Its effectiveness as the primary agent in patients with advanced neurological disease or in those with severe hepatic decompensation is uncertain.

Oral zinc salts have been used successfully in asymptomatic patients and in some patients with neurological disease. Their efficacy and safety in patients with liver disease is not yet established[16].

The role of tetrathiomolybdate, a compound extensively used by veterinarians for the treatment of ovine copper toxicosis, is currently under investigation[17,18].

By now more than 120 patients with Wilson's disease have obtained liver transplants mainly for fulminant hepatitis with haemolysis, hepatic insufficiency not responding to pharmacological therapy, or for hepatic failure developing after an interval of non-compliance with D-penicillamine or trientine therapy[19,20]. Liver transplantation is clearly life-saving. It carries an acceptable risk, considering that most of these patients would not have survived otherwise.

References

1. Wilson SAK. Progressive lenticular degeneration. A familial disease associated with cirrhosis of the liver. Brain. 1912;34:295–509.
2. Cumings JN. The copper and iron content of brain and liver in the normal and in hepatolenticular degeneration. Brain. 1948;71:410.
3. Frommer DJ. Defective biliary excretion of copper in Wilson's disease. Gut. 1974;15:125–9.
4. Walshe JM. Penicillamine, a new oral therapy for Wilson's disease. Am J Med. 1956;21:487–95.
5. Sternlieb I, Scheinberg IH. Prevention of Wilson's disease in asymptomatic patients. N Engl J Med. 1968;278:352–9.
6. Frydman M, Bonne-Tamir B, Farrer LA *et al.* Assignment of the gene for Wilson disease to chromosome 13. Proc Natl Acad Sci USA. 1985;82:1819–1821.
7. Scheinberg IH, Sternlieb I. Wilson's disease. Philadelphia: Saunders; 1984.
8. Scheinberg IH, Gitlin D. Deficiency of ceruloplasmin in patients with hepatolenticular degeneration. Science. 1952;116:484–5.
9. Wiebers DO, Hollenhorst RW, Goldstein NP. The ophthalmologic manifestations of Wilson's disease. Mayo Clin Proc. 1977;52:409–16.
10. Bearn AG, McKusick VA. Azure lunulae. An unusual change in the fingernails in two patients with hepatolenticular degeneration (Wilson's disease). J Am Med Assoc. 1958;166:904–6.
11. Kaushansky A, Frydman M, Kaufman H, Homburg R. Endocrine studies of the ovulatory disturbances in Wilson's disease (hepatolenticular degeneration). Fertil Steril. 1987;47:270–3.
12. Sternlieb I, Scheinberg IH. Wilson's disease. In: Millward-Sadler GH, Wright R, Arthur MJP, editors. Wright's liver and biliary disease. 3rd edn. Philadelphia: Saunders; 1992:965–75.
13. Walshe JM. Wilson's disease. New oral therapy. Lancet. 1956;1:25–6.
14. Stremmel W, Meyerrose KW, Niederau C, Hefter H, Kreuzpaintner G, Strohmeyer G. Wilson's disease: clinical presentation, treatment and survival. Ann Intern. Med. 1991;115:720–6.
15. Scheinberg IH, Jaffe ME, Sternlieb I. The use of trientine in preventing the effects of interrupting penicillamine therapy in Wilson's disease. N Engl J Med. 1987;317:209–13.
16. Brewer GJ, Yuzbasiyan-Gurkan V. Wilson disease. Medicine. 1992;71:139–64.

17. Walshe JM. Tetrathiomolybdate (MoS_4) as an 'anti-copper' agent in man. In: Scheinberg IH, Walshe JM, editors. Orphan diseases, orphan drugs. Manchester: Manchester University Press; 1986:76–85.
18. Brewer GJ, Dick RD, Yuzbasiyan-Gurkan V, Tankanow R, Young AB, Kluin KJ. Initial therapy of patients with Wilson's disease with tetrathiomolybdate. Arch Neurol. 1991;48:42–7.
19. Sternlieb I. Wilson's disease. Indications for liver transplant. Hepatology. 1984;4:15S–17S.
20. Schilsky ML, Scheinberg IH, Sternlieb I. Hepatic transplantation for Wilson's disease: indications and outcome (Abstract). Hepatology. 1992;16:50A.

27

Clinical manifestation of genetic haemochromatosis: pathophysiological aspects of iron overload disease

W. STREMMEL, C. NIEDERAU and G. STROHMEYER

DEFINITION, INCIDENCE AND GENETIC DEFECT

Genetic haemochromatosis is a common inherited disorder of iron metabolism. The mode of inheritance of the haemochromatosis trait is autosomal recessive. The gene defect has been localized to chromosome 6 in proximity to the HLA-A3 histocompatibility locus[1]. Based on pedigree analyses and HLA typing carried out in Europe, USA and Australia it was shown that HLA-A3 occurred in about 75% of patients with haemochromatosis compared to 28–30% in controls[1]. In various studies it was estimated that the gene frequency is 5–7% and that about 0.3–0.45% of the population is homozygous for haemochromatosis[1,2].

Despite the success in localizing the haemochromatosis gene on the short arm of chromosome 6 in very close physical proximity (1 centimorgan) to the HLA-A locus[1], the structural genetic mutation is still unknown. The resulting biochemical defect is also not defined. Several observations indicate that in genetic haemochromatosis iron absorption is 2–4-fold increased due to a regulatory defect of a membrane transport system in duodenal mucosal cells[3,4]. The net pathophysiological effect of homozygosity for the haemochromatosis allele is iron overload of the organism. In advanced symptomatic disease total-body storage iron may be increased to 20–40 g, compared with approximately 1 g of storage iron in normal subjects[5].

Pathological deposition of excessive iron in the parenchymal cells of many organs leads to cellular toxicity and damage followed by functional insufficiency.

When the condition is genetically determined by inappropriate high absorption of iron by the intestinal mucosa, the term genetic or inherited haemochromatosis is used. Due to the autosomal recessive trait of inheritance the full disease is expressed only in homozygotes. The clinical features of advanced symptomatic haemochromatosis are characteristic. Patients usually present with lethargy, loss of libido, upper abdominal pain, joint pain or symptoms related to the onset of diabetes mellitus. Hepatomegaly, skin pigmentation, testicular atrophy/amenorrhoea, and arthropathy are the most prominent physical signs[6]. The clinical and biochemical expression of the disease varies, depending on such factors as age, sex, and chronic blood loss. The lower prevalence of symptomatic diseases among females (1:10) is attributed to physiological iron losses and lower intake of dietary iron. Young patients identified by family screening are often asymptomatic[6]. They rarely present with advanced haemochromatosis. In these cases cardiomyopathy is a relatively frequent clinical feature.

Heterozygous carriers of the haemochromatosis gene may reveal minor biochemical expression of the disease with a slightly increased level of iron absorption in 20–32% of the cases[7–9]. However, progressive iron overload with full clinical and biochemical expression is not a feature of heterozygous subjects, even in subjects who have an excessive intake of alcohol. Secondary iron overload syndromes (secondary haemochromatosis) are characterized by increased absorption promoted by disordered or ineffective erythropoiesis or increased availability of dietary iron[10]. Both genetic and secondary haemochromatosis are distinguished from transfusional iron overload, which leads to excessive iron deposition initially confined to the reticuloendothelial (RE) system[10]. Transfusional iron overload adds an additional iron burden in secondary haemochromatosis due to disordered erythropoiesis with RE cell and parenchymal iron deposition[10].

CONSEQUENCES OF IRON OVERLOAD

Increased iron absorption leads to a positive iron balance and accumulation of excess body iron in genetic haemochromatosis. It is interesting that only specific organs are affected by iron loading. These include liver and pancreas and to a lesser extent endocrine glands, particularly the pituitary, as well as heart and joints.

The dark pigmentation of the *skin*, although a typical clinical feature, is not alone due to iron deposits. The epidermis of the skin is thin, and increased melanin is found in the cells of the basal layer.

Deposits of iron are observed around the synovial lining cells of *joints* and calcium pyrophosphate crystals may be seen within deposits of calcium embedded in the synovial tissue. This arthropathy develops in 25–30% of patients at any stage of the disease[6]. The small joints of the hands (second and third metacarpophalangeal joints) are the first joints to be involved. A progressive polyarthritis involving wrists, hips, and knees may ensue. Roentgenological manifestations consist of subchondral sclerosis and cystic changes, loss of articular cartilage, diffuse demineralization, hypertrophic bone proliferation and calcification of the synovium.

The parenchymal deposits of iron in the *liver* of patients with genetic haemochromatosis are in the form of ferritin and haemosiderin. In early stages these deposits are found in the periportal parenchymal cells, especially within lysosomes in the pericanalicular cytoplasm of the hepatocytes. This stage progresses to perilobular fibrosis and deposition of iron in the bile duct epithelium, Kupffer cells, and fibrous septa. In advanced disease the pattern of cirrhosis is characterized by broad fibrous septa surrounding large areas of comparatively normal parenchyma. Hepatocellular carcinoma without iron deposition in tumour cells is observed in about 30% of cirrhotic patients, even after removal of excess body iron stores by phlebotomy therapy[6]. The pathogenesis of hepatocellular carcinoma is uncertain. One hypothesis suggests a relation to increased oxidative stress produced by iron with oxidant damage to the DNA, acting as initiator or promotor of carcinogenesis[11–13].

Although iron deposits in the *pancreas* are predominantly localized in the exocrine parenchyma with development of tissue fibrosis, functional impairment is a rare clinical feature. However, the selective accumulation of iron in B-cells of the endocrine pancreas in advanced disease contributes to the diabetes often observed in these patients[6]. Along with the component of impaired insulin secretion by damaged B-cells, there is an almost obligatory insulin resistance observed in iron overload disease[14]. This is due to an insulin receptor/postreceptor defect in the iron loaded liver, which is – in contrast to the destruction of the B-cells – reversible after completion of the phlebotomy therapy[14].

Iron deposition in the *heart* is observed in 15% of patients. Those deposits are more extensive in ventricular than in atrial myocardium, resulting in intracellular disruption[15]. The ensuing haemodynamic derangement is generally designated as dilated cardiomyopathy, but some patients have a pattern of myocardial restriction[15].

Another cell type which selectively accumulates iron in genetic haemochromatosis is the hypogonadotropic cell of the *pituitary gland*. Iron-induced cell damage leads to impaired secretion of FSH and LH, which results in the clinical manifestations of hypogonadotrophic hypogonadism with impotence in males and amenorrhoea in females[14]. Despite secondary low testosterone levels in male patients, peripheral sexual hormone metabolism remains unaltered[14].

Why certain organs and cells are particularly affected by excessive iron accumulation remains unclear. It is not the expression of transferrin or ferritin receptors which is responsible for the specific distribution of excessive iron deposition in certain cell types. Very interesting is the observation that in patients with haemochromatosis there is a significant fraction of non-transferrin bound iron in plasma, which gradually decreases during the course of phlebotomy treatment[17,18]. It represents iron ions liganded to low-molecular mass organic molecules such as citrate which do not exchange to a significant extent with the free binding sites on the transferrin molecule[17]. This source of iron is not obviously correlated with the concentration of total plasma non-haem iron, with the exception that it is present only when plasma iron[17] is greater than 40 μmol/l. Although this non-transferrin bound iron does not strongly correlate with the transferrin saturation in plasma, there may be a correlation to the serum ferritin concentration. It has been implied that, in haemochromatosis, this low-molecular mass iron complex enters the circulation from gut[19]. Studies in rats and mice have shown that the liver has an effective uptake system for these non-transferrin bound iron ions[20,21]. As candidate carrier protein for cellular uptake of this non-transferrin bound iron, the recently identified membrane iron binding protein (MIBP) could be suggested[22,23]. This membrane iron transporter was shown to be enriched in those organs which are affected in genetic haemochromatosis[4]. However, these preliminary data need to be confirmed in further studies.

MECHANISM OF IRON-INDUCED CELLULAR TOXICITY

Why does iron overload of cells induce cell damage and cell death with the consequence of functional impairment and structural organ damage? Several mechanisms whereby excess iron causes cellular injury have been proposed. Iron-induced peroxidative injury to phospholipids of organelle membranes, in particular of lysosomes and mitochondria, is the key pathogenetic factor[24,25]. Additional mechanisms may represent iron-stimulated depletion of vitamin E and C stores[26,27] and possibly low glutathione levels[28], as well as a direct stimulation of collagen synthesis by iron in the liver[29,30]. It is well established that ionic iron forms highly reactive free radicals, especially from oxygen. In order to exert potent oxidizing effects, iron must be present in a reactive and presumably low molecular weight form because ferritin bound or transferrin bound iron is relatively unreactive[12,31]. One candidate of this source of iron may be the non-transferrin bound iron which is complexed, e.g. to citrate. It is present in significant concentration in the circulation of haemochromatotic patients[17].

This non-transferrin bound iron is assumed to be taken up by the above-described membrane iron transport protein into hepatocytes and other cell types which are affected in genetic haemochromatosis[4]. Alternatively it is possible that cellular reductants are capable of enhancing the mobilization of iron from cellular ferritin stores[32]. Such low molecular chelate or free ionic iron may play a catalytic role in the initiation of peroxidative injury, either by the Fenton reaction:

$$Fe^{2+} + O_2 \rightarrow Fe^{3+} + \cdot O_2$$

$$\cdot O_2 + O_2 \xrightarrow{+2H+} H_2O_2$$

$$Fe^{2+} + H_2O_2 \rightarrow Fe^{3+} + OH^- + \cdot OH$$

or by the iron catalysed Haber–Weiss reaction:

$$Fe^{3+} - \text{complex} + O_2^- \rightarrow Fe^{2+} - \text{complex} + O_2$$

$$Fe^{2+} - \text{complex} + H_2O_2 \rightarrow F^{3+} - \text{complex} + OH^- + \cdot OH$$

$$\text{Net reaction: } O_2 + H_2O_2 \xrightarrow{Fe - \text{complex}} O_2 + OH^- + \cdot OH$$

The derived hydroxyl radical (·OH) is highly reactive and capable of initiating numerous free radical cascades and oxidations.

Others[33] have questioned the involvement of hydroxy radicals and proposed the initiation of lipid peroxidation by Fe^{2+} and H_2O in a reaction mediated by an oxidant requiring both Fe^{3+} and Fe^{2+}. Regardless of the initiating species the consequence is a peroxidative decomposition of polyunsaturated fatty acids of organelle membrane phospholipids. This damage to cellular organelle membranes causes loss of fluidity, changes in membrane potential, increased permeability to ions, and eventual rupture leading to release of cell and organelle contents[24,25]. Increased lability of iron loaded lysosomes leads to increased autophagy of cells[34]. In mitochondria iron-induced lipid peroxidation impairs particularly the activity of cytochrome oxidase, the terminal enzyme of the mitochondrial electron transport chain[24]. Microsomal lipid peroxidation is associated with a decrease in the level and activity of cytochrome P-450[28].

In addition, tissue concentrations of vitamin C and E, two physiological antioxidants, are often decreased in haemochromatosis, perhaps due to increased vitamin oxidation catalysed by iron[25–27].Therefore it is conceivable that the deficiency of these two antioxidants may be of relevance perpetuating the lipid peroxidation process. Moreover, glutathione, the key compound in protecting cells against numerous toxins and oxidative stress, was found to be significantly decreased in experimentally iron overloaded rats[28]. However, this could not be detected in liver biopsy specimens of patients with genetic haemochromatosis[35].

ACKNOWLEDGEMENTS

This work was supported by grants STR 92/4-3 and STR 216/4-1 from the Deutsche Forschungsgemeinschaft. The authors are very much indebted to Mrs Ch. Scheil for accurate preparation of the manuscript.

References

1. Simon M, LeMignon L, Fauchet R, Yaouanq J, Dabid V, Edang G, Bourel M. A study of 609 HLA haplotypes marking the hemochromatosis gene (1) mapping of the gene near the HLA-A locus and characters required to define a heterozygous population and (2) hypothesis concerning the underlying cause of hemochromatosis HLA association. Am J Hum Genet. 1987;41:89–105.
2. Edwards CQ, Griffen LM, Goldgar D, Drummond C, Skolnick MH, Kushner JP. Prevalence of hemochromatosis among 11,065 presumably healthy blood donors. N Engl J Med. 1988;318:1355–62.
3. Powell LW, Halliday JW. Iron absorption and iron overload. Clin Gastroenterol. 1981;10:707–35.
4. Stremmel W, Teichmann R, Strohmeyer G. Carrier mediated cellular uptake of nontransferrin bound iron: significance and regulation of a membrane iron binding protein. J Hepatol. 1991;13:574.
5. Bomford A, Williams R. Long term results of venesection therapy in idiopathic haemochromatosis. Q J Med. 1976;45:611–23.

6. Niederau C, Fischer R, Sonnenberg A, Stremmel W, Trampisch HJ, Strohmeyer G. Survival and causes of death in cirrhotic and noncirrhotic patients with primary hemochromatosis. N Engl J Med. 1985;313:1256–62.
7. Beaumont C, Simon M, Fauchet R. Serum ferritin as a possible marker of the hemochromatosis allele. N Engl J Med. 1979;301:169–74.
8. Cartwright G, Edwards C, Kravitz K. Hereditary hemochromatosis: phenotypic expression of the disease. N Engl J Med. 1979;301:175–9.
9. Valberg LS, Lloyd DA, Ghent CN. Clinical and biochemical expression of the genetic abnormality in idiopathic hemochromatosis. Gastroenterology. 1980;79:884–92.
10. Tavill AS, Bacon BR. Hemochromatosis: iron metabolism and the iron overload syndromes. In: Zakim D, Boyer TD, editors. Hepatology: a textbook of liver disease. Philadelphia: Saunders; 1989:1273–99.
11. Gutteridge JMC, Rowley DA, Griffiths E, Halliwell B. Low-molecular-weight iron complexes and oxygen radical reactions in idopathic haemochromatosis. Clin Sci. 1985;68:463–71.
12. Halliwell B, Gutteridge JMC. The importance of free radicals and catalytic metal ions in human diseases. Molec Aspects Med. 1985;8:89–95.
13. Halliwell B, Gutteridge JMC. Oxygen free radicals and iron in relation to biology and medicine. Some problems and concepts. Arch Biochem Biophys. 1986;246:501–11.
14. Stremmel W, Niederau C, Berger M, Kley HK, Krüskemper HL, Strohmeyer G. Abnormalities in estrogen, androgen, insulin metabolism in idiopathic hemochromatosis. Ann NY Acad Sci. 1988;526:209–23.
15. Buja LM, Roberts WC. Iron in the heart, etiology and clinical significance. Am J Med. 1971;51:209–21.
16. Dabestani A, Child JS, Henze E, Perloff JK, Schon H, Figueroa WG, Schelbert HR, Thessomboon S. Primary hemochromatosis: anatomic and physiologic characteristics of the cardiac ventricles and their response to phlebotomy. Am J Cardiol. 1984;54:153–9.
17. Okezie IA, Bomford A, Polson RJ, Halliwell B. Nontransferrin-bound iron in plasma from hemochromatosis patients: effect of phlebotomy therapy. Blood. 1988;72:1416–19.
18. Grootveld M, Bell JD, Halliwell B, Okezie IA, Bomford A, Sadler PJ. Non-transferrin-bound iron in plasma or serum from patients with idiopathic hemochromatosis. J Biol. Chem. 1989;264:4417–22.
19. Batey RG, Fong LC, Shamir S, Sherlock S. A non-transferrin-bound serum iron in idiopathic hemochromatosis. Dig Dis Sci. 1980;25:340–9.
20. Wright TL, Brissot P, Ma WL, Weisiger RA. Characterization of non-transferrin-bound iron clearance by rat liver. J Biol Chem. 1986;261:10909–19.
21. Craven CM, Alexander J, Eldridge M, Kushner JP, Bernstein S, Kaplan J. Tissue distribution and clearance kinetics of non-transferrin-bound iron in the hypotransferrinemic mouse: a rodent model for hemochromatosis. Proc Natl Acad Sci USA. 1987;84:3457–64.
22. Teichmann R, Stremmel W. Iron uptake by human upper small intestine microvillous membrane vesicles. J Clin Invest. 1990;86:2145–53.
23. Stremmel W, Lotz G, Niederau C, Teschke R, Strohmeyer G. Iron uptake by rat duodenal microvillous membrane vesicles: evidence for a carrier mediated transport system. Eur J Clin Invest. 1987;17:136–45.
24. Bacon BR, Britton RS. The pathology of hepatic iron overload: a free radical-mediated process? Hepatology. 1990;11:127–37.
25. Britton RS, Bacon BR, Recknagel RO. Lipid peroxidation and associated hepatic organelle dysfunction in iron overload. Chem Phys Lipids. 1987;45:207–39.
26. Bacon BR, Britton RS, O'Neill R. Effects of vitamin E deficiency on hepatic mitochondrial lipid peroxidation and oxidative metabolism in rats with chronic dietary iron overload. Hepatology. 1989;9:398–404.
27. Mak IT, Weglicki WB. Characterization of iron-mediated peroxidative injury in isolated hepatic lysosomes. J Clin Invest. 1985;75:58–63.
28. Bacon BR, Healey JF, Brittenham GM, Park CH, Nunnari J, Tavill AS, Bonkovsky HL. Hepatic microsomal function in rats with chronic dietary iron overload. Gastroenterology. 1986;90:1844–53.
29. Okazaki I, Brinckerhoff CE, Sinclair JF, Sinclair JR, Bonkowsky HL, Harris ED Jr. Iron increases collagenase production by rabbit synovial fibroblasts. J Lab Clin Med. 1981;396–402.

30. Weintraub LR, Goral A, Grasso J. Pathogenesis of hepatic fibrosis in experimental iron overload. Br J Hematol. 1985;59:321–31.
31. Aruoma OI, Halliwell B. Superoxide-dependent and ascorbate-dependent formation of hydroxyl radicals from hydrogen peroxide in the presence of iron. Are lactoferrin and transferrin promoters of hydroxyl radical generation? Biochem J. 1987;241:273–85.
32. O'Connell MJ, Ward RJ, Baum H. The role of iron in ferritin and hemosiderin-mediated lipid peroxidation in lysosomes. Biochem J. 1985;229:135–9.
33. Minotti G, Aust SD. The requirement of iron III in the initiation of lipid peroxidation by iron III and hydrogen peroxide. J Biol Chem. 1987;262:1098–104.
34. Seymour CA, Peters TJ. Organelle pathology in primary and secondary haemochromatosis with special reference to lysosomal changes. Br J Haematol. 1978;40:239–53.
35. Selden C, Seymour CA, Peters TJ. Activities of some free-radical scavening enzymes and glutathione concentrations in human and rat liver and their relationship to the pathogenesis of tissue damage in iron overload. Clin Sci. 1980;58:211–19.

28

Advances in gene therapy for genetic liver diseases

G. Y. WU and C. H. WU

We have shown previously that cell-surface receptors have been used as natural internalization sites for targeting bacterial genes to hepatocytes[1,2]. This targeting is based on the fact that parenchymal liver cells possess unique receptor activity that can recognize galactose-terminal (asialo-) glycoproteins. Binding of the glycoprotein by the receptor leads to invagination of the plasma membrane and internalization of the ligand–receptor complex in membrane-bound vesicles.

In order to deliver DNA via asialoglycoprotein receptors, a carrier system was developed consisting of two components: (1) an asialoglycoprotein ligand covalently bound to (2) a polymer containing multiple positive charges, a polycation. The asialoglycoprotein component provided the recognition signal for hepatocyte targeting, while the positively charged polycation served to bind DNA in a strong, non-damaging electrostatic manner to form a soluble protein–DNA complex. To determine whether normal genes could be targeted *in vivo* to correct a metabolic dysfunction in genetically defective animals, the Nagase analbuminaemic rat model was used. This animal possesses a defect in splicing of messenger RNA for serum albumin. As a result, circulating albumin protein is virtually undetectable[3,4]. A plasmid containing the structural gene for the human serum albumin under the control of mouse albumin enhancer–rat albumin promoter sequences was constructed and complexed with the targetable conjugate[5]. The resulting soluble complex was injected intravenously into Nagase rats and two-thirds partial hepatectomies were performed. Two weeks after injection, densitometric quantitation revealed an average number of 1000 copies of the plasmid/diploid genome[5]. Most of the foreign DNA was in plasmid form. Evidence for transcription of the targeted DNA using an RNase protection assay estimated the level of human albumin mRNA to be between 0.01% and 0.1% of the normal level of rat albumin in normal rats[4]. The presence of circulating human albumin was determined by Western blot analysis which showed the appearance of human albumin in the serum within 48 h. Human serum albumin was first detectable at a level of 0.05 μg/ml, but increased in concentration to a peak level of 34 μg/ml by 2 weeks post-injection. This level remained stable through 4 weeks. No antibodies directed against the human albumin were detected during the 4 weeks of the study[5].

Another model was used to further illustrate the possibility of targeted gene delivery in the correction of genetic metabolic defects. The WHHL rabbit possesses defective receptors for LDL[6]. As a consequence, these animals have hypercholesterolaemia and suffer the consequences of advanced coronary artery disease early in life. The rabbit serves as a model for familial hypercholesterolaemia in humans.

A plasmid carrying a full-length cDNA for the human low-density lipoprotein (LDL) receptor was constructed[7]. Transcriptional regulatory elements from the mouse albumin gene were inserted upstream to drive the LDL receptor gene. These were previously shown to result in liver-specific expression in transgenic animals. The plasmid was complexed with the conjugate and injected intravenously into rabbits. Liver tissue was harvested 10 min after injection. Cellular DNA extracted and analysed for the presence of human LDL receptor sequences demonstrated approximately 1000 copies of plasmid per cell. These levels decreased progressively, and by 48 h plasmid DNA was less than 0.1 copies/cell[7].

To study the transcriptional activity of the recombinant gene, total RNA was extracted and analysed by RNase protection assay for the presence of human LDL receptor transcripts. Exogenous LDL receptor mRNA was detected at 4 h, reached a peak at 24 h and decreased to undetectable levels by 72 h after transfection[7]. Maximal levels of recombinant LDL receptor mRNA occurring at 24 h were estimated to be 2–4% of normal endogenous levels. In order to determine the metabolic effects of hepatocyte-directed gene transfer *in vivo*, WHHL rabbits injected with complexed LDL receptor gene or CAT gene were analysed for changes in total serum cholesterol. After administration of the LDL receptor gene complex there was a rapid but transient decline in serum cholesterol which lasted 6 days. The drop in cholesterol levels was maximal at 2 days post-injection and was 25–30% of pretreatment values. It was further documented that the decline in serum cholesterol was due primarily to a decrease in LDL. To control for possible non-specific effects of any protein–DNA complex, a targetable complex was prepared containing a plasmid completely unrelated to LDL metabolism. In this case the plasmid contained the gene for the bacterial enzyme, chloramphenicol acetyltransferase. Injection of this CAT gene complex in a cross-over experiment in the same animals had no effect on serum cholesterol[7].

We have described, above, experiments demonstrating that a soluble DNA carrier system can result in targeted gene delivery and expression of double-stranded DNA in hepatocytes. We wondered whether the carrier system could target single-stranded DNA in the form of antisense oligomers. Because of the remarkable specificity of the action of antisense DNA in the inhibition of the synthesis of specific proteins based on hybridization of antisense to target mRNA, we hypothesized that receptor-mediated delivery of antisense DNA specific for hepatitis B viral (HBV) mRNA sequences could inhibit viral gene expression in target cells. A 21-mer oligo DNA sequence complementary to the polyadenylation signal for human hepatitis B virus (HBV) was complexed to a soluble DNA-carrier system. A cell line, HepG2 (2.2.15) that possesses asialoglycoprotein receptors and which is permanently transfected with hepatitis B virus (ayw subtype) was exposed to complexed antisense DNA or controls.

The first objective was to determine whether a single-stranded DNA oligonucleotide could be bound by an asialoglycoprotein-based carrier, and whether it could be specifically targeted to asialoglycoprotein receptor-bearing cells. Two cell lines were used: SK Hep1, human hepatoma cells that are asialoglycoprotein receptor (−) cells, and HepG2, asialoglycoprotein receptor (+) cells. The oligo DNA sequence was radiolabelled and administered to cells either alone or in the form of a targetable complex. The average uptake of antisense DNA *alone* by SK Hep1 [receptor (−) cells] was less than 0.05 pmol/h per million cells over 4 h of exposure[8]. Incubation with the oligo DNA in the form of a complex did not improve the uptake in these cells. Similarly, uptake of antisense DNA *alone* by HepG2 [receptor (+) cells] was as low as observed in receptor (−) cells over the course of the 4 h. However, in the receptor (+) cells, *complexed* antisense DNA was taken up nearly linearly at an average rate more than 10 times faster than antisense DNA alone through the 4 h of incubation. Accumulation of *complexed* antisense was also 12 times greater than antisense DNA alone after 4 h of exposure. The uptake of complexed DNA was virtually completely blocked by administration of a large molar excess of free carrier protein, asialoorosomucoid, to compete for receptor binding. This confirmed the involvement of asialoglycoprotein receptors in the differential delivery of the antisense DNA[8].

In order to determine whether the internalized antisense DNA was functional, HepG2 cells (stably transfected with hepatitis B virus) were exposed to complexed antisense DNA. Because these cells normally produce infectious virus, measurement of the production of surface antigen as a fucntion of time provided a simple means of monitoring the effects of antisense DNA on viral gene expression. In the presence of complexed antisense DNA the concentration of hepatitis B surface antigen in medium was *decreased* by 80% by day 1, and by *greater* than 95% through the 6th day compared to untreated cells. There was *no* significant increase in surface antigen concentrations in the presence of complexed antisense DNA after the first day of exposure. Treatment of the cells with a complex containing a random oligo sequence of the same size, prepared identically and in the same concentration, had no effect on the surface antigen concentration. Furthermore, the inhibition induced by the complexed antisense was blocked by competition with an excess of free asialoglycoprotein[8].

To demonstrate that the observed inhibitory effect was not due to a block in the secretion of proteins from the cells, dishes were exposed to complexed antisense DNA in the presence of a radiolabelled amino acid to monitor the production of new protein. If an impairment of surface antigen secretion was responsible for the decreased concentration in the medium after treatment with complexed antisense, it would be predicted that there should be an accumulation of antigen in the cells. Immunoprecipitation of newly synthesized surface antigen in the medium and in the cell layers showed a nearly identical decrease in radioactive protein, indicating that impaired secretion could not account for the observed decline in surface antigen concentration mediated by the complexed antisense[4].

To prove that the observed inhibition of surface antigen production was not simply a reflection of toxicity, or a general decrease in all protein synthesis, total protein synthesis was studied by precipitation with trichloroacetic acid. From these experiments, protein synthesis remained unchanged by exposure to complexed antisense sequences.

Finally, to determine whether this particular antisense sequence also affected viral replication, Southern analysis was performed to search for hepatitis B viral replicative forms using an HBV-specific radiolabelled probe. HBV DNA in the medium and cell layers after 24 h exposure to complexed antisense sequences was found to be 80% lower than in controls. Exposure of cells to a random 21-mer oligo DNA sequence under identical conditions failed to alter HBV surface antigen concentration or HBV DNA in medium or cells[8].

The data indicate that antisense oligonucleotides complexed by a soluble DNA-carrier system can be targeted to cells via asialoglycoprotein receptors resulting in specific inhibition of hepatitis B viral gene expression and replication.

References

1. Wu G, Wu C. Receptor-mediated *in vitro* gene transfection by a soluble DNA carrier system. J Biol Chem. 1987;262:4429–32.
2. Wu CH, Wilson JM, Wu GY. Targeting genes: delivery and persistent expression of a foreign gene driven by mammalian regulatory elements *in vivo*. J Biol Chem. 1989;264:16985–7.
3. Nagase S, Shimamune S, Shumiya S. Albumin-deficient rat mutant. Science. 1979;205:590–1.
4. Shalaby F, Shafritz DA. Exon skipping during splicing of albumin mRNA precursors in Nagase analbuminemic rats. Proc Natl Acad Sci USA. 1990;87:2652–6.
5. Wu GY, Wilson JM, Shalaby F, Grossman M, Shafritz DA, Wu CH. Receptor-mediated gene delivery *in vivo*: partial correction of genetic analbuminemia in Nagase rats. J Biol Chem. 1991;266:14338–42.
6. Watanabe Y. Serial inbreeding of rabbits with hereditary hyperlipidemia (WHHL-rabbit). Atherosclerosis. 1980;36:261–8.
7. Wilson JM, Grossman M, Wu CH, Chowdhury NR, Wu GY, Chowdhury JR. Hepatocyte directed gene transfer *in vivo* leads to transient improvement of hypercholesterolemia in LDL receptor-deficient rabbits. J Biol Chem. 1992;267:963–7.
8. Wu GY, Wu CH. Specific inhibition of hepatitis B viral gene expression *in vitro* by targeted antisense oligonucleotides. J Biol Chem. 1992;267:12436–9.

Section IX
Regeneration, immunology

29

Liver growth factors (hepatotrophic factors)

N. FAUSTO

The liver, both in humans and in laboratory animals, has the capacity to regulate its growth and size[1]. This property is demonstrated by the restoration of liver mass after partial hepatectomy in experimental animals and patients, and by the growth of transplanted livers which are small relative to the body size of the new host[2,3]. Compensatory growth of hepatic tissue does not exceed a relatively fixed ratio between body mass and liver mass. In cases of heterotopic liver transplantation where excess hepatic functional capacity may occur due to the maintenance of function in both the natural and the transplanted liver, the excess capacity does not persist. Instead, a process of apparent functional competition between the natural and the transplanted liver takes place, making one of them atrophic and non-functional[4].

Hepatocytes in the adult liver have a very low rate of cell replication. Yet when the liver functional mass is disrupted either by tissue removal (partial hepatectomy) or cell death (chemical or viral injury) hepatocytes proliferate and rapidly restore the original functional mass. The restoration of liver mass and function that occurs after partial hepatectomy is known as liver regeneration. It is important to keep in mind that liver regeneration is actually a process of compensatory growth in which the removed parts do not grow back. Instead, the growth response consists of the increase in mass of the remaining lobes through a process of hypertrophy and hyperplasia of their cellular elements.

Several models can be proposed to explain how optimal hepatic functional mass is achieved and maintained both in humans and experimental animals[5]. It is logical to assume that liver growth might be regulated by both humoral factors and factors produced in the hepatic tissue itself. These different types of stimuli are generated as the liver interacts with the external environment and other organs. In addition, liver growth and regeneration involve not only hepatocytes but all other elements of the tissue including non-parenchymal cells and extracellular matrix components. Hepatocytes, non-parenchymal cells, matrix components, vascular and biliary elements interact and form a 'microecological' system of their own, as discussed by Rojkind and Greenwell[6] (Fig. 1). All of these elements react to and generate stimuli responsible for liver growth. Indeed, hepatocyte replication is in great part dependent on factors (both positive and negative) produced by non-parenchymal cells. Thus, the establishment of optimum liver size reflects a dynamic equilibrium between extrahepatic and intrahepatic influences. Whenever the equilibrium is disrupted, it is rapidly restored by hepatocyte replication.

On the basis of these considerations it is possible to formulate at least three types of models to account for the stimuli that are responsible for the start of the liver regenerative response[5] (Fig. 2). Model 1 relies on the view that there is a linkage between the functional demands placed on the liver after partial hepatectomy and the initiation of the cascade leading to DNA synthesis[7]. Model 2 stipulates that the start of regeneration is the consequence of the increase in the level of a blood factor which acts as an hepatocyte mitogen[8]. Model 3 is a combination of the two previous models and assumes that the functional demands imposed on the liver modify the sensitivity of hepatocytes to mitogenic factors[5].

HEPATOTROPIC FACTORS – GROWTH FACTORS WHICH ACT ON THE LIVER

Recent work has demonstrated that during liver regeneration the expression of proto-oncogenes, transcription factors and the activity of several growth factors constitute an important link in the chain of events connecting the

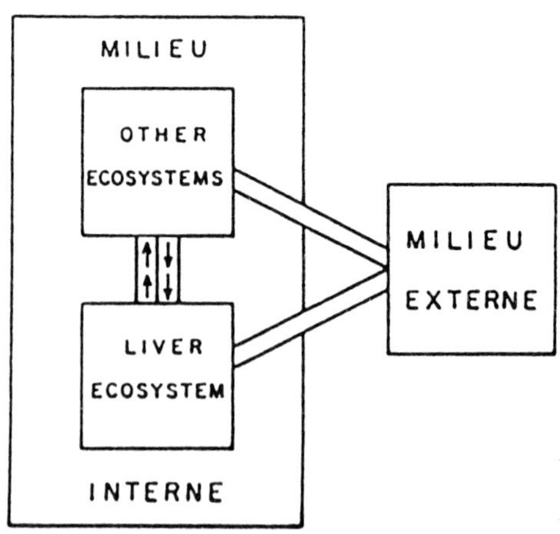

Fig. 1 Interactions between the liver, other organs and the external environment. The liver is represented as an ecosystem consisting of hepatocytes, non-parenchymal cells, matrix components and vascular elements. Hepatocyte functional capacity and growth activity is regulated by both extrahepatic and intrahepatic stimuli. From ref. 6, with permission

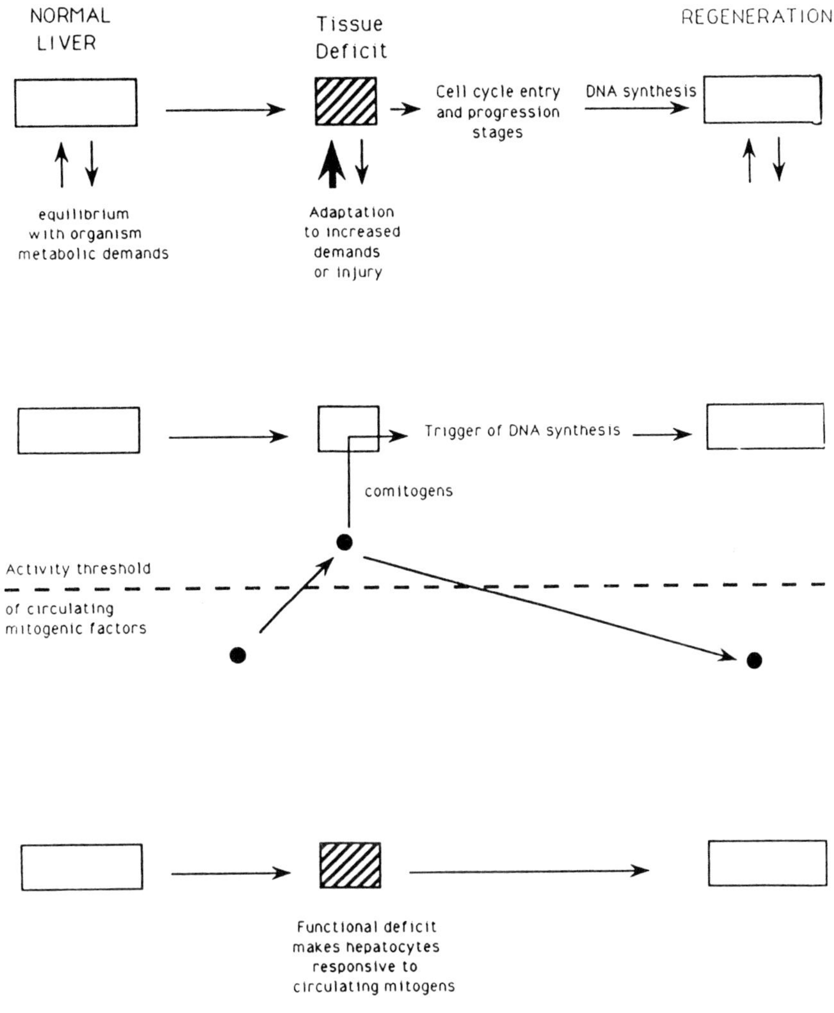

Fig. 2 Models of liver regeneration. The figure represents three general mechanisms for liver regeneration discussed in the text (reprinted from ref. 5)

stimulus provided by partial hepatectomy with the wave of DNA synthesis that starts at 12 h and reaches a maximum 24 h after the operation[9–11].

In light of the present research on growth regulation in the liver and other tissues, the term 'hepatotropic factor' should refer to those growth factors (cytokines) that can influence liver growth. These factors may have a stimulatory or inhibitory effect on liver cell replication. They may be complete mitogens, function as adjuvants or act only at specific steps of the mitogenic response. Growth factors operate by three general mechanisms[12] (Fig. 3):

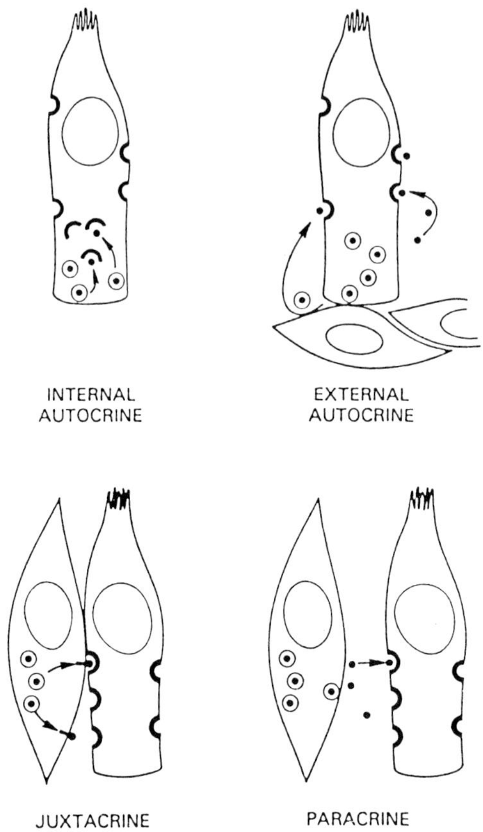

Fig. 3 Mechanisms of action of growth factor. The figure represents: internal autocrine mechanism in which there is no secretion of the growth factor and the factor binds to the receptor intracellularly; external autocrine mechanism in which the growth factor is secreted but acts on cells that produce the factor and have specific cell surface receptors (after secretion the factor may be activated by other cell types before it binds to the receptor); juxtacrine mechanism in which one cell contains a growth factor anchored at the cell membrane and links with another cell containing the receptor; paracrine mechanism in which the producer cell releases the factor which acts on another cell type that contains the specific receptor but does not produce the factor (reprinted from ref. 12)

1. *Autocrine activity.* The growth factor acts on its own producer cell. For this effect the peptide interacts with a specific receptor either externally (secreted factor in the intercellular environment) or internally (intracellular mechanism that bypasses the need for secretion). A variation of the non-secretory type of activity is called a juxtacrine effect. In this case a non-secreted growth factor anchored at the cell membrane interacts with a specific receptor located in an adjacent cell.
2. *Paracrine activity.* The growth factor acts on a cell type which is different from the cell producing the factor. The producer cell lacks the specific receptor for the growth factor while the responder cell has membrane receptors which can bind the factor.

3. *Endocrine activity*. This is the classic mode of action described for hormones which circulate in the blood and may have systemic effects. Some growth factors, although they may not be produced by an endocrine gland, function in a manner analogous to that of circulating hormones.

Several peptide growth factors act on the liver and may have important roles in the regulation of liver regeneration. These factors include: transforming growth factor alpha (TGF-α), epidermal growth factor (EGF), transforming growth factor beta (TGF-β), hepatocyte growth factor (HGF) and acidic fibroblast growth factor (aFGF). This is only a partial list, which is likely to expand as new factors are identified and purified[13]. In addition, substances such as insulin, glucagon, norepinephrine and some hormones can function as adjuvants for the regenerative response[8,9]. These substances are likely to influence the timing and extent of the process, but by themselves cannot elicit a growth response. TGF-α, EGF and HGF are complete liver mitogens that can on their own stimulate DNA synthesis of hepatocytes in primary culture. Of the three, HGF is the most potent while TGF-α is generally more active than EGF. TGF-β has the opposite effect on hepatocytes; that is, it is a very strong inhibitor of DNA synthesis for hepatocytes in culture. aFGF has by itself only weak effects on DNA synthesis of cultured hepatocytes, but it can modulate the effect of complete liver mitogens. In this chapter we examine the properties and effects of two principal liver mitogens, TGF-α and HGF.

INVOLVEMENT OF TGF-α IN LIVER GROWTH REGULATION

TGF-α is a 50 amino acid peptide synthesized as a part of a larger precursor. When the precursor migrates to the cell membrane the peptide is cleaved from the precursor by elastase-type enzymes acting at two alanine–valine junctions[14]. However, partially cleaved forms of the precursor which are still anchored to the cell membrane show biological activity. A cell which contains these partially cleaved forms of TGF-α at its surface can induce a growth stimulus in an adjacent cell that has the receptor for TGF-α (juxtacrine effect). In this manner TGF-α can function both to stimulate growth and to facilitate cell adhesion. TGF-α has 30–40% homology with EGF and binds to the same receptor as EGF (EGF/TGF-α receptor).

TGF-α is developmentally regulated in rat liver[15]. Hepatic levels of both the peptide and its mRNA are high at the end of gestation and the first few days of life, but decrease rapidly during the following 10–14 days. TGF-α mRNA increases after partial hepatectomy in rats starting at 4 h and reaching a peak at around 24 h, the time of maximum DNA synthesis[16]. *In vivo* and in culture hepatocytes stimulated to undergo DNA synthesis produce TGF-α mRNA and secrete the peptide[16,17]. These and other studies indicate that TGF-α is an autocrine factor for hepatocyte proliferation, and that it has a physiological role on liver growth and regeneration[10,16] (Table 1).

Further demonstration of the role of TGF-α on liver growth regulation was obtained in transgenic mouse lines that overexpress human TGF-α[18–21]. In these animals liver weight is 25–40% higher than normal[21] (Webber *et*

Table 1 Evidence for the involvement of TGF-α in liver growth regulation

I. Expression of TGF-α mRNA and peptide
1. developmentally regulated
2. increase during liver regeneration
3. increase after toxic liver injury
4. increased in replicating hepatocytes in culture
5. blockage with TGF-α antisense oligonucleotides inhibit hepatocyte DNA replication in culture

II. TGF-α overexpression in transgenic mice
1. larger livers with centrilobular hypertrophy
2. increased proliferative activity of hepatocytes
3. focal dysplasia leading to development of liver tumours in most animals

III. TGF-α overexpression in cultured hepatocytes
1. hepatocytes from TGF-α transgenic mice maintained in serum free medium in the absence of growth factors undergo DNA synthesis
2. in these cells, DNA replication is not stimulated by EGF and HGF
3. stable differentiated lines can be established from TGF-α hepatocytes

IV. Inhibition of TGF-α by antisense genes
1. TGF-α mRNA and peptide increase in transformed liver epithelial cells which serves precursors to HCC
2. stable transfection of these cells with TGF-α antisense genes leads to drastic decrease in TGF-α production
3. transformed cells transfected with a TGF-α antisense gene have low tumorigenicity in nude mice

V. TGF-α expression in human liver
1. correlates with cell proliferation in chronic liver disease
2. detected in 80% of HCC
3. expression in adjacent non-tumorous liver correlates with HBsAg
4. increased excretion in HCC patients

al., unpublished) and hepatocytes have high mitotic activity, particularly in young animals (two or three times higher than normal values). Livers of transgenic mice show distinct areas of centrilobular hypertrophy, similar to that present in livers of animals treated with phenobarbital and hepatocytes are generally larger than normal[19]. In the TGF-α transgenic mice the constitutive expression of the TGF-α transgene causes a very high incidence of liver tumours (approximately 85%) in male animals between 12 and 15 months of age[18–20]. The development of the tumours is not associated with mutations of *ras* family genes and apparently does not involve alterations in the p53 gene[20]. Further indication of the role of TGF-α as an autocrine stimulator of hepatocyte replication was demonstrated in cultures of hepatocytes isolated from livers of the TGF-α transgenic mice (Wu *et al.*, submitted for publication). These cells grow in culture in serum-free medium in the absence of any other growth factor and are not stimulated by the addition of EGF or HGF. Several cell lines have been established from these cells. These lines have been maintained for over a year in culture and express many of the differentiated traits of hepatocytes (Table 1).

Work with TGF-α in human livers has shown that the expression of the mRNA for the factor generally correlates with the degree of cell proliferation in chronic liver disease[22]. More recent work shows that more than 80% of human hepatocellular carcinomas stain for TGF-α and that the presence of TGF-α in adjacent non-tumorous portions of the liver corresponds to the expression of HBsAg[23,24]. There are also several reports demonstrating that excretion of TGF-α but not of EGF is high in patients with HCC, and that TGF-α might serve as a marker for the tumour in conjunction with alpha-fetoprotein measurements[25]. These and other findings on the role of TGF-α in the liver are summarized in Table 1. All of the evidence listed indicates that TGF-α is a physiological stimulator of hepatocyte proliferation in both animals and humans, and that it acts through an autocrine mechanism.

EGF, which has a considerable degree of homology with TGF-α and shares the same receptor, is a potent mitogen for hepatocytes in culture. However, it has been difficult to establish a physiological role for the factor in rat liver regeneration. Nevertheless, EGF may play a significant role as a regulator of liver regeneration after partial hepatectomy in mice. Noguchi *et al.*[26] have shown that salivary gland removal (sialoadenectomy) causes a decrease in plasma EGF levels and a considerable delay in the timing of DNA replication after partial hepatectomy. Administration of EGF to sialoadenectomized mice corrects this defect, suggesting that, in mice, EGF may have an endocrine effect on liver growth regulation.

ROLE OF HGF IN LIVER GROWTH REGULATION

This factor was initially isolated from plasma, platelets and the liver in animals and humans[8,27,28]. It has been cloned in several laboratories and shown to be identical to a previously described factor known as scatter factor (SG), named because of its capacity to stimulate the motility of epithelial cells[29,30]. A single factor (HGF/SC) exhibits mitogenic properties for liver, most epithelial cells and other cell types (endothelial cells and melanocytes) and can act as a motility and/or differentiation agent for epithelial cells. HGF has a structure similar to that of plasminogen and other coagulation factors. It is synthesized as a 728 amino acid precursor which is cleaved into two chains referred to as α or heavy and β or light chains. The heavy chain contains four kringle domains characteristic of blood coagulation proteins[27]. The light chain has the primary structure of a serine protease but has no proteolytic activity because of a change in two amino acids that form the catalytic site of active proteases.

HGF is present in plasma, placenta, liver and many other normal tissues[31]. In all of these sites it appears to be produced mostly by fibroblasts and other mesenchymal cells. The major source for HGF in the liver is the Ito cell[32]. Hepatocytes do not produce the factor but contain the HGF receptor which was identified as the c-*met* proto-oncogene[33,34]. These receptors are absent in liver non-parenchymal cells that are capable of synthesizing HGF. Thus, one mechanism for the mitogenic effect of HGF on hepatocytes is a paracrine effect of the factor which is secreted by non-parenchymal cells.

Plasma concentrations of HGF increase in the first 3 h after partial hepatectomy and also after CCl_4 injury[35]. Because of the very early rise in blood HGF levels in these conditions it has been proposed that HGF in conjunction with norepinephrine may constitute an early stimulus for liver regeneration[8]. In this case HGF would act through an endocrine mechanism to initiate hepatocyte replication. In liver regeneration after partial hepatectomy there is also an increase in HGF mRNA in the liver at about 12–18 h after the operation, probably as a result of the production of the mRNA by non-parenchymal cells[36,37]. This increase is much more pronounced during liver regeneration after CCl_4 and galactosamine injury[38]. In these types of injury, maximal levels of HGF mRNA are reached at about 15 h after the administration of the agent. A more detailed analysis of the physiological role of HGF as a triggering agent for liver regeneration, and of the specific effects of circulating and intrahepatic HGF on liver cells, requires work using experimental systems in which HGF is either overexpressed or blocked. Furthermore, the regulation of the biological effect of HGF may reside in part on receptor modification. Studies exploring these questions are in progress in several laboratories.

Serum HGF reaches very high levels in patients with fulminant liver[39,40] failure, and it has been suggested that serum HGF concentration may have prognostic value as it has been found to inversely correlate with patient survival. This finding is somewhat paradoxical, as it may be expected that patients with the highest blood level of a liver mitogen would have a better capacity for liver regeneration and better chance of survival. It is possible, however, that blood HGF levels reflect the degree of liver injury, in which case the highest levels of HGF would be found in patients with more severe hepatic injury. In fulminant hepatic failure, release of HGF from non-parenchymal cells may be greatly increased while the uptake of HGF produced in other tissues would be decreased because of diminished liver function. Among the many different organs in which HGF is synthesized, the lung may be a particularly important source for the production and regulation of circulating HGF. It has been proposed that after liver injury the liver releases a substance ('injurin'), which may induce the synthesis and release of HGF by lung mesenchymal cells[41].

Serum HGF levels are moderately increased in patients with chronic hepatic failure and show a relatively minor elevation in acute hepatitis[39,40]. It has been suggested that the extent of the increase in serum HGF may be clinically useful to distinguish between fulminant and chronic hepatic failure, and may reflect the degree of hepatocellular necrosis in these two conditions. Serum HGF levels are also elevated in patients with chronic renal failure and increase even further after haemodialysis[40].

SUMMARY AND PERSPECTIVES

In this chapter we reviewed some general mechanisms of liver growth regulation and growth factor activity and focused on two important factors, TGF-α and HGF. Both are complete liver mitogens, HGF being the most potent. *In vivo*, HGF, which is not synthesized by hepatocytes, can apparently act by both endocrine and paracrine mechanisms. TGF-α, which is made by hepatocytes, functions as an autocrine factor in hepatocyte proliferation.

Although much more information is needed for the formulation of hypotheses, a plausible view is that HGF may act as a triggering agent while TGF-α acts on cells that have already reached the G1 phase of the cycle. Further work on the role of HGF as a potential triggering agent for liver regeneration is needed to ascertain whether the rise in HGF in the blood after partial hepatectomy is fast enough to account for changes in transcription factor activity (DNA binding) which occur 10–15 min after the operation[11]. It is also important to determine why only the liver undergoes a mitogenic response after partial hepatectomy despite the increase in serum HGF, which is a mitogen for epithelial cells in kidney, skin and other organs.

References

1. Fausto N. Hepatic regeneration. In: Zakim D, Boyer TD, editors. Hepatology: a textbook of liver disease. Philadelphia: Saunders; 1990:49–62.
2. Van Thiel DH, Gavaler JS, Kam I, Francavilla A, Polimeno L, Schade RR, Smith J, Diven W, Penkrot RJ, Starzl TE. Rapid growth of an intact human liver transplanted into recipient larger than the donor. Gastroenterology. 1987;93:1414–19.
3. Broelsch CE, Emond JC, Whitington PF, Thistlethwaite JR, Baker AL, Lichtor JL. Application of reduced-size liver transplants as split grafts, auxiliary orthotopic grafts, and living related segmental transplants. Ann Surg. 1990;212:368–75.
4. Willemse PJA, Ausema L, Terpstra OT, Krenning EP, ten Kate FWJ, Schalm S. Graft regeneration and host liver atrophy after auxiliary heterotropic liver transplantation for chronic liver failure. Hepatology. 1992;15:54–7.
5. Fausto N. Liver regeneration: models and mechanisms. In: Bernuau D, Feldman G, editors. Liver regeneration. Paris: John Libbey Eurotext; 1992:1–6.
6. Rojkind M, Greenwell P. The liver as a bioecological system. In: Arias I, Jakoby WB, Popper H, Schachter D, Shafritz DA, editors. The liver biology and pathobiology, 2nd edn. New York: Raven Press; 1988:1269–85.
7. Mead JE, Braun L, Martin DA, Fausto N. Induction of replicative competence ('priming') in normal liver. Cancer Res. 1990;50:7023–30.
8. Michaelopoulos GK. Liver regeneration: molecular mechanism of growth control. FASEB J. 190;4:176–87.
9. Fausto N, Mead JE. Regulation of liver growth: protooncogenes and transforming growth factors. Lab Invest. 1989;60:4–13.
10. Fausto N. Growth factors in liver development, regeneration and carcinogenesis. Prog Growth Factor Res. 1991;3:219–34.
11. Tewari M, Dobrzanski P, Mohn KL, Cressman DE, Hsu JC, Bravo R, Taub R. Rapid induction in regeneration liver of RL/1F-1 (an lkB that inhibits Nf-kb, Rel B-p50 and c-Rel-p50) and PHF, a novel kB site-binding complex. Mol Cell Biol. 1992;;12:2898–908.
12. Sporn MB, Roberts AB. Autocrine secretion – 10 years later. Ann Intern Med. 1992;117:408–14.
13. Woodman AC, Selden CA, Hodgson HJF. Partial purification and characterization of an inhibitor of hepatocyte proliferation derived from nonparenchymal cells after partial hepatectomy. J Cell Physiol. 1992;151:405–14.
14. Brachman R, Lindquist PB, Nagashima M, Kohr W, Lipari T, Napier M, Derynck R. Transmembrane TGF-α precursors activate EGF/TGF-α receptors. Cell. 1989;56:691–700.
15. Brown PI, Lam R, Lakshmanan J, Fisher DA. Transforming growth factor alpha in developing rats. Am J Physiol. 1990;259:E256–60.
16. Mead JE, Fausto N. Transforming growth factor α may be a physiological regulator of liver regeneration by means of an autocrine mechanism. Proc Natl Acad Sci USA. 1989;86:1558–62.
17. Evarts RP, Nakatsukasa H, Marsden ER, Hu Z, Thorgeirsson S. Expression of transforming growth factor-alpha in regenerating liver and during hepatic differentiation. Mol Carcinogen. 1992;5:15–31.

18. Jhappan C, Stahle C, Harkins RN, Fausto N, Smith GH, Merlino GT. TGFα overexpression in transgenic mice induces liver neoplasia and abnormal development of the mammary gland and pancreas. Cell. 1990;61:1137–46.
19. Lee G-H, Merlino G, Fausto N. Development of liver tumors in transforming growth factor α transgenic mice. Cancer Res. 1992;52:5162–70.
20. Takagi H, Sharp R, Hammermeister C, Goodrow T, Bradley MO, Fausto N, Merlino G. Molecular and genetic analysis of liver oncogenesis in transforming growth factor α transgenic mice. Cancer Res. 1992;52:5171–7.
21. Sandgren EP, Luetteke NC, Palmiter RD, Brinster RL, Lee DC. Overexpression of TGFα in transgenic mice induces liver neoplasia and abnormal development of the mammary gland and pancreas. Cell. 1990;61:1137–46.
22. Castilla A, Prieto J, Fausto N. Transforming growth factors β1 and α in chronic liver disease: effects of interferon alpha therapy. N Engl J Med. 1991;324:933–40.
23. Hsia CC, Axiotis CA, DiBisceglia AM, Tabor E. Transforming growth factor-alpha in human hepatocellular carcinoma and coexpression with hepatitis B surface antigen in adjacent liver. Cancer. 1992;70:1049–56.
24. Collier JD, Guo K, Gullick WJ, Challen C, Burt AD, Bassendine MF. Transforming growth factor alpha (TGF-α): a role in human hepatocarcinogenesis by an autocrine mechanism? Hepatology. 1991;14:110A.
25. Yeh Y-C, Tsai J-F, Chuang L-Y, Yeh H-W, Tsai J-H, Florine DL, Tam JP. Elevation of transforming growth factor α and its relationship to the epidermal growth factor and α-fetoprotein levels in patients with hepatocellular carcinoma. Cancer Res. 1987;47:896–901.
26. Noguchi S, Obha Y, Oka T. Influence of epidermal growth factor on liver regeneration after partial hepatectomy in mice. J Endocrinol. 1991;128:425–31.
27. Nakamura T, Nishizawa T, Hagiya M, Seki T, Shimonishi M, Sugimura A, Tashiro K, Shimizu S. Molecular cloning and expression of human hepatocyte growth factor. Nature. 1989;163:967–73.
28. Miyazawa K, Tsubouchi H, Naka D, Takahashi K, Okigaki M, Arakaki H, Nakayama H, Hirono S, Sakiyama O, Gohda E, Daikuhara Y, Kitamura N. Molecular cloning and sequence analysis of cDNA for human hepatocyte growth factor. Biochem Biophys Res Commun. 1989;163:967–73.
29. Weidner KM, Arakaki N, Hartmann G, Vandekerckhove J, Weingart S, Rieder H, Fonatsch C, Tsubouchi H, Hishida T, Daikuhara Y, Birchmeier W. Evidence for the identity of human scatter factor and human hepatocyte growth factor. Proc Natl Acad Sci USA. 1991;88:7001–5.
30. Gherardi E, Stoker M. Hepatocytes and scatter factor. Nature. 1990;346:228.
31. Zarnegar RS, Muga S, Rahija R, Michalopoulos G. Tissue distribution of HPTA: a heparin-binding polypeptide growth factor for hepatocytes. Proc Natl Acad Sci USA. 1990;87:1252–6.
32. Schirmacher P, Geerts A, Pietrangelo A, Dienes HP, Rogler CE. Hepatocyte growth factor/hepatopoietin A is expressed in fat-storing cells from rat liver but not myofibroblast-like cells derived from fat-storing cells. Hepatology. 1992;15:5–11.
33. Bottaro DP, Rubin JS, Faletto DL, Chan AM, Kmiecik TE, Vande Woude GF, Aaronson SA. Identification of the hepatocyte growth factor receptor as the c-*met* protooncogene produce. Science. 1991;251:802–4.
34. Naldini L, Vigna E, Narsimhan RP, Gaudino G, Zarnegar R, Michalopoulos GK, Comoglio PM. Hepatocyte growth factor (HGF) stimulates the tyrosine kinase activity of the receptor encoded by the proto-oncogene c-*met*. Oncogene. 1991;6:501–4.
35. Lindroos PM, Zarnegar R, Michalopoulos GK. Hepatic growth factor (hepatopoietin A) rapidly increases in plasma before DNA synthesis and liver regeneration stimulated by partial hepatectomy and carbon tetrachloride administration. Hepatology. 1991;13:743–50.
36. Kinoshita T, Hirao S, Matsumoto K, Nakamura T. Possible endocrine control by hepatocyte growth factor of liver regeneration after partial hepatectomy. Biochem Biophys Res Commun. 1991;177:330–5.
37. Zarnegar R, DeFrances MC, Kost DP, Lindroos P, Michalopoulos GK. Expression of hepatocyte growth factor mRNA in regenerating rat liver after partial hepatectomy. Biochem Biophys Res Commun. 1991;177:559–65.

38. Okajima A, Miyazawa K, Kitamura N. Primary structure of rat hepatocyte growth factor and induction of its mRNA during liver regeneration following hepatic injury. Eur J Biochem. 1990;193:375–81.
39. Tsubouchi H, Niitani Y, Hirono S, Nakayama H, Gohda E, Arakaki N, Sakiyama O *et al*. Levels of the human hepatocyte growth factor in serum of patients with various liver diseases determined by an enzyme-linked immunosorbent assay. Hepatology. 1991;13:1–5.
40. Tomiya T, Nagoshi S, Fujiwara K. Significance of serum human hepatocyte growth factor levels in patients with hepatic failure. Hepatology. 1992;15:1–4.
41. Matsumoto K, Tajima H, Hamanoue M, Hohno S, Kinoshita T, Nakamura T. Identification and characterization of 'injurin', an inducer of expression of the gene for hepatocyte growth factor. Proc Natl Acad Sci USA. 1992;89:3800–4.

30
Liver and unspecific defence reactions

W. GEROK

Higher organisms respond to disturbances of homeostasis or to disturbed integrity of their cells and tissues with specific and unspecific defence reactions. Both cellular and humoral components are involved in the specific as well as the unspecific defence reactions (Table 1). In specific reactions T-lymphocytes represent the cellular, antibodies the humoral components. In the unspecific defence reactions the cellular components are macrophages and probably natural killer cells, whereas complement system and acute-phase proteins the humoral components. The unspecific defence reactions are independent of the cause of the disturbance; they are observed after bacterial, parasitic or viral infections, invasion of foreign material, traumatic or anoxic injury of cells and tissues as well as reactions against tumour cells. The significance of the liver in unspecific defence reactions is based on two facts:

1. The liver is extremely well endowed with macrophages, 80–90% of sessile macrophages in the organism are localized in the liver.
2. The liver is the most important organ for the synthesis of the proteins of the complement system, and acute proteins are synthesized exclusively in the liver.

Table 1 Defence reactions of the organism

Components	*Unspecific (constitutive)*	*Specific (acquired)*
Cellular	Macrophages (NK cells)	T-lymphocytes
Humoral	Complement system Acute-phase proteins	Immunoglobulins

In the following the role of the liver for the unspecific defence mechanisms is described under four aspects:

1. Role of Kupffer cells in unspecific defence reactions.
2. Liver and complement system in unspecific defence reactions.
3. Liver and acute-phase proteins in unspecific defence reactions.
4. Clinical consequences: significance of disturbed liver function for unspecific defence reactions.

FUNCTION OF KUPFFER CELLS WITH REGARD TO UNSPECIFIC DEFENCE REACTIONS

Kupffer cells are predominantly located within the lumen of the sinusoids. They are anchored to endothelial cells of the sinusoidal wall by long cytoplasmic processes. Occasionally thin evaginations from Kupffer cells penetrate between endothelial cells into the Disse space. Within the hepatic acinus Kupffer cells are preferentially located in the periportal region. With other cells, qualified for phagocytosis, circulating in the blood (e.g. monocytes, granulocytes) or present in tissues or body cavities (e.g. histiocytes, alveolar macrophages, peritoneal macrophages) the Kupffer cells belong to the mononuclear phagocyte system (MPS) (for review see refs 1–4).

According to their number – Kupffer cells represent 10–15% by cell number and 3% by cell mass in the rat liver – their strategic location in the portal system between intestine and systemic circulation, and particularly by their specific functions Kupffer cells play an important role in unspecific defence. Blood entering the sinusoids is monitored for microorganisms, altered cells and foreign material. The following functions are essential in the defence reactions:

1. endocytosis;
2. secretion of cytotoxic or antimicrobial substances;
3. release of signal and mediator substances;
4. processing and presentation of antigens.

The latter function is an important process in specific (immunological) defence and is therefore not discussed in this chapter.

These functions are not performed continuously, but only after 'activation' of the Kupffer cells by exogenous and endogenous signals. The most effective exogenous signal is mediated by lipopolysaccharides (LPS) of Gram-negative bacteria, as endogenous signal interferon-γ (IFN-γ) plays a prominent role. The activation is a two-stage process with transformation of the macrophage from basal state to the triggered macrophage as the first step, followed by the formation of the completely activated macrophage in the second step. Most forms of activation include precise de-emphasis or down-regulation of certain characteristics, as well as emphasis or up-regulation of others, probably dependent on the type and combination of activation signals[2–4].

Endocytosis

The uptake and intracellular ingestion of macromolecules and particles are well known functions of macrophages since the beginning of this century; the term 'macrophage' derives from this function. The substance to be taken up and ingested is progressively enclosed by a small portion of the plasma membrane, which invaginates and then pinches off to form an intracellular vesicle containing the material to be ingested. Two types of endocytosis can be distinguished: pinocytosis and phagocytosis. Pinocytosis ('cell drinking') involves uptake and ingestion of fluid and/or solutes via small vesicles. Phagocytosis ('cell eating') means uptake and ingestion of insoluble macromolecules or particles, such as microorganisms or cell debris, via large vesicles. In both processes the first step involves recognition of the substance or particle and its binding to a specific binding site (receptor) within the cell membrane, followed by its invagination (for review see ref. 5).

Pinocytosis is generally induced by the lectin-like interaction of the carbohydrate moiety of the macromolecule with a glycoprotein or glycolipid of the cell membrane. Kupffer cells have like various other cell receptors for mannose/fucose-, mannose-6-phosphate- or galactose-terminal glycoproteins. The modification of the carbohydrate moiety of the macromolecule, for instance the cleavage of the terminal *N*-acetyl-neuraminic acid, makes possible the binding to the receptor, which induces pinocytotic uptake[3,4].

Phagocytosis as a rule involves opsonins. The Kupffer cells recognize and bind the material coated with the opsonin via specific receptors. Opsonins are immunoglobulins G (IgG) and the derivatives of the complement component C3, especially C3b.

Three receptors for IgG on macrophages were identified (Table 2). They react with the Fc-domain of the immunoglobulin. The three receptors are different with regard to their molecular weight. Fcγ receptors form a subgroup of the immunoglobulin supergene family with closest homology to class II histocompatibility antigens. The special role of the three types of Fcγ receptors is unclear as yet. It was supposed that each of the three receptors reacts with subtypes of IgG. The Fcγ receptor, with molecular weight 50–70 kDa, preferentially binds immunocomplexes; the regulation of the three Fcγ receptors is probably also different; only the Fcγ R72 is induced by IFN-γ (for review see ref. 6). The intracellular signal transduction after interaction between receptor and IgG is unclear. Depolarization with opening of ion

Table 2 Receptor for immunoglobulins (FcγR) on Kupffer cells

FcγR$_{72}$	Binding mediated by carbohydrates Induced by IFN-γ
FcγR$_{50-70}$	Only in tissue macrophages Preferentially binding of immune complexes
FcγR$_{p40}$	Polymorphism Target for NK cell activity

channels and an inward Na^+ flow was described, and may be a part of the chain of intracellular signal transduction.

Two complement receptors in the membrane of Kupffer cells were identified and characterized: CR1 and CR3. CR1 recognizes and binds the complement component C3b. Native, uncleaved C3 is not recognized, nor is the degradation product C3dg. In contrast, the complex of C3b with an inhibitor protein (C3bi) is recognized. CR1 functions not only as a receptor, but also as a cofactor in the degradation of its ligand. CR1 is a glycosylated protein with a molecular weight between 160 and 250 kDa. Four allelic forms of CR1 have been described. The gene of CR1 has been cloned and partially sequenced.

CR3 recognizes the complement component C3bi, but does not recognize the precursor C3b, or the product of further cleavage C3dg. The receptor is composed of two polypeptides. The region of the C3bi molecule that is recognized by the receptor has been identified as the triplet Arg–Gly–Asp (RGD). This triplet also serves as a recognition structure for receptors in the family of cell-adhesion molecules (integrins). The recognition of the lipid-A region in LPS, zymosan, and the membrane of various microorganisms is mediated by CR3. The function of these complement receptors, especially CR3, is to mediate the uptake of infectious microorganisms without the intervention of antibodies, and possibly without complement, presumably forming a novel mechanism by which macrophages may recognize and destroy pathogens before the onset of adaptive immunity. This conclusion is underlined from observations of patients who are genetically deficient in CR3 and suffer recurrent, life-threatening infections caused by a variety of microorganisms.

The regulation of complement receptors CR1 and CR3 is performed in an unexpected fashion. IFN-γ, but not IFN-α, causes a striking decrease in the binding capacities of C3 receptors. This behaviour contrasts with that of Fcγ receptors in that IFN-γ causes dramatically enhanced expression and function of FcγR. The depression of binding activity of CR1 and CR3 by IFN-γ appears to be caused by reversible changes in conformation of existing receptors, and is not associated with a reduced number of receptor molecules at the cell surface. Activation of C3 receptors is observed after the contact of macrophages (Kupffer cells) with matrix proteins, such as fibronectin or laminin. The rapid switch from inactive to active state of the receptor and vice-versa may be controlled by phosphorylation, followed by the formation of clusters of six to ten receptors on the surface of the macrophages (for review see ref. 6).

Production and secretion of cytotoxic and antimicrobial substances

Kupffer cells, like some other sessile macrophages, can destroy a wide range of microorganisms, and a variety of isogenic and allogenic cells, such as erythrocytes, aged or injured tissue cells, and tumour cells. A prerequisite is the recognition of the intruder or the noxious cell, which is often, but not always, mediated by receptor–ligand interaction. This is followed by the decision as to whether the microorganism or the noxious cell is retained at the surface of the Kupffer cell or is taken up by endocytosis. The last step is the secretion or intracellular liberation of substances from the Kupffer cells killing the microorganism or the noxious cell (for review see ref. 7). Such killer substances are: (a) reactive oxygen intermediates (ROI); (b) nitric oxide (NO); (c) peptides (TNF-α, defensins).

Reactive oxygen intermediates

Kupffer cells in contact with foreign material, microorganisms or noxious cells show a rapid uptake of molecular oxygen ('oxidative burst'). Catalysed by NADPH oxidase residing in the plasma membrane of Kupffer cells, the superoxide anion radical O_2^- is produced. This reactive oxygen intermediate ('oxygen radical') can inactivate and destroy phagocytosed microorganisms or noxious cells, but can also be released on the outside, where it destroys retained cells or material at the surface. Superoxide production by Kupffer cells is probably regulated by protein kinase C and IFN-γ, but not suppressible by glucocorticoids. Reactive oxygen intermediates are extremely unstable, therefore they act as 'chemical weapons for immediate use' in the intimate surrounding of the production site and secretion[8,12].

Nitric oxide

After activation Kupffer cells are able to synthesize and excrete nitric oxide. This was demonstrated for rat Kupffer cells activated by LPS; for human Kupffer cells NO production is not proven as yet. The source for NO is L-arginine. Nitric oxide does not act through a receptor in the membrane of target cells, but can pass the lipid bilayer of biomembranes by diffusion. In the intracellular space NO reacts with enzymes containing a prosthetic iron group for which NO has a strong avidity. The result is an activation of some enzymes and inactivation of others (Table 3). The activation of soluble guanylate cyclase is involved in the relaxation of vascular smooth muscle, inhibition of platelet adherence and aggregation and also in neutrophil chemotaxis. For these actions NO acts as a signalling molecule. Inactivation of enzymes involved in the Krebs cycles, electron transport chain and DNA synthesis, is the basis for the cytotoxic and antimicrobial effect of NO[9,10,12].

The generation of NO is regulated by glucocorticoids and cytokines. Glucocorticoids inhibit the induction of the NO synthase. Whereas the cytokines IFN-γ, IL-1, IL-6, TNF and GM-CSF induce the NO-synthase, other cytokines (IL-8, IL-10, TGF-β and PDGF) are inhibitors of the induction. NO in aqueous solution and in the presence of oxygen has a very short lifespan (timed in seconds); it is rapidly oxidized to nitrite (NO_2^-) and nitrate (NO_3^-); so NO plays an ambiguous role: it is on the one hand a signal or mediator for reactions in the process of unspecified defence, and on the other hand has a direct cytotoxic and antimicrobial effect.

Table 3a Action of nitric oxide (NO)

Enzyme activation
Guanylate cyclase
ADP-ribosyltransferase
Enzyme inactivation
Aconitase
NADPH ubiquinon: oxidoreductase
Succinate ubiquinon: oxidoreductase
Ribonucleotide reductase

Table 3b Function of nitric oxide

Enzyme activation: mediator effect
Relaxation of vascular smooth muscle
Inhibition of platelet adherence and aggregation
Enzyme inactivation: antimicrobial cytotoxic effect
Inhibition of citrate cycle
Inhibition of DNA synthesis

Peptides

Tumour necrosis factor α (TNF-α) is synthesized in the liver by Kupffer cells, but not by hepatocytes or sinusoidal endothelial cells. TNF released from the producing Kupffer cells binds to a plasma membrane receptor of target cells. It is not yet clear whether the membrane-associated TNF-α of Kupffer cells is an obligatory intermediate in the release of the soluble peptide or has a specific function. TNF-α has various effects at various target cells. Cytotoxicity, especially against tumour cells, is based on the katabolic effect and induction of necrosis. TNF-α synthesis is elicited by LPS and viruses, but not by phagocytosis; it is instantly suppressed by dexamethasone or prostaglandin E_2. TNF-α mediates most (if not all) effects of LPS[11–13].

Defensins are peptides with antimicrobial activity which were isolated from macrophages, granulocytes and neutrophils. Several closely homologous single peptides have been purified to homogeneity and their amino acid sequence has been analysed. Despite their common structural feature, the biological potency of individual peptides varies considerably. Initial binding of the peptide to the microorganism is temperature-independent, reversible, and insufficient for microbicidal activity. Post-binding events are temperature-dependent, but it is unknown how the defensins exert their cytotoxic effect. Some experiments have shown rapid suppression of O_2-consumption and the suggestion of an envelope damage of the target cells[7,17,18].

Kupffer cells also synthesize and release a great number of hydrolases, such as proteases, lipid hydrolases and phospholipases. But evidence is lacking that the enzymatic action of these hydrolases, except lysozyme, can be effectively microbicidal for pathogenic microorganisms. However, several reports suggest that certain combinations of hydrolytic enzymes have synergistic antimicrobial effects, but not necessarily by virtue of their catalytic activity (for reviews see ref. 7).

Signal and mediator substances

Activated Kupffer cells synthesize and release different types of signal and mediator substances (Table 4).

Lipid signals. Prostanoids are synthesized from arachidonic acid on the cyclooxygenase pathway. Rate-limiting is the cleavage of arachidonic acid from phospholipids by phospholipase A_2. The activity of this enzyme in Kupffer cells is regulated by phosphorylation of the enzyme directed by protein kinase C, or of regulatory proteins. In the liver the major producers of prostanoids are the Kupffer cells. A small contribution, mainly thromboxane, prostacyclin and PGE_2, comes from the sinusoidal endothelial cells. In contrast, hepatocytes do not produce substantial amounts. None of the eicosanoids have been found to accumulate or to be stored within the liver cells. Their half-life in the circulation is very short, ranging from seconds to minutes, because of rapid degradation in the hepatocytes (preferentially by a small portion of perivenous hepatocytes) and excretion into bile of both intact and degraded prostaglandins. The synthesis of prostaglandin E_2 in Kupffer cells is stimulated by LPS, TNF-α and some viruses. PGE_2 inhibits its own production in Kupffer cells (autoregulation).

Leukotrienes are synthesized on a second route of arachidonate metabolism: the lipoxygenase pathway. Kupffer cells are the main producers, whereas hepatocytes have only the enzymes for degradation, not for the synthesis of leukotrienes. The inactivation of peptide leukotrienes in the hepatocytes is catalysed by peptidases. Another pathway of inactivation is a cytochrome P-450-dependent hydroxylation followed by ω-oxidation. Finally leukotrienes can be excreted into bile by an ATP-dependent transport system in the canalicular membrane.

Platelet activating factor (PAF) is synthesized in Kupffer cells. An inactive precursor is accumulated within the cells with release of the active PAF after stimulation with Ca^+. Rat Kupffer cells exposed to PAF produce superoxides and eicosanoids. Furthermore, their inositol phosphate production and cytosolic Ca^{2+} concentration increase. The hepatic action of PAF is mediated by this release of eicosanoids (TXA_2 and PGE_2) from Kupffer cells.

The numerous effects of lipid signals on hepatic metabolism, haemodynamic, bile secretion, ion fluxes and secretion of other mediator substances, cannot be presented in this chapter.

Table 4 Signal and mediator substances of Kupffer cells

Lipids
Prostanoids
Leukotrienes
Platelet-activation factor (PAF)
Peptides
IL-1, IL-6
TNF-α
IFN-γ, IFN-β

Peptide signals (cytokines). Kupffer cells are both target cells and cells of production of various cytokines. In the process of unspecific defence the cytokines IL-1, IL-6, TNF-α and IFN-α/β play a predominant role. All cytokines have two peculiar properties: the pleiotropic action of a single cytokine and network interaction of different cytokines. Pleiotropic action means that each signal substance induces a variety of effects and has several target organs (Fig. 1); so IL-6 stimulates the release of ACTH, neural differentiation, haematopoiesis in bone marrow, transformation of lymphocytes to plasma cells and protein synthesis in the liver. Network action means the manifold interactions between different cytokines. Such interactions exist with regard to the synthesis or degradation of mediators, but also with respect to their action on specific receptors at the target organ. For instance, the synthesis of IL-6 in Kupffer cells is stimulated by IL-1 and TNF-α[15,16].

Synthesis and effects of cytokines can be regulated at various levels[12–16] (Fig. 2):

1. *Autostimulation.* The positive feedback loop consists of the production and release of a single substance and the receptor for this signal on the same cell. In most instances the signal has to pass through the extracellular space; so TNF-α secreted by Kupffer cells induces in the same cells the production of TNF-α, IL-1 and IL-6.
2. *Regulation by interaction of signals.* PGE_2 inhibits the synthesis and secretion of TNF-α, whereas IL-1 and TNF-α stimulate the synthesis and secretion of IL-6 by the Kupffer cell. The result in the first process is a regulatory circuit with negative feedback; in the second with positive feedback.

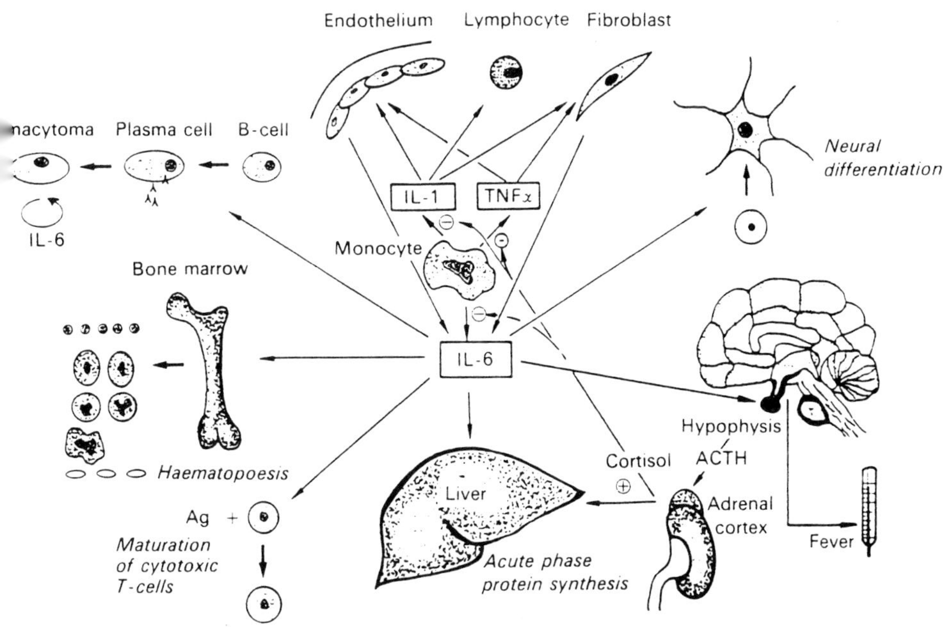

Fig. 1 Pleiotropic action of IL-6

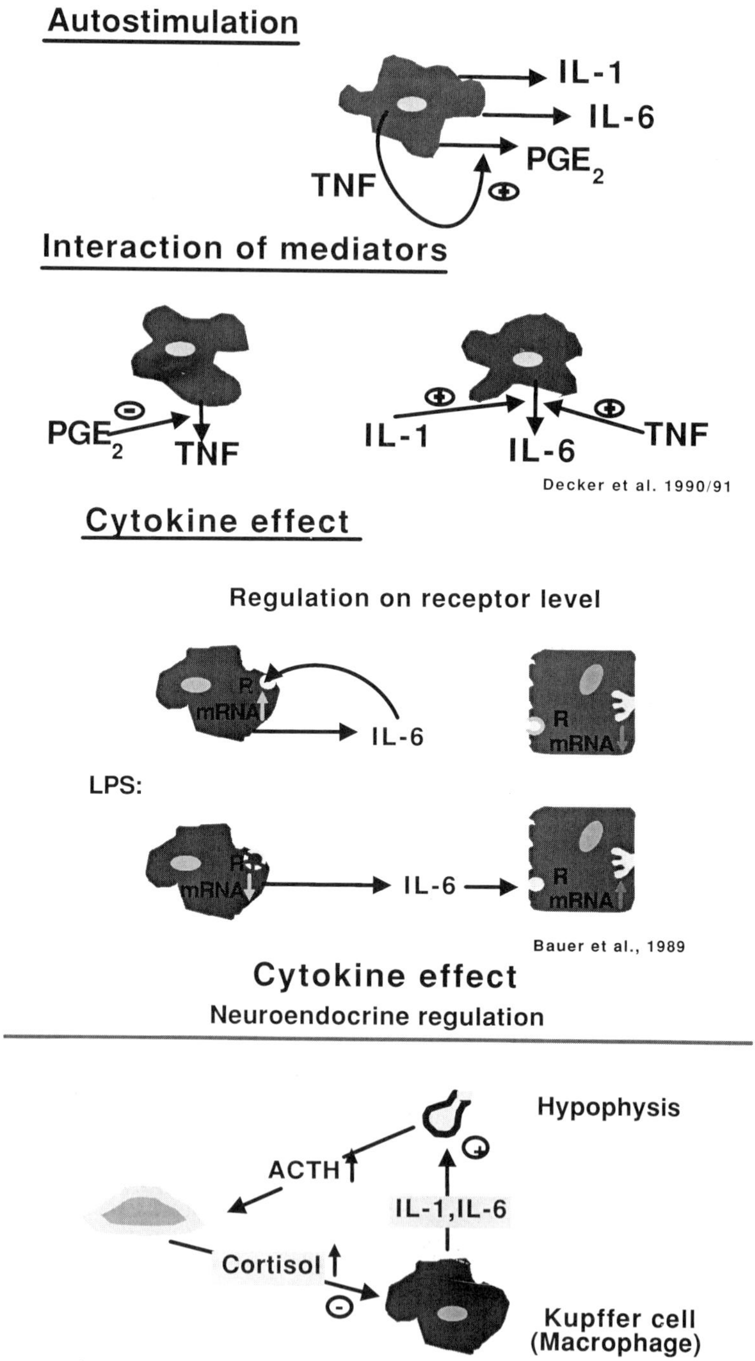

Fig. 2 Regulation of cytokine effect: (**a**) autostimulation, (**b**) interaction of mediators, (**c**) regulation on receptor level, (**d**) neuroendocrine regulation

3. *Regulation at the receptor level.* IL-6 is released by monocytes, which also synthesize the protein of the IL-6 receptor. In monocytes under normal conditions the mRNA concentration of the receptor protein is high. In contrast, hepatocytes synthesize under normal conditions only minimal receptor protein; the corresponding mRNA is low. In acute inflammation induced by LPS the synthesis of the receptor protein in monocytes is reduced, shown by low concentration of mRNA for the IL-6 receptor, whereas in hepatocytes the synthesis of the receptor protein is up-regulated with increase of the mRNA. So, in acute inflammation self-stimulation of the monocytes by self-produced IL-6 is prevented, whereas the IL-6 effect on the hepatocytes is augmented[15].
4. *Neuroendocrine regulation.* IL-1 and IL-6 produced by Kupffer cells stimulate the hypophysis to increased secretion of ACTH. The result is an increase of cortisol secretion from the adrenal cortex. Cortisol inhibits the production of the two cytokines in the Kupffer cells. The result is a regulatory circuit with negative feedback.

For the function of cytokines as coordinates of immune and inflammatory responses see ref. 13.

LIVER AND COMPLEMENT SYSTEM

The complement system plays an important role in unspecific defence mechanisms, especially in the inflammatory process against infectious agents. It consists of two proteolytic cascades, designated 'classical' and 'alternative' pathway. Their end-products activate the cytolytic pathway of membrane attack complex. This complex, consisting of five hydrophilic proteins, binds to the membranes of target cells owing to hydrophobic interaction with the lipid bilayer. Finally, unfolding and polymerization of the complement component C9 within the membrane cause weakening of membrane structure and formation of transmembrane channels (pores) with the consequence of cell death. But not only the membrane attack complex, also intermediates of the proteolytic cascades are essential for unspecific defence. So proteolytic cleavage of the complement components C3, C4 and C5 results in anaphylatoxins. One of these peptides, C5a, is a particularly potent mediator of inflammation, causing chemotaxis, cell adhesion, production of eicosanoids and release of reactive oxygen intermediates (for reviews see refs 19–22).

For unspecific defence the alternative pathway plays a predominant role since it does not require antibodies for its activation. It exists in an activated state at all times due to the spontaneous hydrolysis of C3. In contrast, the classical pathway is antibody-dependent; binding of an antibody to a foreign particle results in its activation.

The 20 proteins of the complement system circulating in blood plasma are mainly synthesized in the liver. Evidence is based on studies in patients who have received liver transplants. After transplantation the allotypes of several complement components became those of the donor. Furthermore, *de novo* synthesis of the components has been demonstrated in isolated hepatocytes and hepatoma cells (for review see ref. 20). Extrahepatic cells shown to synthesize complement factors are monocytes, tissue macrophages, fibroblasts, and cells of gastrointestinal and urogenital tract; but the functional importance of an extrahepatic source of complement components has been established only for mononuclear phagocytes. Complement factors produced by these cells alter locally vascular permeability, smooth muscle tone and migration of leucocytes, but probably have no systemic effect.

Synthesis of complement factors in the liver is preferentially regulated at the level of transcription[21]. There is some evidence for additional translational and post-translational modification of synthesis rate (processing of mRNA, cleavage of signal peptides or glycosylation), but these modifications are of minor significance for the regulation of synthesis. In general, variations in the rate of synthesis and mRNA in the liver correspond to variations in the serum concentration of complement factors. Cytokines are mediators of hepatic complement synthesis. So IL-1 and TNF mediate, time- and dose-dependently, the increase in the rate of synthesis of C3 and factor B with corresponding increase of their mRNAs, but have no effect on the synthesis of C2 and C4. In contrast, IFN-γ regulates time- and dose-dependently the synthesis of C2 and C4. So the regulation of classical and alternative pathways of the complement system depends on different patterns of cytokines. LPS has direct and indirect effects on the synthesis of complement proteins. The indirect effect may be mediated through IL-1, IL-6, TNF or IFN-γ. LPS also directly increases the synthesis of C2, C3 and factor B in human mononuclear phagocytes by a tissue-specific, pretranslational and translational effect. In macrophages complement synthesis is also stimulated by neuropeptides (substance P) and regulated by the concentrations of complement proteins in the extracellular medium. It is unclear whether both these types of regulation are also effective for complement synthesis in the liver.

The importance of the liver for the complement system is also based on the synthesis of regulator proteins; so the biological activities of surface-bound C3b are regulated by proteins H and I, which are synthesized in the liver. Factor H attaches to C3b and renders it susceptible to the action of Factor I, a serin proteinase. Factor I cleaves the α-chain of C3b. Another example is the regulation of anaphylatoxins: peptides derived from the complement components C3, C4 and C5, designated C3a, C4a and C5a respectively. The anaphylatoxins have a broad spectrum of biological activities, essential for unspecific defence. Among human anaphylatoxins the rank order of potency is C5a > C3a > C4a. The anaphylatoxin C5a is rapidly inactivated in serum by an inactivator protein, which appears to be identical with carboxypeptidase N and cleaves an arginine residue. On the other hand, human plama contains a heat-stable polypeptide (molecular weight 60 kDa), termed cochemotaxin and produced by the liver, which restores chemotactic activity of C5a-des-Arg. It forms a physical complex with native C5a-des-Arg by attaching to the sialic residue of the oligosaccharide chain. Finally, there is evidence for an inhibitor of cochemotaxin. This inhibitor, which is chemically and antigenically similar to the Bb fragment of factor B in the alternative pathway and is synthesized in the liver, has no effect on the chemotactic activity of C5a but abolishes the chemotactic activity exhibited by mixtures of C5a-des-Arg and cochemotaxin (Fig. 3) (for review see ref. 22).

So the complement system is regulated by hepatic synthesis of complement factors under the influence of cytokines. Furthermore, biologically active intermediates are regulated with regard to their activity by the net balance of proteases and antiproteases, predominantly synthesized and secreted by the liver.

LIVER AND ACUTE-PHASE PROTEINS

The term 'acute-phase response' was introduced in 1941 by Abernethy and Avery. It means the answer of the organism to disturbances of its homeostasis due to infection, tissue injury, neoplastic growth or traumatic lesions. The aim of this response is to restore the disturbed homeostasis. Within the acute-phase response one can discriminate between a local reaction at the site of injury and a systemic reaction (for review see refs 23–27).

The systemic reaction is characterized by fever, leucocytosis, cortisol secretion, negative nitrogen balance, decreased plasma concentration of iron and zinc, and alteration of the cellular and humoral components of the immune system. It is a well-known phenomenon also that the concentration of several plasma proteins increases. They are called 'acute-phase proteins'. Dependent on the grade of increase in plasma concentration three groups of acute-phase proteins can be differentiated (Table 5). This pattern is species-specific. In humans CRP and serum amyloid A show the highest increases, whereas in the rat, α_2-macroglobulin and α_1-acid glycoprotein are the acute-phase proteins showing the most prominent changes. Simultaneously, plasma concentrations of albumin and transferrin decrease ('negative acute-phase proteins').

The acute-phase proteins are synthesized exclusively in the liver. Their changes in plasma concentration are preceded by corresponding alterations in mRNA concentrations; therefore the increased synthesis is based on increased rate of transcription. An increased secretion has been observed for

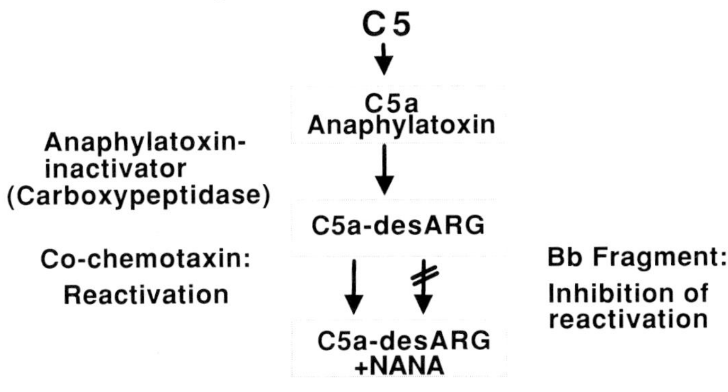

Fig. 3 Regulation of C5a anaphylatoxin

some acute-phase proteins, but has minor importance compared to the increase of synthesis by increased transcription[28].

IL-6 is the major signal substance which induces the synthesis and secretion of acute-phase proteins[29,30]. In rat hepatocytes and hepatoma cells this cytokine stimulates, time- and dose-dependently, the synthesis and secretion of acute-phase proteins with the species-specific pattern. IL-6, a phosphoglycoprotein, is produced at the site of local injury by monocytes, macrophages and, to a smaller extent, also by endothelial cells and fibroblasts. The synthesis of IL-6 is supported by IL-1 and TNF, and is suppressed by glucocorticoids. The cytokine reaches the liver with the blood and stimulates IL-6 synthesis in Kupffer cells. This could mean an amplification of the IL-6 effect (for reviews see refs 14, 16 and 26–32).

The IL-6 receptor in the plasma membrane consists of two glycoproteins with molecular weights of 80 and 130 kDa, respectively[33]. The 80 kDa glycoprotein has the specific binding site for IL-6. Although the protein is endowed with an intracellular domain, no intracellular signal transfer can be induced by this protein alone. Binding of IL-6 to the 80 kDa glycoprotein triggers the association with a non-ligand-binding 130 kDa membrane glycoprotein[33–35]. Only after association of the two proteins the intracellular signal transduction can start. From the 80 kDa glycoprotein a subunit can be cleaved and released in the extracellular fluid. This soluble receptor protein binds IL-6, can be reintegrated in the membrane, and induces the expression of acute-phase proteins[36].

The intracellular signal transmission pathway is as yet unclear. The subsequent activation of a tyrosine kinase is probably involved[33]. In contrast, there is no evidence for the involvement of protein kinase C, inositol triphosphate or cAMP. Enhancer regions responsible for the IL-6 mediated

Table 5 Acute-phase plasma proteins in human and rat

	Increase				
Species	*10–100-fold*	*2–10-fold*	*≤ 2-fold*	*No change*	*Decrease*
Human	C-reactive protein	α_1-Proteinase inhibitor	Caeruloplasmin	α_2-Macroglobin	Inter-α-antitrypsin
	Serum amyloid A	α_1-Acid glycoprotein	C3 of complement	Haemopexin	Transferrin
		α_1-Antichymotrypsin	α_2-Antiplasmin	Serum amyloid P	α_1-Lipoprotein
		Fibrinogen	C_1 inactivator	Prothrombin	Prealbumin
		Haptoglobin			Albumin
Rat	α_2-Macroglobulin	Fibrinogen	α_1-Proteinase inhibitor	α_1-Macroglobulin	α_1-Inhibitor 3
	α_1-Acid glycoprotein	Haptoglobin	Caeruloplasmin	Antithrombin III	Transferrin
		Cysteine proteinase inhibitor	Prekallikrein	Serum amyloid P	Prealbumin
			Haemopexin	Prothrombin	Albumin
			C-reactive protein		

increased transcription rate of acute-phase proteins have been identified[25,37,38]. In the case of rat α_1-acid glycoprotein gene this enhancer element with 142 bp sequence is located 5300–5150 bp upstream of the transcriptional start site. The IL-6 responsive elements of various genes for acute-phase proteins (α_1-acid glycoprotein, α_2-macroglobulin, haptoglobin) contain a common sequence motive (Fig. 4). This consensus sequence in the enhancers, in combination with appropriate transaction factors, mediates the IL-6-induced increase of transcription for the whole set of genes for acute-phase proteins. The signal is switched off by internalization of the 80 kDa receptor glycoprotein with bound IL-6[39].

The functions of acute-phase proteins in unspecific defence are predominantly based on their antiproteolytic effect, opsonization effect and immunomodulation effect.

Antiproteolytic effect. An antiproteolytic effect applies to several acute-phase proteins. These protease inhibitors are directed not only towards the active forms of proteases normally circulating in the plasma, but also towards proteases released from different cells and tissues under pathological conditions, such as inflammation or necrosis. The protease inhibitory capacity of plasma is normally much higher than proteolytic activity. Only under specific conditions is there a local predominance of proteases, e.g. at the site of traumatic or vascular injury, infection or necrosis.

The acute-phase proteins with the property of antiproteases and their biological substrates are summarized in Table 6. With the exception of α_2-macroglobulin all acute-phase proteins are inhibitors of serine proteases. α_2-Macroglobin has a wide spectrum of protease inhibitory activity. It inhibits proteases of all four catalytic classes: serine-, cysteine-, aspartic- and metallo-proteases. Within the inhibitors of serine proteases each acute-phase protein has a main target substrate. Other serine proteases are also inhibited with less effectivity. So the acute-phase proteins are antiproteases with broad and overlapping substrate specificity. This function is extremely important in unspecific defence, because the proteolytic cascades induced during inflammation would result in severe disturbances of homeostasis and shock if not controlled by the antiproteolytic effect of acute-phase proteins (for review see refs 40 and 41).

Opsonization effect (removal of foreign material). C-reactive protein (CRP) binds to phosphorylcholine with high affinity in the presence of calcium ions[42,43]. Phosphorylcholine is widely distributed in biological material as an integral constituent of the mammalian and bacterial cell membranes.

−176 −159

5′ ATCCTT | CTGGGA | ATTCTG 3′

3′ TAGGAA | GACCCT | TAAGAC 5′

Fig. 4 Consensus sequence of the enhancer region for IL-6-induced synthesis of acute-phase proteins

Furthermore, CRP binds to chromatin and fragments of DNA, which arise in connection with cell necrosis[44,45] and, like lectins, to the carbohydrate moeity in glycoproteins and glycolipids of cell membranes[46]. CRP thereby mediates precipitation, agglutination and capsular swelling of bacteria. Inflammatory cells, such as neutrophils, appear to have a surface receptor for CRP with the consequence of binding and phagocytosis. After coating of a foreign particle with CRP the complement component C3b can also be attached to it with high affinity. This allows phagocytosis by macrophages through their C3b receptor (for review see ref. 47).

Serum amyloid A (SAA) is associated with plasma lipoproteins of the HDL class, and this complex is rapidly cleared from the plasma. Therefore SAA could also increase the clearance of foreign or toxic materials bound to HDL. Indeed, LPS have been found to be bound to HDL[48].

Immunomodulation. Several acute-phase proteins are immunomodulators; α_1-acid glycoprotein inhibits the proliferation of lymphocytes stimulated by mitogens or by allogenic cells. Further effects of α_1-acid glycoprotein are the inhibition of antibody formation and the induction of cytotoxic lymphocytes[49].

CRP activates monocytes[50]. Serum amyloid A and α_1-antiprotease suppress antigen-dependent reactions of lymphocytes[51,52].

In summary, a mutual interaction exists between the site of local extrahepatic injury and the liver. At the site of local injury proteolytic cascades are induced. Their overshoot would result in tissue destruction and shock. Signal substances, especially IL-6, produced at the site of local injury, induce hepatic synthesis and secretion of acute-phase proteins. These proteins inhibit proteases and proteolytic cascades, they favour the removal of cells, bacteria and their degradation products by macrophages, and they modulate the specific defence reaction by the immune system.

Table 6 Acute-phase proteins with function of antiproteases

Acute-phase protein	*Type of inhibited protease*	*Main target protease*	*Other inhibited proteases*
α_1-Antitrypsin	Serine protease	Granulocyte elastase	Chymotrypsin, cathepsin G, trypsin, plasmin, thrombin
α_1-Antichymotrypsin	Serine protease	Cathepsin G	Mast cell chymase
Inter-α-trypsin inhibitor	Serine protease	Trypsin, chymotrypsin	
α_2-Antiplasmin	Serine protease	Plasmin	Trypsin, chymotrypsin, kallikrein, thrombin, Factor Xa, XIa
α_2-Macroglobulin	Serine, cysteine proteases, aspartic, metalloproteases	Majority of proteases	

CLINICAL CONSEQUENCES

The experimental results demonstrate that the liver is an important organ for the unspecific defence reaction; therefore one can expect that liver diseases leading to a reduced hepatic organ function influence the grade and the course of an acute extrahepatic injury with disturbance of homeostasis.

Indeed, the incidence of bacterial infections in patients with decompensated cirrhosis is increased. In the study of Rimola *et al.*[53], 46% of the patients with decompensated cirrhosis were infected at admission to hospital, or developed bacterial infection during the early hospital stay. This incidence is nearly four times greater than that occurring in the general hospitalized population (12%). Hospital-acquired infections are significantly more frequent in patients with cirrhosis (38%) than in a control group without liver diseases (2–11%). Probably dysfunction of Kupffer cells, their partial exclusion from the portal blood stream by portacaval anastomoses, reduced synthesis of complement factors and of regular proteins for the complement system, and finally the diminished production and release of acute-phase proteins may be causes of the reduced unspecific defence reaction in liver diseases.

References

1. van Furth R. Phagocytic cells: development and distribution of mononuclear phagocytes in normal steady state and inflammation. In Gallin JI, Goldstein IM, Snydermann R, editors. Inflammation: basic principles and clinical correlates. New York: Raven Press; 1988:281–95.
2. Jones EA, Summerfield J. Kupffer cells. In: Arias IM, Jakoby WB, Popper H, Schachter D, Shafritz DA, editors. The liver: biology and pathobiology. New York: Raven Press;1988:683–704.
3. Decker K. Biologically active products of stimulated liver macrophages (Kupffer cells). Eur J Biochem. 1990;192:245–61.
4. Adams DO, Hamilton TA. Phagocytic cells: cytotoxic activities of macrophages. In: Gallin JI, Goldstein IM, Snyderman R, editors. Inflammation: basic principles and clinical correlates. New York: Raven Press; 1988:471–92.
5. Wileman TH, Harding C, Stahl P. Receptor-mediated endocytosis. Biochem J. 1985;232:1–14.
6. Unkeless JC, Wright SD. Phagocytic cells: Fcy and complement receptors. In: Gallin JI, Goldstein IM, Snyderman R, editors. Inflammation: basic principles and clinical correlates. New York: Raven Press; 1989:343–62.
7. Elsbach P, Weiss J. Phagocytic cells: oxygen-independent antimicrobial systems. In: Gallin JI, Goldstein IM, Snyderman R, editors. Inflammation: basic principles and clinical correlates. New York: Raven Press; 1989:445–70.
8. Sies H. Oxidative stress: from basic research to clinical application. Am J Med. 1991;91:3C–31S.
9. Monacada S, Palmer RMJ, Higgs EA. Nitric oxide: physiology, pathophysiology and pharmacology. Pharm Rev. 1991;43:109–42.
10. Billiar TR, Hoffmann RA, Curran RD, Langrehr JM, Simmons RL. A role for inducible nitric oxide biosynthesis in the liver in inflammation and in alogeneic immune response. J Lab Clin Med. 1992;120:192–7.
11. Beutler B, Cerami A. The biology of cachectin TNF – a primary mediator of the host response. Ann Rev Immunol. 1989;7:625–55.
12. Decker K. Basic mechanisms of the inflammatory response. Molecular aspects of inflammation. Heidelberg: Springer Verlag; 1991:1–23.
13. Arai K, Lee F, Miyajima A, Miyatake S, Arai N, Yokota T. Cytokines: coordinators of immune and inflammatory responses. Ann Rev Biochem. 1990;59:783–836.

14. Bauer J. Interleukin 6 and its receptor during homeostasis, inflammation, and tumor growth. Klin Wochenschr. 1989;67:697–706.
15. Bauer J, Lengyel G, Bauer T, Acs G, Gerok W. Regulation of interleukin-6 receptor expression in human monocytes and hepatocytes. FEBS Lett. 1989;249:27–30.
16. Andus T, Bauer J, Gerok W. Effects of cytokines on the liver. Hepatology. 1991;13:364–75.
17. Selsted ME, Harwig SSL, Ganz T, Schilling JW, Lehrer RI. Primary structures of three human neutrophil defensins. J Clin Invest. 1985;76:1436–9.
18. Ganz T, Selsted ME, Szklarek D, Harwig SSL, Daher K, Bainton DF, Lehrer RI. Natural peptides antibiotics of human neutrophils. J Clin Invest. 1985;76:1427–35.
19. Müller-Eberhard H. Molecular organization and function of the complement system. Ann Rev Biochem. 1988;57:321–47.
20. Campbell RD, Law SKA, Reid KBM, Sim RB. Structure, organization and regulation of the complement genes. Ann Rev Immunol. 1988;6:161–95.
21. Perlmutter DH, Colten HR. Molecular immunobiology of complements biosynthesis: a model of single-cell control of effector–inhibitor balance. Ann Rev Immunol. 1986;4:231–51.
22. Goldstein IM. Complement: biologically active products. In: Gallin JI, Goldstein IM, Snyderman R, editors. Inflammation: basic principles and clinical correlates. New York: Raven Press; 1988:55–74.
23. Kushner I. The phenomenon of the acute phase response. Ann NY Acad Sci. 1982;389:38–48.
24. Koj A. Definition and classification of acute phase proteins. In: Gordon AH, Koj A, editors. The acute phase response to injury and infections. Amsterdam: Elsevier; 1985:139–232.
25. Castell JV, Andus T, Kunz D, Heinrich PC. Interleukin-6. The major regulator of acute-phase protein synthesis in man and rat. Ann NY Acad Sci. 1989;557:87–99.
26. Heinrich PC, Castell JV, Andus T. Interleukin-6 and the acute phase response. Biochem J. 1990;269:621–36.
27. Andus T, Heinrich PC, Castell JC, Gerok W. Interleukin-6: Ein Schlüsselhormon der Akutphase-Reaktion. Dtsch Med Wochenschr. 1989;114:1710–16.
28. Castell JV, Gomez-Lechon MJ, David M, Fabra R, Trullenque R, Heinrich PC. Acute-phase response of human hepatocytes: Regulation of acute-phase protein synthesis by interleukin-6. Hepatology. 1990;12:1179–86.
29. Gauldie J, Richards C, Harnish D, Landsdorp P, Baumann H. Interferon β_2/B-cell stimulatory factor type 2 shares identity with monocyte-derived hepatocytes-stimulating factor and regulates the major acute phase protein response in liver cells. Proc Natl Acad Sci USA. 1987;84:7251–5.
30. Andus T, Geiger T, Hirano T, Northoff H, Ganter U, Bauer J, Kishimoto T, Heinrich PC. Recombinant human B cell stimulatory factor 2 (BSF-2/IFNβ2) regulates β-fibrinogen and albumin mRNA levels in Fao-9 cells. FEBS Lett. 1987;221:18–22.
31. Snick J. Interleukin 6: an overview. Ann Rev Immunol. 1990;8:253–78.
32. Kishimoto T. The biology of interleukin-6. Blood. 1990;74:1–10.
33. Taga T, Hibi M, Hirata Y, Yamasaki K, Yasukawa K, Matsuda T, Hirano T, Kishimoto T. Interleukin 6 triggers the association of its receptor with a possible signal transducer gp 130. Cell. 1989;58:573–81.
34. Rose-John S, Hipp E, Lenz D, Legres LG, Horr H, Hirano T, Kishimoto T, Heinrich PC. Structural and functional studies on the human interleukin-6 receptor. J Biol Chem. 1991;266:3841–6.
35. Schooltink H, Stoyan T, Lenz D, Schmitz H, Hirano T, Kishimoto T, Heinrich PC, Rose-John S. Structural and functional studies on the human hepatic interleukin-6 receptor. Molecular cloning and overexpression in Hep G 2 cells. Biochem J. 1991;277:659–64.
36. Mackiewicz A, Schooltink H, Heinrich PC, Rose-John S. Complex of soluble human IL-6-receptor up regulates expression of acute phase proteins. J Immunol. 1992 (in press).
37. Fey GH, Fuller GM. Regulation of acute phase gene expression by inflammatory mediators. Mol Biol Med. 1987;4:323–8.
38. Oliviero S, Cortese R. The human haptoglobin gene promoter: interleukin-6-responsive elements interact with a DNA-binding protein induced by interleukin-6. EMBO J. 1989;8:1145–51.
39. Zohlnhöfer D, Graeve L, Rose-John S, Schooltink H, Dittrich E, Heinrich PC. The hepatic interleukin-6 receptor. Down-regulation of the interleukin-6 binding subunit (gp 80) by its ligand. FEBS Lett. 1992;306:219–22.

40. Gerok W. Clinical implications of infections with respect to the liver. In: Bianchi L *et al.*, editors. Infectious diseases of the liver. Lancaster: Kluwer; 1990:91–106.
41. Gerok W, Gross V. Secretory proteins; synthesis, secretion, and function. In: McIntyre N, Benhamou JP, Bircher J, Rizzetto M, Rodes J, editors. Oxford textbook of clinical hepatology. Oxford: Oxford University Press; 1991:174–98.
42. Andersen JK, Stroud RM, Volonakis JE. Studies on the binding specificity of human CRP for phosphorylcholine. Fed Proc. 1978;37:1495.
43. Volonakis JE, Narkates AJ. Interaction of CRP with artificial phosphatidylcholine bilayers and complement. J Immunol. 1981;126:1280.
44. Robey RA, Jones KD, Tanaka T, Liu TY. Binding of CRP to chromatin and nucleosom cor particles. J Biol Chem. 1984;259:7311–16.
45. Shepard EG, Van Helden PD, Strauss M, Böhm L, De Beer FC. Functional effects of CRP binding to nuclei. Immunology. 1986;58:489–94.
46. Soelter J, Uhlenbruck G. The role of phosphate groups in the interaction of human CRP with galactan polysaccharides. Immunology. 1986;58:139–44.
47. Pepys MB. C-reactive protein. A review of its structure and function. Eur J Rheumatol Inflam. 1982;5:386–97.
48. Coetzee GA, Strahan F, Van Der West-Huyzen DR, Hoppe HC, Jeenah MS, De Beer FC. Serum amyloid A-containing human high density lipoprotein 3. J Biol Chem. 1986;261:9644–51.
49. Cheresh DA, Haynes DH, Distasio JA. Interaction of an acute phase reactant, alpha-1-acid glycoprotein with the lymphoid cell surface: a model for non-specific immune suppression. Immunology. 1984;51:541–8.
50. Zahedi K, Mortensen RF. Macrophage tumoricidal activity induced by human CRP. Cancer Res. 1986;46:5077–83.
51. Benson MD, Aldo-Benson M. Effect of purified protein SAA in immune response *in vitro*: mechanisms of suppression. J Biol Chem. 1979;122:2077.
52. Aroba PK, Miller HC, Aronson LD. Alpha-1-antitrypsin is an effector of immunological stasis. Nature. 1978;274:589–90.
53. Rimola A, Arroyo V, Rodes J. Infective complications in acute and chronic liver failure: basis and control. In: Williams R, editor. Liver failure. Edinburgh: Churchill Livingstone; 1986:93–111.

31
Liver and immune response

K.-H. MEYER ZUM BÜSCHENFELDE

INTRODUCTION

During recent years cell biology, biochemistry, molecular biology and immunology have formed a more complete picture of the physiological functions of the various components of the liver[1–4]. The importance of all elements of the liver, as well as of structural–functional relationships between all liver cells and matrix components, has been realized. The interactions among cells and between cells on the one hand, and the matrix components on the other hand, play an important role in determining the phenotypic and functional expression of cells. In particular cytokines, hormone-like factors and metabolites produced by the cells within the liver are responsible for maintaining the specific functions of the liver. In this context a good balance between regulatory factors produced by hepatocytes and non-parenchymal liver cells is of great importance, but factors coming from other parts of the body may also have a regulatory function. Disturbances of this balance will produce changes in the amount and type of cells, and in the nature of the matrix components produced by these cells. The alterations in cell–cell and cell–matrix interaction will lead to abnormalities in liver structure and function.

LIVER AND IMMUNOLOGICAL HOMEOSTASIS

Among the different physiological functions of the liver the crucial role in maintaining the immunological homeostasis of the body is of central importance. Evidence for this comes from experimental studies and some clinical observations.

Tolerance against orally applied antigens can be prevented through portacaval shunting. Experimental transplantations of heart, kidney and bone marrow have shown that rejection without application of immunosuppressive drugs can be retarded through anastomoses of the venous vessels of the transplanted organs with the portal vein, or direct implantation of bone marrow cells in the liver. Kamada's group from Japan[5,6] could demonstrate in special rat strains not only a better acceptance of liver transplants but also a better tolerance of other organ transplants such as kidney and skin after liver transplantation. Furthermore immune reactions against skin transplants could be abolished after liver transplantation. Finally it is well known that an impaired filter function of the sinusoidal cells of the liver results in increased production of IgM and IgG. In chronic active hepatitis and cirrhosis of the liver hypergammaglobulinaemia, circulating autoantibody and antibodies to enteric bacteria and dietary antigens are frequently observed[7,8].

SINUSOIDAL CELLS IN HOST DEFENCE MECHANISMS

Due to its unique position at the interface between blood and hepatocytes the sinusoidal cells, together with hepatocytes[9–11], are responsible for several cell-specific host defence mechanisms. In this process Kupffer cells (KC), sinus endothelial cells (SEC), liver-associated lymphocytes (LAL) and probably to a lesser extent Ito cells, are involved.

Kupffer cells

The KC[12] – 30% of the non-parenchymal liver cell population – form a protective barrier for the systemic circulation (Table 1). Harmful materials such as bacterial endotoxins, microorganisms, immune complexes, dietary antigens, etc., are being removed from the blood by a highly developed filter mechanism of KC; for this KC contain various receptor systems[12]. Besides their clearance function of immunogens coming from the gut via the portal vein, the KC play an important role in the induction of specific tolerance to these antigens. KC, like other macrophages, express MHC class II antigens and CD4 molecules[13], and are able to present antigens[14,15]. The uptake and processing of alloantigens by KC is probably the crucial step in the development of tolerance against immunogens coming from the gut[16]. Furthermore KC can present antigens to primed T cells, but in contrast to other macrophages they are insufficient for stimulating unprimed T cells.

Table 1 Kupffer cell function

Clearance of foreign material, endotoxin, cell debris, enzymes and modified LDLs
Clearance of immune complexes
Modulation of immune response to portal antigens
Phagocytosis of erythrocytes and microorganisms
Involved in iron metabolism

Sinus endothelial cells

Sinus endothelial cells (SEC)[17] comprise about 6.3% of the total liver volume. Among the non-parenchymal liver cells they are the most common cell type. The significance of the SEC in host defence is not completely clear, and needs to be studied in greater depth. So far it has been demonstrated that SEC, like KC, are actively engaged in the clearance of harmful substances from the circulation. For this SEC process a number of different receptors (Table 2)[17]. Concerning host defence functions the lectin-like receptor, the Fc receptor, as well as the phagocytic and endocytic function of SEC, are of major importance.

In 1979 receptors for specific carbohydrates[18], so-called 'lectin-like receptors', were found to be present on SEC. They showed specificity for mannose or *N*-acetylglucosamine-terminated glycoproteins. In this respect SEC are more active than KC. The physiological substrates of these receptors are lysosomal enzymes and tissue plasminogen activator. This fact illustrates the important function of this receptor for the removal of potentially harmful endogenous substances from the circulation.

Receptors for the Fc part of IgG are characteristic for SEC. They are not present on endothelial cells of other organs. Via this receptor small soluble IgG–antigen complexes are removed from the circulation without the interaction of complement. In contrast to KC the SEC are not able to phagocytose via this receptor, for instance IgG-coated erythrocytes. In cirrhosis of the liver the length and number of Fc receptor-positive SEC is

Table 2 Receptor-specific endocytosis of sinusoidal endothelial cells

Receptor	*Ligands*	*Comments*
Mannose (M_r 175 000)	Glycoproteins terminating with fucose, *N*-acetyl-glucosamine, mannose	Uptake via coated pits; rapid internalization and lysosomal degradation
Fc	Soluble immune complexes (IgG)	Degradation occurs more slowly than in Kupffer cells
Scavenger (M_r 250 000)	Aldehyde modified proteins, AGE proteins, modified LDL	Uptake via coated pits; rapid internalization and lysosomal degradation
ApoE (M_r 60 000)	VLDL	No internalization
ApoB/E	HDL	
Hyaluronan	Hyaluronan chondroitin sulphate	Uptake via coated pits; lysosomal degradation
Collagen	Denatured collagens I, II, III, IV, V, VI gelatin	
P-III-NP	N-terminal propeptide of collagen type III	
Caeruloplasmin (M_r 32 000)	Caeruloplasmin	Transcytosis and desialylation
Insulin	Insulin	
Glucagon	Glucagon	Transcytosis
CD4 (M_r 54 000)	Human immunodeficiency virus	Present also on Kupffer cells

considerably reduced, explaining the increased occurrence of circulating immune complexes in chronic liver diseases.

Under certain circumstances SEC can replace destroyed or functionally inactive KC and can phagocytose particles as large as 1 μm[19]. Finally SEC are able to endocytose by specific receptors transferrin, caeruloplasmin, transcobalamin, insulin and glucagon. Some studies provide evidence that these proteins are desialylated during their transport across the endothelial lining, and then can be taken up by hepatocytes via their galactosyl receptors[18].

Liver-associated lymphocytes

Liver-associated lymphocytes (LAL) are now considered as a hepatic intrasinusoidal cell population. They consist of the Pit cell[20] or large granular lymphocytes (LGL) and of agranular lymphocytes (about 67% of the LAL)[21]. The agranular lymphocytes share some charactertistics of Pit cells, except the granules. All types of LAL are in close contact with KC and SEC. Data from rats, mice and humans have shown that LAL differ phenotypically from peripheral blood lymphocytes (PBL) (Table 3)[21]. The percentage of CD8 and $CD56^+$ cells is higher in LAL than in PBL. Among the $CD56^+$ cells the percentage with typical natural killer (NK) phenotypes ($CD56^+/CD3^-/CD16^+$) is very low in LAL, compared to PBL. The percentage of $CD56^+/CD3^-/CD16^-$ cells is very high, and that of cells with the phenotype $CD56^+/CD3^+/CD16^-$ increased in comparison to PBL. Data mainly from studies in rats and mice indicate that LAL have an anticancer and antiviral function. In humans LAL have been proposed to act as a natural resistance mechanism to hepatic tumours and hepatic metastases. Few data indicate that LAL may have an antiviral function in hepatitis A and B. Their role in the killing of viral infected hepatocytes is unclear. Since LAL are in close contact to KC and SEC within the sinusoid, cell–cell interactions influenced by a variety of cytokines produced by these cells (Table 4) may induce a special microenvironment that may keep LAL continuously in an activated state. In the same way as peripheral blood large granular lymphocytes (LGL) to vascular endothelial cells, LAL seem to be

Table 3 Phenotype markers on human LAL and PBL

	LAL	*PBL*
CD_3	49	68
CD_2	83	79
CD_4	19	49*
CD_8	52	28*
CD_{16}	4	12**
CD_{56}	53	29*
$CD_{56^+}/CD_{3^-}/CD_{16^+}$	6	41†
$CD_{56^+}/CD_{3^-}/CD_{16^-}$	55	39†
$CD_{56^+}/CD_{3^+}/CD_{16^-}$	39	20†

* $p < 0.001$; ** $p < 0.05$
† Percentage of CD_{56^+} cells

Table 4 Cytokines produced by LAL, KC, SEC

LAL	*SEC*	*KC*
IL-1/2/3	IL-1/6	IL-1/6
IFN-α/γ	GM-CSF	IFN-α/β
TNF-α	M-CSF	TNF-α
	G-CSF	PDGF
GM-CSF	PDGF	TGF-β
M-SCF	Chemotactic F_s	

in contact with SEC and KC through cellular adhesion molecules (CAM). As shown by perfusion experiments cytokines, in particular interleukin 2, can increase the number of LAL, but also of KC and mononuclear cells coming from outside the liver, indicating that LAL may represent one of the most important mechanisms of host defence against diseases[22]. Their role in the immunopathology of liver diseases needs to be clarified[23].

SINUSOIDAL CELLS AND IMMUNE RESPONSE

The sinusoidal cells are not only responsible for several cell-specific host defence mechanism, but may also play a central role in the immunopathogenesis of many inflammatory liver diseases. Immediately after an injury of the liver by viruses, xenobiotics, autoimmune mechanisms, etc., or in a case of liver transplantation, the number of non-parenchymal liver cells increases. In part this is due to proliferation of endogenous cells. In addition new cells, e.g. leucocytes, macrophages, lymphocytes, etc., arrive from the circulation in response to chemotactic substances. The incoming cells modify the normal cell–cell interactions and also may produce cytokines that increase the proliferation and synthetic capacity of the cells. Foreign and self-antigenic material originating in the liver tissue is internalized by sessile macrophages. Together with MHC class II antigens which are constitutively expressed on most macrophages, processed antigens are presented to lymphocytes. Interferon-γ secreted by activated lymphocytes[24] stimulates local macrophages but also SEC, which then also express MHC class II antigens and may function as antigen-presenting cells[25–27]. Furthermore macrophages produce the cytokines TNF-α and interleukin-1 which alter the function of sinus endothelial cells in two important ways: a switch from an anticoagulatory to a procoagulatory state and an expression of adhesion molecules for neutrophils (ELAM-1)[28–30] and intercellular adhesion molecules (ICAM-1/2), vascular cellular adhesion molecules (VLAM-1)[31,32] and platelet-activation-dependent granule external membrane protein (PADGEM)[17]. These are adhesion proteins for PMN which may move across the endothelium or secrete reactive oxygen and enzymes to destroy SEC, the matrix of the Disse space or hepatocytes. IL-1 and TNF-α may enhance the expression of ICAM-1 on SEC. Via ICAM-1, MHC-class II, CD58 and probably VCAM-1 on SEC, lymphocytes are attracted to the liver sinusoid. By diapedesis they obtain access to the hepatocytes which express ICAM-1, MHC-class II and CD58 *de novo*.

Interferon-γ secreted by lymphocytes is a known mediator, besides IL-1 and TNF-α, for the expression of these adhesive molecules. Some of these receptors can also be used by monocytes (VCAM-1, PADGEM, ICAM-1), and may be crucial for the influx of this cell type in the injured livers[17] (Fig. 1).

Due to the expression of MHC class II antigens, adhesion molecules, and the secretion of cytokines, SEC, KC, LAL and mononuclear cells arriving from outside the liver promote and amplify the local immune response. Thus, lymphocytes, whether of $CD4^+$ or $CD8^+$ phenotype, must meet several prerequisites in order to act as cytotoxic effector cells[33]. First a close topographic contact between target structures and effector cells is necessary, followed by several steps[34–36] of interactions between effector and target cells before the actual killing of the target cell can take place. The components of the effector/target cell-binding complex are demonstrated schematically in Figs 2 and 3; Fig. 2 shows the structure of the molecules on the target and effector cellside; Fig. 3 demonstrates the frequency of events in the cytotoxic process.

LIVER AND IMMUNE-MEDIATED DISEASE

The concept of the local immune response stems mainly from experimental studies, but there is now substantial evidence that these mechanisms may also operate in the liver sinusoid in patients with viral, autoimmune, and drug-induced liver diseases and in liver transplantation[37,38]. This is based

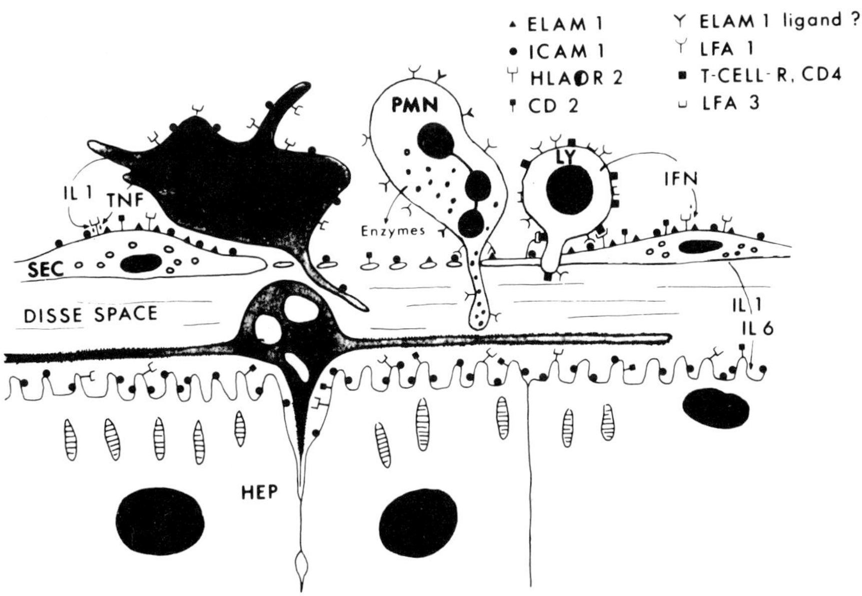

Fig. 1 Cellular interactions of sinusoidal endothelial cells of the liver with leucocytes and other liver cells. Taken from ref. 17; for explanation see text

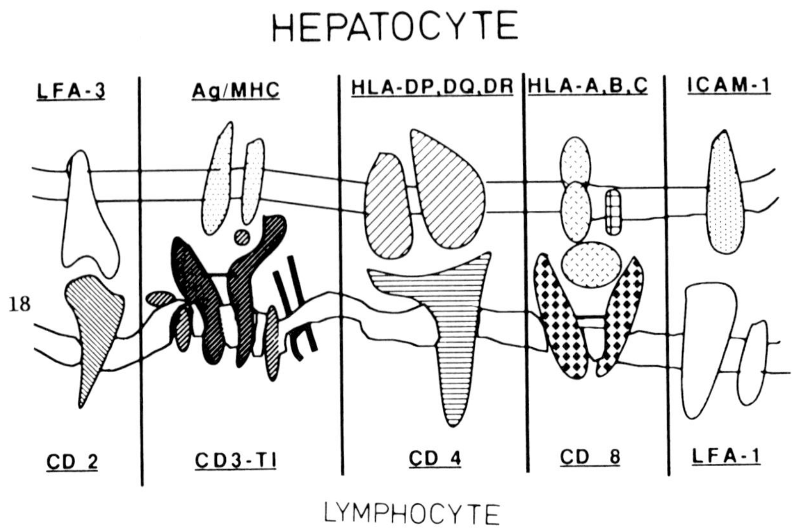

Fig. 2 Schematic structure of molecules on the surface of effector and target cells[34]

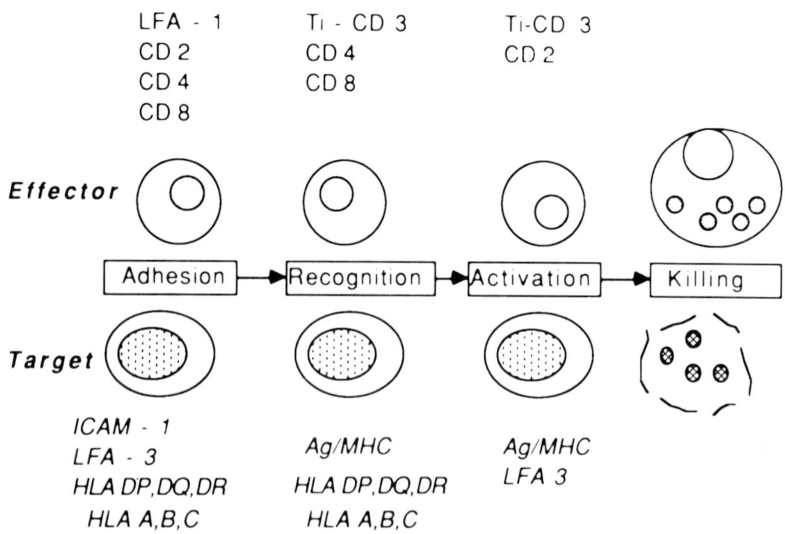

Fig. 3 Sequence of events in the cytotoxic process[34]

on immunohistological, ultrastructural and immunological studies in patients with various forms of liver disease. Phenotype, antigen specificity, and function of liver infiltrating lymphocytes, type, distribution, and cellular expression of adhesion peptides and of inter- and vascular cellular adhesion molecules, as well as the expression of HLA class I and II antigens on target[39] and antigen-presenting cells are the basis of our knowledge of the local immune response of the liver[40].

Two pathways of T cell activation may play a role[41,42].

1. The antigen-specific pathway via T-cell receptor, the natural ligand of the MHC/antigen complex. An activation signal can also be induced by alloantigens and lectins.
2. The alternative antigen unspecified pathway via CD2. The natural activating ligand of CD2 is unknown. Monoclonal antibodies against CD2, but also lectins are shown to operate as stimulators of CD2 in *in vitro* systems.

Ultrastructural analyses of the immune response in human liver diseases clearly indicate that after an antigen-specific initiation of an immune response by virus, drugs and probably also autoantigens, the interaction between target cells and lymphocytes via the CD2/LFA3 complex seems to play a dominant role[43].

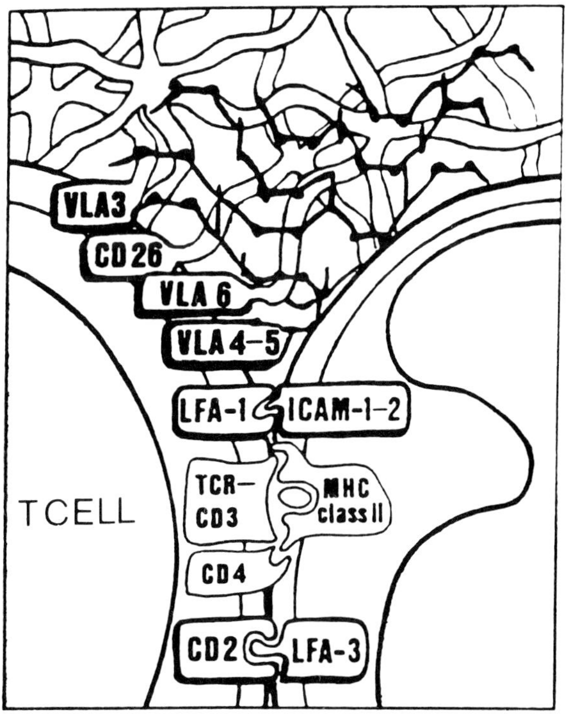

Fig. 4 Interaction between target cell and lymphocyte via the CD2/LFA3 binding complex; schematic demonstration of the involved molecules[43a]

Based on studies in active diseases such as viral hepatitis, autoimmune liver diseases, drug-induced allergic hepatitis and in liver transplantation, an increased expression of the adhesion molecule ICAM-1 and LFA3, the natural ligand of the CD2 molecule of the T cell receptor[42], is displayed on hepatocytes, SEC, and KC[43]. Through these adhesion molecules, CD2 and LFA1-positive lymphocytes of $CD4^+$ or $CD8^+$ phenotype will be retained in the liver sinusoid, and their migration through the sinusoidal endothelium will be initiated, before the sequence of events in the target–effector–cell interaction can take place. In a further step β_1 integrins (very late activation chains = VLA chains) bind to the extracellular matrix and complete the effector–target–cell interaction. Volpes *et al.*[40] have shown a change of the pattern of VLA chain expression in the inflamed liver on sinusoidal lining cells and hepatocytes (Fig. 4).

Studies in viral-induced liver diseases such as hepatitis A and B, have shown clearly that the antigen-specific T cell activation and the cytotoxic effect of $CD8^+$ viral-specific lymphocytes are of major importance[44–46]. In autoimmune hepatitis[47] and in drug-induced allergic hepatitis the inflammatory tissue destruction seems to be caused by $CD4^+$ T cell activation[48,49]. This can be concluded from our own studies on tissue-derived T lymphocytes in autoimmune hepatitis[50] and from a recently published observation by Tsutsui *et al.*[51] in a drug-induced allergic hepatitis. Furthermore Tiegs *et al.*[52] were recently able to induce a T cell-dependent experimental liver injury in mice using lectin concanavalin A (con-A), when an i.v. dosage greater than 1.5 mg/kg con-A was given. The authors could show clearly that the disease

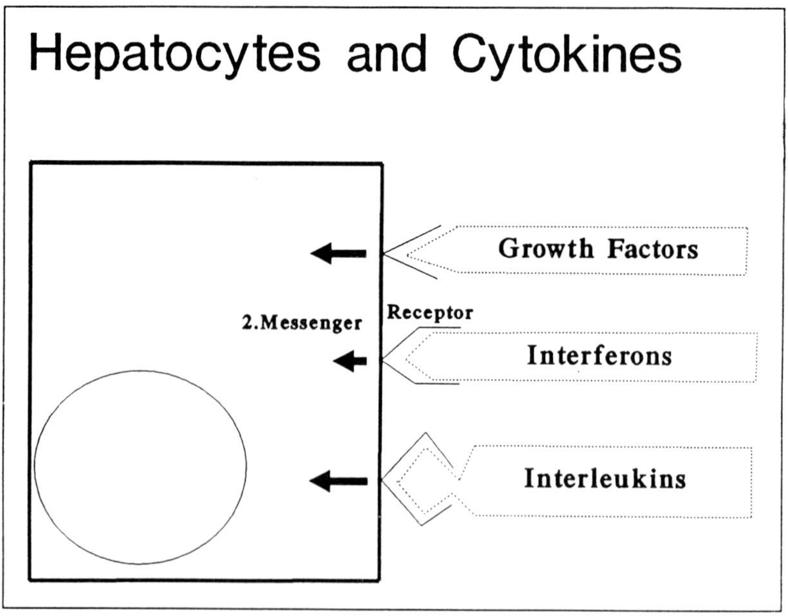

Fig. 5 Hepatic protein synthesis induced by cytokines and regulated by second messenger mechanisms such as G-protein binding and phosphorylation

depends on the activation of CD4$^+$ T lymphocytes by macrophages in the presence of con-A in a dose-dependent manner. The con-A hepatitis is a very interesting model, and of considerable interest as to the pathophysiology of autoimmune liver diseases, or generally of autoimmune diseases. It might be possible that under special genetic conditions self-antigen presentation by macrophages and recognition of CD4$^+$ cells can be mimicked by the lectin con-A at the final step of a common activation pathway.

The hepatocyte reacts dramatically to changes of its cytokine environment. Several cytokines are capable of binding to its specific receptors which are expressed on the hepatocellular surface in small numbers. Hepatic receptors have been described, for example, for insulin-like growth factors, epidermal growth factors, IFN-α, IFN-γ and some interleukins such as IL-1 and IL-6. The hepatic protein synthesis is then regulated by second messenger mechanisms such as G-protein binding and phosphorylation. Both transcriptional and post-transcriptional pathways of protein synthesis are affected (Fig. 5).

In more detail we could demonstrate that a hepatocyte-specific molecule, the asialoglycoprotein receptor, is affected by cytokine action. Tumour necrosis factor-α, IFN-α, IFN-γ and, surprisingly, IL-2, totally inhibit the ASGPR function which normally mediates uptake of galactose-terminating glycoproteins into the liver cell. In particular, hepatocytes were shown to express the β-chain of the IL-2 receptor. Further experiments have shown that the cell membrane-associated ASGPRs were hyperphosphorylated due to IL-2.

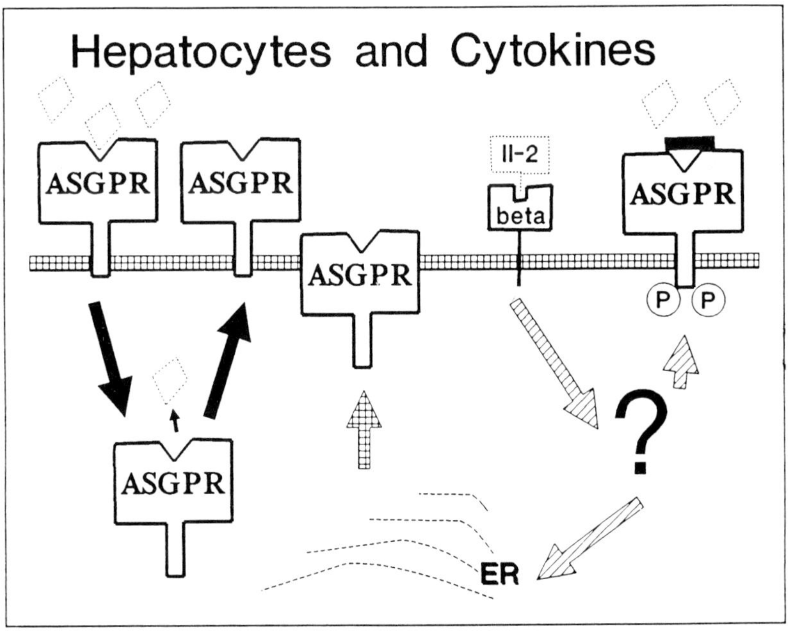

Fig. 6 Physiological regulation of the hepatocyte-specific ASGPR (left part); interruption of the normal pathway of the ASGPR through IL-2 (right part)

Looking at the results with a schema (Fig. 6), the T-lymphocyte-derived cytokine IL-2 regulates the hepatocyte-specific ASGPR in a differential manner. The normal ASGPR pathway – ligand binding, hepatic endocytosis and recirculation to the cell surface – is interrupted by IL-2-induced phosphorylation of the ASGPR. Moreover, new synthesis of the receptor is suppressed due to IL-2 binding to the hepatocyte. Therefore, whenever a change of the microenvironment of the hepatocyte involves the cytokine milieu the cell surface of the liver cell will probably react with a striking remodelling of its organization and function[53].

CONCLUDING REMARKS

In summary, the liver plays a crucial role in maintaining the immunological homeostasis of the body. Due to its unique position at the interface between blood and hepatocytes the sinusoidal cells are of central importance for the cell-specific host defence mechanisms, but immediately after an organ-specific injury by viruses, xenobiotics, autoantigens, or in a case of liver transplantation, the physiological interactions among and between the sinusoidal cells and hepatocytes and the balance between the regulatory factors produced by these cells will become unstable or may be disturbed. This leads to changes in the amount and type of cells within the sinusoid. These changes are in part due to proliferation of endogenous cells; in addition new mononuclear cells arrive from the circulation in response to chemotactic factors. These changes in the internal environment of the liver form the basis for a local immune process induced by foreign and self-antigens or by lectins which can probably mimic self-antigen presentation via macrophages, sinus endothelial cells or probably also hepatocytes.

References

1. Arias I, Popper H, Schachter D, Schafritz DA. The liver: biology and pathobiology. New York: Raven Press; 1982.
2. Gressner AM, Ramadori G. Molecular and cell biology of liver fibrogenesis. Dordrecht/Boston/London: Kluwer; 1992.
3. Knook D, Sefferlaar AM, DeLeeuw AM. Fatstoring cells of rat liver their isolation and purification. Exp Cell Res. 1982;139:468–71.
4. Knook DL, Sleyster ECh. Separation of Kupffer and endothelial cells of the rat liver by centrifugal elutriation. Exp Cell Res. 1976;99:444.
5. Kamada N. Transplantation tolerance and immunosuppression following liver grafting in rats. Immunol Today. 1985;6:336–42.
6. Kamada N, Teramoto K, Baguerio A, Ishikawa M, Sumimoto R, Ohkouchi Y. Cellular basis of transplantation tolerance induced by liver grafts in the rat: extent of clonal deletion among thoracic duct lymphocytes, spleen and lymph node cells. Transplantation. 1988;46:165–7.
7. Meyer zum Büschenfelde KH. Hepatologie in Klinik und Praxis. Stuttgart/New York: Thieme; 1989:32–46.
8. Souhami R, Addison I, Bradfield J. Increased antibody production following depression of hepatic phagocytosis. J Exp Med. 1975;20:155–9.
9. Praaning-van Dalen DP, Brouwer A, Knook DL. Clearance capacity of rat liver Kupffer, endothelial, and parenchymal cells. Gastroenterology. 1981;81:1036.

10. Tomana M, Kulhavy R, Mestecky J. Receptor-mediated binding and uptake of immunoglobulin A by human liver. Gastroenterology. 1988;94:762–70.
11. Wisse E, De Zanger R, Charels K, Van der Smissen P, McCuskey RS. The liver sieve: considerations concerning the structure and function of endothelial fenestrae, the sinusoidal wall and the space of Disse. Hepatology. 1985;5:683.
12. Toth CA, Thomas P. Liver endocytosis and Kupffer cells. Hepatology. 1992;16:255–66.
13. Scoazer JY, Feldmann G. Both macrophages and endothelial cells of the human hepatic sinusoid express the CD4 molecule, a receptor for the human immunodeficiency virus. Hepatology. 1990;12:505–10.
14. Rogoff T, Lipsky P. Role of the Kupffer cells in local and systemic immune responses. Gastroenterology. 1981;80:854–60.
15. Rubenstein D, Roska A, Lipsky P. Liver sinusoidal lining cells express class II major histocompatibility antigen gut are poor simulators of fresh allogenic T lymphocytes. J Immunol. 1986;137:1803–8.
16. Callery M, Kamei T, Flye M. Kupffer cell blockade inhibits induction of tolerance by the portal venous route. Transplantation. 1988;46:1092–3.
17. Rieder H, Meyer zum Büschenfelde KH, Ramadori G. Functional spectrum of sinusoidal endothelial liver cells – Filtration, endocytosis, synthetic capacities and intercellular communication. J Hepatol. 1992;15:237–50.
18. Ashwell G, Harford J. Carbohydrate-specific receptors of the liver. Ann Rev Biochem. 1982;51:531–54.
19. Steffan A, Genrault J, McCluskey P, Kirn A. Phagocytosis an unrecognized property of murine endothelial liver cells. Hepatology. 1986;6:830–6.
20. Bouwens L, Wisse E. Pit cells in the liver. Liver. 1992;12:3–9.
21. Winnock M, Garcia-Barcina M, Dubuisson L, Bernard P, Lefebvre P, Bioulac-Sage P, Balabaud C. Are pit cells involved in fibrogenesis? In: Gressner AM, Ramadori G, editors. Molecular and cell biology of liver fibrogenesis. Dordrecht/Boston/London: Kluwer; 1992:439–53.
22. Lukosmka B, Pienkowska B, Andrezejewski W, Olszewski WL. Liver sinusoidal cytotoxic cells are recruited from blood and divide locally. J Hepatol. 1991;12:332–5.
23. Aronson FR, Libby P, Brandon EP, Janicka MW, Mier JW. IL-2 rapidly induces natural killer cell adhesion to human endothelial cells. A potential mechanism for endothelial injury. J Immunol. 1988;141:158–63.
24. Volpes R, van den Oord JJ, De Vos R, Depla E, De Ley M, Desmet VJ. Expression of interferon-gamma receptor in normal and pathological human liver tissue. J Hepatol. 1991;12:195–202.
25. Cotran RS, Pober JS. Effects of cytokines on vascular endothelium. Their role in vascular and immune injury. Kidney Int. 1989;35:969–75.
26. Kirn A, Steffan AM, Kochren F. Interaction between viruses and primary cultures of murine and human liver endothelial cells. In: Knook DL, Wisse E, editors. Sinusoidal liver cells. Amsterdam: Elsevier; 1982:413–19.
27. McCloskey TW, Todaro JA, Laskin DL. Lipopolysaccharide treatment of rats alters antigen expression and oxidative metabolism in hepatic macrophages and endothelial cells. Hepatology. 1992;16:191–203.
28. Bevilaqua MP, Stengelin S, Gimbrone MA, Seed B. Endothelial leucocyte adhesion molecule-1: an inducible receptor for neutrophils related to complement regulatory proteins and lectins. Science. 1989;243:1160–5.
29. Osborn L. Leucocyte adhesion to endothelium in inflammation. Cell. 1990;62:3–6.
30. Smedly LA, Tonnesen MG, Sandhaus RA. Neutrophil-mediated injury to endothelial cells. Enhancement by endotoxin and essential role of neutrophil elastase. J Clin Invest. 1986;77:1233–43.
31. Damle NK, Doyle LV, Bender JR, Bradley EC. Interleukin 2-activated human lymphocytes exhibit enhanced adhesion to normal vascular endothelial cells and cause their lysis. J Immunol. 1987;138:1779–85.
32. Pober JS, Gimbrone MA Jr, Collius T. Interactions of T lymphocytes with human vascular endothelial cells: role of endothelial cell surface antigens. Immunobiology. 1984;168:483–8.
33. Ramadori G, Moebius C, Dienes HP. Lymphocytes from hepatic inflammatory infiltrate kill rat hepatocytes in primary culture. Virchows Arch B. 1990;59:263.

34. Dienes HP, Autschbach F, Gerber MA. Ultrastructural lesion in autoimmune hepatitis and steps of the immune response in liver tissue. Sem Liver Dis. 1991;11:197–204.
35. Krensky AM, Sanchez-Madrid F, Robbins E. The functional significance, distribution, and structure of LFA-1, LFA-2, and LFA-3: Cell surface antigens associated with CTL-target interactions. J Immunol. 1983;131:611–16.
36. Wawryk SD, Novotny JR, Wicks JP. The role of the LFA-1/ICAM-1 interaction in human leucocyte homing and adhesion. Immunol Rev. 1989;108:135–61.
37. Baradin KA, Scheuer PJ. Endothelial cell changes in acute hepatitis. A light and electron microscopic study. J Pathol. 1984;144:213–20.
38. Steinhoff G, Behrend M, Pichlmayr P. Induktion von ICAM-1 auf Hepatozytenmembranen und Gallengängen nach Leber-transplantation Z Gastroenterol. 1990;28:69.
39. Lobo-Yeo A, Senaldi G, Portmann B, Mowat A, Mieli-Vergani G, Vergani D. Class I and Class II major histocompatibility complex antigen expression in hepatocytes: a study in children with liver disease. Hepatology. 1990;12:224–32.
40. Volpes R, van den Oord JJ, Desmet VJ. Immunohistochemical study of adhesion molecules in liver inflammation. Hepatology. 1990;12:59–65.
41. Meuer S, Hauer M, Deusch K. Two pathways of T cell activation. Behring Inst Mitt. 1987;81:15–30.
42. Selvaraj P, Plunkett ML, Dustin M. The T lymphocyte glycoprotein CD2 binds the cell surface ligand LFA-3. Nature. 1987;326:400–3.
43. Autschbach F, Meuer SC, Moebius U, Manns M, Hess G, Meyer zum Büschenfelde KH, Thoenes W, Dienes HP. Hepatocellular expression of lymphocyte function-associated antigen 3 in chronic hepatitis. Hepatology. 1991;14:223–30.
43a. De Sousa M, Tilney NL, Kupriec-Weglinski. Recognition of self within self: specific lymphocyte positioning and the extra cellular matrix. Immunol Today. 1991;12:262–6.
44. Bertoletti A, Ferrari C, Fiaccadori F, Penna A, Margolskee R, Schlicht HJ, Fowler P, Guilhot S, Chisari FV. HLA class I-restricted human cytotoxic T cells recognize endogenously synthesized hepatitis B viral nucleocapsid antigen. Proc Natl Acad Sci USA. 1991;88:10445–9.
45. Penna A, Chisari FV, Bertoletti A, Missale G, Fowler P, Guiberti T, Fiaccadori F, Ferrari C. Cytotoxic T lymphocytes recognize an HLA-A2-restricted epitope within the hepatitis B virus nucleo-capsid antigen. J Exp Med. 1991;174:1565–70.
46. Penna A, Fowler P, Bertoletti A, Guilhot S, Moss B, Margolskee RF, Cavalli A, Valli A, Fiaccadori F, Chisari FV, Ferrari C. Hepatitis B virus (HBV)-specific cytotoxic T-cell (CTL) response in humans: characterization of HLA class II-restricted CTL that recognize endogenously synthesized HBV envelope antigens. J Virol. 1992;66:1193–8.
47. Meyer zum Büschenfelde KH, Lohse AW, Manns M, Poralla T. Autoimmunity and liver disease. Hepatology. 1990;12:354–63.
48. Löhr H, Manns M, Kyriatsoulis A, Lohse AW, Trautwein C, Meyer zum Büschenfelde KH, Fleischer B. Clonal analysis of liver-infiltrating T cells in patients with LKM-1 antibody-positive autoimmune chronic active hepatitis. Clin Exp Immunol. 1991;84:297–302.
49. Löhr H, Treichel U, Poralla T, Manns M, Meyer zum Büschenfelde KH, Fleischer B. Liver-infiltrating T helper cells in autoimmune chronic active hepatitis stimulate the production of autoantibodies against the human asialoglycoprotein receptor in vitro. Clin Exp Immunol. 1992;88:45–9.
50. Meyer zum Büschenfelde KH, Poralla T. Immunology and autoimmune liver diseases. Curr Opin Gastroenterol. 1992;8:320–87.
51. Tsutsui H, Terano Y, Sakagami C, Hasegawa I, Mizoguchi Y, Morisawa S. Drug-specific T cells derived from patients with drug-induced allergic hepatitis. J Immunol. 1992;149:706–16.
52. Tiegs G, Hentschel J, Wendel A. A T cell-dependent experimental liver injury in mice inducible by concanavalin A. J Clin Invest. 1992;90:196–203.
53. Treichel U, Poralla T. The asialoglycoprotein receptor (ASGPR) as hepatic autoantigen (Submitted).

Closing remarks

R. SCHMID

Ladies and Gentlemen,
Over the past $2\frac{1}{2}$ days, we have discussed a vast panoply of extrahepatic manifestations of liver disease, too many to remember all, and most of them still incompletely understood in terms of pathogenesis. I want to assure you that I have no intention – nor the ability or time – to summarize what has been presented in this symposium. But I would like to express one or two thoughts which surfaced during these intellectually rich days.

It has been amply demonstrated that the liver is central to the body's normal function. Virtually every organ is somehow connected to the liver and each thereby may be secondarily affected by hepatic dysfunction.

Although all cells of the body have complete sets of genetic information, few of them express phenotypically more than a very small fraction of it. The liver is unique in that it expresses much more of its genetic information than any of the other organs or tissues. This undoubtedly is one of the reasons why hepatic integrity is so essential for the proper function of the body. Think for a moment how many of the organism's constituents are formed in the liver – and only in the liver – from albumin and cholesterol to most clotting factors and many cell components. And some organs are critically dependent on the liver for their energy provision, for example the brain on the glucose synthesized and released by the liver, or muscle on the creatine and carnitine formed only in the liver. No wonder, then, that chronic liver disease may appear in the disguise of a variety of ailments which at first sight seem to have little relevance to the liver. We have encountered many such examples during the past 2 days.

But what we have not discussed here in any depth are the patients with chronic liver disease – hepatitis or cirrhosis – who fail to exhibit clinical symptoms or signs that would suggest hepatic impairment. There are large numbers of such patients whose chronic liver disease has remained undetected, and may never be diagnosed, simply because their clinical manifestations are too subtle to be recognized, or their laboratory findings too unspecific or uncharacteristic to arouse the physician's suspicion. Every so often there appears in the skin clinic a patient with therapy-resistant pruritus whose underlying occult cholestasis has been overlooked; or we are called to the neurological service to consult on a comatose patient with evident metabolic encephalopathy in whom an unmistakable hint of chronic liver disease has been missed, for example an isolated arterial spider naevus, an unusually hard liver edge, or a fetor hepatis.

This of course is the art of medicine: the looking, feeling, touching, smelling and listening, particularly the listening to the patient trying to tell his or her story that often contains the diagnostically critical information. This is the art of medicine, the invariable of the practice of medicine, which increasingly is being displaced, if not replaced, by the relentless progress of modern medical science and particularly medical technology. Whereas we, of course, welcome and embrace the latter with enthusiasm, we may not neglect or demean the art of medicine, for the sake of our patients as well as our spiritual sanity as physicians.

This brings me to the conclusion of this symposium. I would like to thank all the members for their contributions, which made this event such a memorable one. Once more, I express our deep gratitude to Dr Falk for his enduring generosity, and to his incomparable staff for a job superbly done.

Thank you.

Index